Evidence-Based Asthma Management

J. Mark FitzGerald, MD, FRCPC, FRCPI
Respiratory Physician,
Respiratory Clinic,
Vancouver General Hospital
Vancouver, British Columbia

Pierre Ernst, MD, MSc, FRCPC
Professor of Medicine,
Division of Clinical Epidemiology,
Royal Victoria Hospital
Montreal, Québec

Louis-Philippe Boulet , MD, FRCPC
Professor of Medicine,
Centre de Pneumologie Hôpital Laval
Ste-Foy, Québec

Paul M. O'Byrne, MB, FRCPI, FRCPC
Professor of Medicine,
Firestone Chest and Allergy Clinic,
St. Joseph's Hospital
Hamilton, Ontario

2001
B.C. Decker Inc.
Hamilton • London

B.C. Decker Inc.
20 Hughson Street South
P.O. Box 620, L.C.D. 1
Hamilton, Ontario L8N 3K7
Tel: 905-522-7017; 1-800-568-7281
Fax: 905-522-7839
E-mail: info@bcdecker.com
Website: www.bcdecker.com

00 01 / UTP / 9 8 7 6 5 4 3 2 1

ISBN 1-55009-114-X

Printed in Canada

Sales and Distribution

United States
B.C. Decker Inc.
P.O. Box 785
Lewiston, NY 14092-0785
Tel: 905-522-7017 / 1-800-568-7281
Fax: 905-522-7839
E-mail: info@bcdecker.com
Website: www.bcdecker.com

Canada
B.C. Decker Inc.
20 Hughson Street South
P.O. Box 620, L.C.D. 1
Hamilton, Ontario L8N 3K7
Tel: 905-522-7017 / 1-800-568-7281
Fax: 905-522-7839
E-mail: info@bcdecker.com
Website: www.bcdecker.com

Japan
Igaku-Shoin Ltd.
Foreign Publications Department
3-24-17 Hongo
Bunkyo-ku,Tokyo, Japan 113-8719
Tel: 3 3817 5680
Fax: 3 3815 6776
E-mail: fd@igaku.shoin.co.jp

U.K., Europe, Scandinavia, Middle East
Harcourt Publishers Limited
Customer Service Department
Foots Cray High Street
Sidcup, Kent
DA14 5HP, UK
Tel: 44 (0) 208 308 5760
Fax: 44 (0) 181 308 5702
E-mail: cservice@harcourt_brace.com

Singapore, Malaysia, Thailand, Philippines,
Indonesia, Vietnam, Pacific Rim
Harcourt Asia Pte Limited
583 Orchard Road
#09/01, Forum
Singapore 238884
Tel: 65-737-3593
Fax: 65-753-2145

Foreign Rights
John Scott & Company
International Publishers' Agency
P.O. Box 878
Kimberton, PA 19442
Tel: 610-827-1640
Fax: 610-827-1671

Notice: The authors and publisher have made every effort to ensure that the patient care recommended
herein, including choice of drugs and drug dosages, is in accord with the accepted standard and practice
at the time of publication. However, since research and regulation constantly change clinical standards,
the reader is urged to check the product information sheet included in the package of each drug, which
includes recommended doses, warnings, and contraindications. This is particularly important with new
or infrequently used drugs.

Contributors

Ellinor Ädelroth, MD, PhD
Department of Respiratory Medicine
  and Allergy
University Hospital
Umeå, Sweden
Cellular and Pathologic Characteristics

Tony R. Bai, MD
UBC Respiratory Division
St. Paul's Hospital
Vancouver, British Columbia
Role of Short-Acting β_2-Therapy Agonists

Allan B. Becker, MD, FRCPC
Section of Allergy and Clinical Immunology
Department of Pediatrics and Child Health
University of Manitoba
Winnipeg, Manitoba
Environmental Control and Immunotherapy

Louis-Philippe Boulet, MD, FRCPC
Professor of Medicine
Centre de Pneumologie Hôpital Laval
Ste-Foy, Québec
Role of Long-Acting β_2-Adrenergic Agents
Role of Asthma Education

Moira Chan-Yeung, MB, FRCPC
Respiratory Division
Department of Medicine
Vancouver, British Columbia
Role of Indoor Aeroallergens

Gerard J. Canny, MD, FRCPC, FAAP, FCCP
Respiratory Department
Children's Hospital
Dublin-12, Ireland
Severe Acute Asthma in Children

André Cartier, MD, FRCP
Chest Department
Sacre-Coeur Hospital
Montreal, Québec
Diagnosis and Management of
Occupational Asthma

Ken Chapman, MD, MSc, FRCPC, FACP
Professor of Medicine
University of Toronto
Asthma Centre and Pulmonary
Rehabilitation Program
Toronto Western Hospital
Toronto, Canada
Asthma Unresponsive to Usual Therapy

Joanne B. Clough, DM, FRCA, MRCP, FRCPCH
Consultant Paediatrician
University Child Health
Southampton General Hospital
Southampton, United Kingdom
Role of Childhood Infection

Donald W. Cockcroft, MD, FRCPC
Royal University Hospital
Saskatoon, Saskatchewan
Principles of Asthma Management in Adults

Christopher J. Corrigan, MA, MSc, PhD, FRCP
Department of Respiratory Medicine & Allergy
Guy's Hospital
London, United Kingdom
Alternate Anti-inflammatory Therapies

Jeffrey M. Drazen, MD
Division of Pulmonary and Critical Care Medicine
Brigham and Women's Hospital
Boston, Massachusetts
Leukotriene Modifiers

Pierre Ernst, MD, MSc, FRCPC
Division of Clinical Epidemiology
Royal Victoria Hospital
Montreal, Canada
Measures of Outcome

Alexander C. Ferguson, MB, ChB, FRCPC
Department of Pediatrics
University of British Columbia
B.C. Children's Hospital
Vancouver, British Columbia
Diagnosis in Children

J. Mark FitzGerald, MD, FRCPC, FRCPI
Respiratory Physician
Respiratory Clinic
Vancouver General Hospital
Vancouver, British Columbia
Acute Life-Threatening Asthma

Peter G. Gibson, MBBS (Hons), FRACP
Staff Specialist
Airway Research Center
Respiratory Medicine
John Hunter Hospital
Newcastle NSW, Australia
Role of Asthma Education

Anton Grunfield, MD, FRCPC
Emergency Room Physician
Department of Surgery
Vancouver General Hospital
Vancouver, British Columbia
Acute Life-Threatening Asthma

Frederick Hargreave MD, FRCPC, FRCP
Firestone Regional Chest & Allergy Unit
St. Joseph's Hospital
Hamilton, Ontario
Role of Inhaled Corticosteroids

Mark D. Inman, MD, PhD
Firestone Regional Chest & Allergy Unit
St. Joseph's Hospital
Hamilton, Ontario
Exercise-Induced Bronchoconstriction

Elliot Israel, MD
Division of Pulmonary and Critical Care
   Medicine
Brigham and Women's Hospital
Boston, Massachusetts
Leukotriene Modifiers

Catherine Lemière, MD
Chest Department
Sacre-Coeur Hospital
Montreal, Québec
Diagnosis and Management of Occupational Asthma

Avi Nahum MD, PhD
University of Minnesota
Regions Hospital
St. Pauls, Minnesota
Management of Asthma in the Intensive Care Unit

Paul M. O'Byrne, MB, FRCPI, FRCPC
Firestone Chest & Allergy Clinic
St. Joseph's Hospital
Hamilton, Ontario
Role of Inhaled Corticosteroids

Brian J. O'Connor, MD
Kings College Hospital
London, England
Use of Theophylline and Anticholinergic Therapy

Clive P. Page, MD
Kings College Hospital
London, England
Use of Theophylline and Anticholinergic Therapy

Peter D. Paré, MD
University of British Columbia
Pulmonary Research Laboratory
Vancouver, British Columbia
Genetics of Asthma

Andrew J. Sandford, PhD
University of British Columbia
Pulmonary Research Laboratory
Vancouver, British Columbia
Genetics of Asthma

Suzanne Schuh, MD, FRCPC, AB PEM
Emergency Pediatrician
Emergency Department
The Hospital for Sick Children
Toronto, Ontario
Severe Acute Asthma in Children

Malcolm R. Sears, MB, ChB, FRACP, FRCPC
Firestone Regional Chest & Allergy Unit
St. Joseph's Hospital
Hamilton, Ontario
Natural History and Epidemiology

F. Estelle R. Simons, MD, FRCPC
Children's Hospital
Winnipeg, Manitoba
Management of Persistent Asthma in Childhood

Samy Suissa, PhD,
Division of Clinical Epidemiology
Royal Victoria Hospital
Montreal, Canada
Measures of Outcome

D. Robin Taylor, MD, MRCP, FRCPC
Department of Medicine
Dunedin School of Medicine
University of Otago
New Zealand
Diagnosis

David V. Tuxen, MBBS, FRACP DipDHM, MD
Department of Intensive Care
Monash University
Victoria, Australia
*Management of Asthma in the Intensive
    Care Unit*

Sverre Vedal, MD, MSc
Respiratory Division
Vancouver Hospital
Vancouver, British Columbia
Role of Outdoor Environment

Tracey D. Weir, BMLSc
University of British Columbia
Pulmonary Research Laboratory
Vancouver, British Columbia
Genetics of Asthma

We would like to dedicate this book to our partners
Trish, Magdalena, Céline, Irene, and our children for all the support
given in this endeavor and our careers in general.

We would also like to thank Dr. Freddy Hargreaves and the late
Dr. Jerry Dolovich for helping us think more clearly about asthma and its
management. Both have contributed greatly as mentors of many of the
chapter authors of this book.

Contents

Introduction

Asthma is a common medical problem, the prevalence of which is increasing. Epidemiologic surveys have confirmed that this increase is real and is associated with significant morbidity, suggesting that the condition is not adequately treated in some patients. Although asthma mortality is declining in many countries, avoidable deaths continue to occur. Asthma guidelines have been developed globally, nationally, and locally. Recently, it has been recognized that these guidelines should be evidence based to provide primary care physicians with a more persuasive argument for their use. Review of the evidence also serves to highlight, for clinical investigators, the important clinical questions that need to be rigorously addressed.

Against this background, we have developed an evidence-based asthma textbook in which appropriate levels of evidence are categorized as follows:

> Level I: Evidence from one or more randomized clinical trials
> Level II: Evidence from one or more well-designed cohort or case-control studies
> Level III: Consensus from expert groups based on clinical experience

In addition, where therapeutic recommendations are being made, authors were given the option to subdivide the evidence, according to the following criteria:*

> A: Good evidence to support a recommendation for use
> B: Moderate evidence to support a recommendation for use
> C: Poor evidence to support a recommendation for or against use
> D: Moderate evidence to support a recommendation against use
> E: Good evidence to support a recommendation against use

We hope you find this textbook useful. We sincerely believe that the quality of life of our patients and control of their asthma will improve significantly if we implement the management strategies outlined. We also hope that investigators will focus their research efforts on those areas for which we do not have robust evidence for our current clinical practice.

Finally this book would not have been possible without the excellent contributions from the chapter authors and assistance from the staff at B.C. Decker Inc., in particular Ms Jennifer Smiley.

J. Mark FitzGerald, MD, FRCPC, FRCPI
Pierre Ernst, MD, MSc, FRCPC
Louis-Philippe Boulet, MD, FRCPC
Paul O'Byrne, MB, FRCPI, FRCPC

---

*These recommendations were adapted from Cook et al. Chest 1995;108:127–230S.

CHAPTER 1

Natural History and Epidemiology

Malcolm R. Sears, MB, ChB, FRACP, FRCPC

Asthma remains a common and troublesome problem affecting a substantial proportion of the childhood and adult population worldwide. Interest in the epidemiology of asthma has increased over recent decades as clinicians and epidemiologists have noted apparent increases in the incidence and prevalence of asthma, together with upward trends in mortality suggesting increasing severity, at a time when morbidity and mortality of other chronic diseases is declining. Interest has been further heightened by suggestions from several studies that lifestyle factors, increasing "westernization," and effects of modern civilization have contributed to these trends. The natural history of asthma, likewise, has been more extensively studied in recent decades, and earlier concepts that most children "grow out of" asthma have been challenged. This chapter summarizes recent studies of the epidemiology and natural history of asthma.

METHODS

Epidemiology does not lend itself to randomized controlled trials, and so most evidence cited is at Level II, arising from well-designed cohort or case-control studies. The strength of such evidence derives from the soundness of epidemiologic and statistical methods, the size of the populations examined, and the tools used to determine the presence and severity of asthma. This has been greatly facilitated by the two recently concluded international studies of the epidemiology of asthma, the International Study of Asthma and Allergies in Childhood (ISAAC)[1] and the European Community Respiratory Health Survey (ECRHS).[2]

DEFINITION

There is no one symptom, physical characteristic, or laboratory test that defines asthma. Rather, asthma is recognized from a pattern of symptoms including wheeze, cough, chest tightness, and dyspnea, and it is confirmed by evidence of variable or reversible airflow obstruction. Increased responsiveness of the airways to nonallergic stimuli usually accompanies asthma symptoms but is not synonymous with asthma.[3] Asthma is characterized by inflammation, but methods for noninvasive detection of airway inflammation using induced sputum[4] have only recently been introduced and are not extensively used in population studies. The most recent international definition of asthma proposed by the Global Initiative on Asthma indicates the difficulty in writing a precise and universally applicable definition.[5] That document describes asthma as

> A chronic inflammatory disorder of the airways in which many cells play a role, in particular, mast cells, eosinophils, and T-lymphocytes. In susceptible individuals this inflammation causes recurrent episodes of wheezing, breathlessness, chest tightness, and cough particularly at night and/or in the early morning. These symptoms are usually associated with widespread but variable airflow limitation that is at least partly reversible either spontaneously or with treatment. The inflammation also causes an associated increase in airway responsiveness to a variety of stimuli.

A working definition of current asthma for epidemiologic purposes was proposed by Toelle et al, namely, recent symptoms (within the last 12 months) with an appropriate degree of airway responsiveness.[6] However, many studies have not included measurements of airway responsiveness, and in those in which it has been included, even among the internationally standardized studies, the measurement has proven more variable than ideal for a "gold standard" test. Hence, the majority of data on the epidemiology of asthma is still symptom based.

PREVALENCE

In Children

In longitudinal studies of children from infancy to age 6 years, the cumulative prevalence of episodic wheezing has been reported as high as 49% (Level II).[7] Much of this early childhood wheezing is not persistent. Prevalence studies of childhood asthma over the last three decades have used various nonstandardized questionnaires and range of objective measurements. The ISAAC study used a standard protocol in two age groups, with parents answering a questionnaire regarding their children aged 6 to 7 years, while 13- to 14-year-old children completed their own questionnaire. The validity of the ISAAC questionnaire item regarding wheezing or

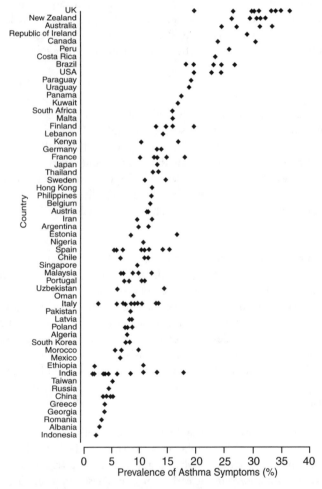

Figure 1–1 12-month prevalence of self-reported asthma symptoms in 13 to 14 year olds completing the ISAAC written questionnaire. (Reproduced with permission from The International Study of Asthma and Allergies in Childhood [ISAAC] Steering Committee. Worldwide variation in the prevalence of symptoms of asthma, allergic rhinoconjunctivitis, and atopic eczema: ISAAC. Lancet 1998;351:1225–32.)

whistling in the chest in the past 12 months was established by comparison with an assessment of a pediatric pulmonologist making a clinical diagnosis of asthma, aided by measurements of airway responsiveness to hypertonic saline (Level II).[8] Results from the ISAAC study, which was conducted in more than 130 centers in more than 50 countries, are summarized in Figure 1–1.[9] Results indicate real differences between countries and also point to the likely underdiagnosis of asthma in many areas previously considered to have low prevalence rates. There are also quite wide variations in prevalence seen within countries, posing further questions with regard to risk factors for asthma (Level II).[10]

Because differences in cultural factors and language barriers may bias answers to written questionnaires, a video questionnaire was included with the ISAAC study for the older age group.[11] This demonstrated five scenes showing mild, moderate, and severe asthma, exercise-induced asthma, and nocturnal symptoms. Responses to the video questionnaire generally gave prevalence rates lower than those reported using the written questionnaire, likely due to the recording of symptoms on the written questionnaire that were less severe than those seen on the video. The agreement between video and written questionnaires is only moderate (Level II).[12]

In Adults

The epidemiology of asthma in adults was not well studied, with relatively few population-based studies being conducted, until the development of the ECRHS. This study has now been completed in 48 centers in 22 countries. In brief, each center recruited 3,000 subjects aged 20 to 44 years, using random population sampling methods, and requested completion of a short postal questionnaire asking about symptoms of wheezing, dyspnea, exercise-related symptoms, and a previous diagnosis of asthma. Related questions including smoking habits, occupational exposures, and symptoms of allergy were added in many centers. In each center, approximately 20% of the sampled population were invited to undergo further investigation, including more detailed questionnaires, measurements of lung function and airway responsiveness, and allergy testing by skin-prick tests and Phadiatop, a serum-based screening test for specific IgE antibody.

Table 1–1 shows a sample of prevalence rates determined by the ECRHS postal questionnaire in different countries (Level II).[2] There are differences within countries and marked differences between countries, some of which were previously identified through nonstandardized studies and are now confirmed by a more rigorous, internationally accepted protocol.[2] The distribution of responses to the questions in the ECRHS questionnaire is further demonstrated in Table 1–2. There was a wide variability in the prevalence of airway responsiveness among centers in the ECRHS study (Level II).[13]

Evidence for Increasing Prevalence

In Children

The increasing acceptance of the label "asthma" has confounded reports of increased prevalence of the disease. Studies that have reported changes in the prevalence of recurrent wheezing, whether labeled as asthma or not, provide more accurate information. As an example of the changing acceptance of the label of asthma, a New Zealand study conducted in 1973 showed that only one-third of the 9-year-old children with a history of recurrent wheezing were labeled as having asthma,[14] whereas, in the ISAAC study conducted in Canada in 1994 to 1995, over 80% of those who had wheezing episodes four or more times per year had been given a label of asthma (Level II).[15] Burney et al reported increased prevalence of "asthma" in the United Kingdom between 1973 and 1986; however, the increase in prevalence of wheeze was much less and was significant only in girls (Level II).[16] A later UK survey found a threefold increase in asthma attacks in 5- to 11-year-old children, a 30 to 60% increase in occasional wheeze, and a 30 to 40% increase in persistent wheeze, between 1982 and 1992,

Table 1-1 *Percentage Prevalence of Positive Responses to Asthma Symptoms by ECRHS Questionnaire Subjects in Selected Countries*

	Wheeze	Wheeze + Breathlessness	Wheeze, No Cold	Chest Tightness	Breathlessness at Night	Cough at Night	Asthma Attack	Asthma Medicine	Diagnosed Asthma
Bergen (Norway)	24.6	13.6	15.8	11.4	5.0	26.1	3.1	3.4	4.3
Göteborg (Sweden)	23.2	12.3	13.5	14.7	7.1	28.2	3.1	4.8	5.8
Tartu (Estonia)	26.8	7.8	12.8	13.9	8.1	42.6	1.8	0.6	2.0
Groningen (Netherlands)	21.1	13.9	14.5	13.1	7.6	28.9	3.0	3.6	4.3
Antwerp City (Belgium)	20.6	10.9	12.9	10.3	6.9	27.2	2.6	3.4	4.6
Hamburg (Germany)	21.1	8.0	13.3	9.6	5.0	25.8	3.0	3.4	4.4
Montpellier (France)	14.4	9.0	8.9	16.9	4.1	25.8	3.6	3.5	5.0
Paris (France)	14.5	9.3	9.0	16.8	4.7	26.0	4.3	3.2	5.1
Cambridge (UK)	25.2	13.9	17.7	17.4	8.4	27.4	5.7	6.8	8.4
Norwich (UK)	25.7	14.2	18.7	18.8	7.9	29.2	5.0	6.3	7.5
Dublin (Ireland)	32.0	15.2	21.6	17.8	9.5	29.1	3.6	3.9	5.0
Athens (Greece)	16.0	9.4	9.8	11.7	5.7	17.8	2.4	2.2	2.9
Turin (Italy)	10.7	4.4	7.6	9.1	8.1	31.7	4.2	2.2	4.5
Barcelona (Spain)	19.2	5.6	10.7	7.2	4.6	28.2	2.1	2.2	3.1
Coimbra (Portugal)	19.0	9.8	12.9	18.8	10.6	25.2	4.3	4.9	6.0
Bombay (India)	4.1	3.0	2.0	7.0	6.8	11.2	2.6	2.8	3.5
Wellington (New Zealand)	27.3	16.0	18.0	18.1	10.4	31.2	8.6	9.8	11.3
Portland, OR (USA)	25.7	10.5	14.9	16.6	7.7	32.5	5.8	4.8	7.1

Adapted with permission from Burney P, Chinn S, Luczynska C, et al. Variations in the prevalence of respiratory symptoms, self-reported asthma attacks, and use of asthma medication in the European Community Respiratory Health Survey (ECRHS). Eur Respir J 1996;9:687–95.

Table 1–2 *Distribution of Responses to Questions in ECRHS Questionnaire**

		Percent Prevalence			
	Minimum	25th Centile	Median	75th Centile	Maximum
Wheeze in past 12 months	4.1	14.9	20.7	25.2	32.0
Wheeze with breathlessness	1.4	7.7	9.8	13.9	16.3
Wheeze without a cold	2.0	9.3	12.7	16.2	21.6
Waking with tightness in the chest	6.2	9.7	13.5	17.5	20.5
Waking with breathlessness	1.5	4.7	7.3	8.9	11.4
Waking with cough	6.0	25.6	27.9	29.5	42.6
Attack of asthma	1.3	2.6	3.1	4.5	9.7
Treatment for asthma	0.6	2.4	3.5	5.0	9.8
Nasal allergies and hayfever	9.5	16.6	20.9	28.2	40.9

*From 45 of 48 centers that responded.
Adapted with permission from Burney P, Chinn S, Luczynska C, et al. Variations in the prevalence of respiratory symptoms, self-reported asthma attacks, and use of asthma medication in the European Community Respiratory Health Survey (ECRHS). Eur Respir J 1996;9:687–95.

suggesting a real increase in the prevalence of asthma (Level II).[17] Similarly, in the United States, reported prevalence among 6- to 11-year-old children increased from 4.8 to 7.6% between the first and second National Health and Nutrition Examination surveys, spanning an interval of approximately 5 years (Level II).[18] In each of these surveys, "asthma" included recurrent wheezing not associated with colds, as well as physician-diagnosed asthma, and so the increase in prevalence is not explained simply by a greater use of the label "asthma."

In Aberdeen, Scotland, the prevalence of wheezing among children surveyed in 1964 and 1989 rose from 10 to 20%, shortness of breath from 6 to 10%, diagnosed asthma from 4 to 10%, eczema from 6 to 12%, and hay fever from 3 to 12%, indicating a generalized increase in atopic diseases, as well as in respiratory symptoms suggesting asthma (Level II).[19] The label of wheezing as "asthma" in this survey increased from 27 to 50% during this time interval. Hence, increasing childhood "asthma" is related both to a true increase in symptoms and a greater use of the diagnostic label.

In Adults

There are few adequate data by which to judge changes in prevalence of adult asthma over the last two or three decades. In Canada, a medical claim insurance database provided some evidence of an increase in adult asthma as judged by first presentations for asthma in any given year between 1981 and 1990 (Level II).[20] Among Belgian army conscripts aged 17 to 31 years, the proportion with reported asthma rose from 2.4% in 1978 to 7.2% in 1991.[21] Throughout this period, approximately half of those reporting asthma had documented airway hyperresponsiveness, suggesting the increase was real and not just an increased reporting of milder symptoms.

Evidence for Increasing Severity

Information gathered concerning hospital admissions for asthma, use of antiasthma drugs, and asthma mortality, suggest that the prevalence or severity of asthma, or both, have increased. The marked increase in use of bronchodilator drugs and inhaled corticosteroids in

New Zealand, Australia, and the United Kingdom between 1975 and 1981 may reflect either increased severity of asthma or increased intensity of treatment of asthma.[22] However, in 1984 a New Zealand community study found that inhaled corticosteroid therapy was underused, with corticosteroids prescribed for only 42% of subjects with daily symptoms of asthma (Level II).[23] In five Scandinavian countries, asthma drug sales doubled over approximately 10 years.[24] More importantly, the number of drugs used per patient increased significantly. These data suggest that the increase in sales of antiasthma drugs are not necessarily just the reflection of improved treatment of asthma, but may also reflect an increase in the prevalence of more severe disease.

The role of asthma treatment in changing severity of the disease has been widely debated over the past decade, following the randomized controlled trial showing that regular use of the inhaled β-agonist fenoterol was associated with increased symptoms, reduced lung function, increased airway responsiveness, and overall less satisfactory control of asthma (Level I).[25] The greatest concern with regard to this finding related to asthma mortality, which increased sharply in New Zealand when fenoterol was introduced and decreased abruptly when it was withdrawn; the implications that high doses or frequent use of potent inhaled β-agonists may worsen the severity of asthma have suggested that this may account for some of the trends seen in the epidemiology of the disease, with regard to both morbidity and mortality.[26] The substantial decrease in hospital admissions, and in mortality in New Zealand when fenoterol was withdrawn, is consistent with a drug-induced increase in asthma and, consequently, morbidity and mortality (Level III).[27]

NATURAL HISTORY OF CHILDHOOD ASTHMA

Several studies have reported the outcome of childhood asthma by examining trends from mid-childhood into adulthood. Only recently have studies addressed the natural history of asthma or wheezing illness occurring in infancy and early childhood. The impact of treatment on the natural history of childhood asthma has not been systematically studied. Population-based longitudinal studies provide the best information as to the course and prognosis of childhood asthma followed to adulthood, even though the natural history may be modified by interventions.

The development and likelihood of persistence or early remission of childhood asthma has been most clearly defined in a cohort of newborns followed to age 6 years (Level II).[7] In this Tucson, Arizona study, 1,246 children born to parents registered in a Health Maintenance Organization were studied by questionnaire. Subgroups within this cohort underwent measurements of serum IgE, at birth and at 9 months, and lung function testing. Follow-up information regarding symptom status at age 3 years and age 6 years was reported for 826 children. Throughout these 6 years, 51% remained symptom free, 20% were characterized as "early wheezers" with development of wheezing before age 3 years and remission by age 6 years, 15% were "late wheezers" with no wheezing by age 3 years but wheezing symptoms developing by age 6 years, while 14% were "persistent wheezers" with wheezing occurring before age 3 years and persisting to age 6 years. Hence, by age 6 years, 49% of children had reported wheezing, but nearly half of these had no wheezing at age 6 years, suggesting remission. Those going into remission were more likely to have low lung function at ages 1 year and 6 years and to be exposed to maternal cigarette smoke, but they were not more likely to have high IgE levels, positive allergy skin tests, or a family history of asthma. Those whose wheezing persisted to age 6 years were more likely to have had a mother reporting asthma, elevated IgE at ages 1 and 6 years, and decreased lung function at age 6 years but not at age 1 year. This study strongly suggests that early wheezing followed by remission was more closely related to airway caliber and irritant than allergic exposures, whereas the dominant factors in the development of late onset and persistent wheezing were genetic and environmental factors related to atopy.

CHILDHOOD ASTHMA FOLLOWED UP TO ADULTHOOD

Three types of "natural history" studies of childhood asthma have been reported: follow-up of patients seen in an office practice, follow-up of patients seen in a specialist asthma clinic, and longitudinal studies of populations. Those followed up from office practices represent a selected population, as do those seen in specialty clinics, and outcomes can be expected to differ from those reported from population-based longitudinal studies. Particularly from specialist clinics, there is a high proportion of persistent disease, predicted by greater severity in early childhood, concomitant allergic disease including eczema and rhinitis, skin sensitivity to pollens and pets, and increased airway responsiveness in childhood. In a study from the Netherlands in which 101 children with asthma were followed up after a mean interval of 16 years, 65% of those with provoking concentration $(PC)_{10}$ histamine <2 mg/mL were asthmatic in adulthood, compared with 40% of those whose PC_{10} histamine had been between 2 and 8 mg/mL, and 33% of those with PC_{10} histamine >8 mg/mL (Level II).[28] In another Dutch university clinic cohort of children aged 8 to 12 years followed up at a mean age of 25 years, persistence of symptoms was more likely among women than men (85% vs 72%), and females had more adult airway responsiveness than males (Level II).[29] The prevalence of airway responsiveness was lowest in the children with the least degree of atopy in childhood.

Longitudinal studies of childhood asthma have been conducted in a number of communities. In Scotland, among 2,511 children selected at primary schools in Aberdeen in 1962 and followed up 25 years later, a history of childhood asthma was associated with adult wheezing (odds ratio 14.4) and sputum production (odds ratio 3.3), as well as a lower FEV_1 and greater airway responsiveness compared with normals (Level II).[30] Those with childhood wheezing not diagnosed as asthma had a better prognosis, with an odds ratio for wheezing in adulthood of 3.8 and for sputum production of 4.4. Lung function and airway responsiveness were similar to normals.

A 35-year follow-up study has been conducted in Melbourne, Australia. The initial cohort was a random sample of children aged 7 years, representative of socioeconomic status and geographic region, including every child with diagnosed asthma or more than five episodes of wheezing associated with infection, every second child with wheezing but less than five episodes associated with infection, and every twentieth normal child.[31] These subjects were seen again at ages 10, 14, 21, 28, and 35 years, with an 86% follow-up at age 35 years.[32] At that age, 32% of those classified as having "asthma" at age 7 years had persistent wheezing at least once per week in the previous 3 months, 18% had wheezing in the previous 3 months but less than once per week, 20% had less frequent symptoms, and only 30% were asymptomatic (Level II). Among those initially classified as having wheezy bronchitis, these figures were respectively 15%, 10%, 12%, and 63%. Hence, the likelihood of persistent symptoms were strongest in those with diagnosed asthma. Risk factors for persistence to age 35 years included multiple episodes occurring before the age of 2 years, the presence of atopy, eczema, and low lung function, but not the age of onset of symptoms.

In another Australian study of 8,600 7-year-old children living in Tasmania, the likelihood of current asthma symptoms as an adult was 25.6% among those who reported asthma at age 7 years, versus 10.0% of those who were asymptomatic at 7 years (Level II).[33] Current asthma as an adult was more likely among those with a later age of onset, more frequent attacks, and a greater total number of attacks. Risk factors for persistence to adult asthma included female gender, eczema, low lung function, maternal and paternal asthma, and the subject's own history of childhood asthma.

In Dunedin, New Zealand, a cohort of 1,037 children born in the city in 1 year had been followed up for 21 years.[34] Airway responsiveness in this cohort, defined as PC_{20} methacholine ≤8 mg/mL, decreased with age from 18% at age 9 years to become stable at 8 to 10% from ages 13 to 21 years. The cumulative prevalence of diagnosed asthma exceeded 20% at age 21 years. There was a wide variability of severity, with relatively few subjects having persistent asthma and many having remissions (but a substantial proportion of those with remissions experienced relapses in later teenage years) (Level II).[35] Persistence of early childhood asthma into adulthood was related to atopy, especially to allergic sensitization to house dust mite. In this cohort, adolescents who took up smoking did not increase the frequency of asthmatic episodes but, rather, developed increased cough and sputum suggesting the development of bronchitis rather than worsening of asthma (Level II).[36]

In the United Kingdom, a birth cohort of 18,559 children born in 1 week in March 1958 have been evaluated at ages 7, 11, 16, 23, and 33 years with respect to the presence of asthma and wheezing symptoms.[37] At age 7 years, experience of asthma or wheeze was reported by 18.2%, decreasing to 12.0% by age 11 years, and 11.5% at age 16 years. The prevalence of asthma or wheezing in the prior 12 months at ages 7, 11, 16, and 23 years was respectively 8.1%, 4.6%, 3.3%, and 4.0%. The incidence of new asthma from ages 17 to 33 years was strongly associated with active cigarette smoking and with a history of hay fever, with weaker associations with female gender, and histories of migraine and eczema. Maternal smoking during pregnancy was an independent predictor of incidence of asthma after age 16 years. Relapse at age 33 years after prolonged remission of childhood wheezing was more common among current smokers and those with atopy (Level II).

Using data from three longitudinal cohort studies, Strachan and Gerritsen reported that children who outgrew wheezing tended to return to normal pulmonary function, whereas those with persistent wheezing had reduced lung function even after administration of β-agonists (Level II).[38] The degree of reduction of pulmonary function was proportional to the duration and persistence of symptoms and was predicted by airway hyper-responsiveness and decreased lung function in childhood.

In the Melbourne cohort, followed up to age 35 years, lung function at age 35 years was related to severity of asthma at ages 7 and 10 years (Level II).[39] Those with childhood asthma had significantly lower mean FEV_1 values and FEV_1/VC ratios in adult life.

Several factors have been clearly identified as contributing to persistence of childhood asthma, including the family history, atopy in childhood, continuing exposure to environmental tobacco smoke, and severity of childhood asthma. The effect of gender on persistence is consistent among studies, with a greater likelihood of persistence in females, even though childhood asthma is more common among males.

The effects of treatment on the natural history of asthma have been little studied. In the Melbourne cohort, prognosis from childhood to adulthood did not appear to be influenced by the management of childhood asthma.[32] However, Agertoft and Pedersen, in a study of children attending a pediatric clinic, noted substantial improvement in lung function with use of inhaled corticosteroid therapy, with more improvement in those receiving early corticosteroid therapy (Level III).[40]

NATURAL HISTORY OF ADULT ASTHMA

There are remarkably few data examining the course and prognosis of adult asthma and the effects of treatment. Studies of occupational asthma show frequent persistence of both symptoms and abnormal pulmonary function, even in subjects removed from exposure, but the outcome does depend on the sensitizing agent and duration of exposure (Level III).[41] Studies from Scandinavia report a very low incidence of remission of adult asthma (Level II).[42] Only 3% of those reporting current asthma in 1986 were asymptomatic in 1996. In a study of younger adults in the Netherlands, retested 25 years after their initial investigations for asthma, 40% had no symptoms in later adult life, but only 21% did not show airway hyper-responsiveness.[43] Remission was more likely to occur in younger subjects, those with less severe disease at initial study, and those in whom treatment was initiated relatively early after the onset. In contrast, among subjects residing in Tucson, Arizona, who were aged over 65 years at enrolment, less than 20% had remission of their asthma over a 7-year follow-up period.[44]

MORTALITY

Overall, mortality rates in asthma are low compared with other chronic diseases. Substantial increases in reported asthma mortality have occurred over the last three decades, in particular in two epidemics: the first involving England, Wales, Australia, and New Zealand between 1964 and 1966;[45] and the second occurring in New Zealand from 1977 to 1988.[46] In these two epidemics, the mortality from asthma, particularly among young people, rose to 3 to 5 times the baseline level. Increases in other countries have been more gradual and have rarely exceeded a twofold increase over the 10-year period.[47]

Accuracy of certification of death due to asthma has been studied in several countries, and while false-negatives and a few false-positives are reported, the identification of true asthma deaths in the younger population appears accurate (Level II).[48,49] In the older population, confusion between asthma and chronic airflow limitation due to bronchitis or other causes has made interpretation of trends more difficult, particularly when there are coding changes between different revisions of the International Classification of Disease. These have little impact on trends in mortality rates in young people.

Risk factors for asthma mortality include young and old age, ethnicity, psychosocial disturbance, a previous history of severe or life-threatening attacks, discontinuity of physician care, and recurrent emergency department visits and previous hospital admissions (Level III).[50–52] In the majority of descriptive studies of asthma mortality, inadequate assessment and treatment of severe asthma was implicated, with excess reliance on bronchodilator treatment and inappropriately low use of corticosteroid therapy. In a prospective study of asthmatic patients in Copenhagen, risk factors for mortality included cigarette smoking, age, atopic status, impairment of lung function, and degree of reversibility to β-agonist, with greater mortality among those with moderate impairments of obstruction and greater reversibility, as compared with more fixed airflow obstruction (Level II).[53]

The role of β-agonist treatment in the epidemics of asthma mortality has been widely debated, but consistent evidence supporting the effect of frequent use of the potent β-agonist fenoterol has been provided from several sources, including three case-control studies in New Zealand,[54–56] and a nested case-control study in Canada (Level II).[57] The use of fenoterol was associated with a significantly higher risk of death than the use of salbutamol, but the risks were similar when adjustment was made for the higher dose per puff in the fenoterol canister. Use of more than two canisters of β-agonist per month increased the risk of mortality over 10-fold.[58] Debate continues as to whether these risks are indicative of severe asthma or a direct deleterious effect of β-agonist on asthma severity.[26] Evidence favouring the latter comes from randomized clinical trials showing that regular use of inhaled β-agonist may be associated with increased airway responsiveness to nonspecific as well as allergen challenge, reduced lung function, shortening of time to first exacerbation, and overall less satisfactory control of asthma (Level I).[25,59,60] On the other hand, use of inhaled corticosteroid therapy in adequate dosage reduces the risk of asthma mortality. In Saskatchewan, subjects using more than one canister per month of low-dose inhaled corticosteroid had an odds ratio for death of 0.1 (Level II).[61]

The withdrawal of fenoterol from use in New Zealand was followed within 1 year by an abrupt fall in both asthma mortality and asthma morbidity as reflected in a reduction in hospital admissions.[27] This argues against the effect of β-agonist on mortality being due to cardiac arrhythmias, and favours an adverse effect on asthma severity (Level III).[62]

In most countries, asthma mortality rates have decreased over the last decade—the exceptions being the United States, which only now appears to be reaching a plateau; and Japan, which has yet to reach a plateau.[63] The overall decline in mortality likely reflects many factors, including increased use of inhaled corticosteroid, decreased reliance on β-agonist, and a greater appreciation of the chronicity and severity of asthma necessitating regular treatment and follow-up.

REFERENCES

1. Asher MI, Keil U, Anderson HR, et al. International Study of Asthma and Allergies in Childhood (ISAAC): rationale and methods. Eur Respir J 1995;8:483–91.

2. Burney P, Chinn S, Luczynska C, et al. Variations in the prevalence of respiratory symptoms, self-reported asthma attacks, and use of asthma medication in the European Community Respiratory Health Survey (ECRHS). Eur Respir J 1996;9:687–95.

3. Sears MR, Burrows B, Flannery EM, et al. Relation between airway responsiveness and serum IgE in children with asthma and in apparently normal children. N Engl J Med 1991;325:1067–71.

4. Pizzichini E, Pizzichini MMM, Efthimiadis A, et al. Indices of airway inflammation in induced sputum: reproducibility and validity of cell and fluid-phase measurements. Am J Respir Crit Care Med 1996;154:308–17.

5. National Institutes of Health, National Heart, Lung and Blood Institute. Global strategy for asthma management and prevention. NHLB/WHO Workshop Report March 1993. Bethesda:NHLBI; 1995 Publication No: 95-3659. p. 6.

6. Toelle BG, Peat JK, Salome CM, et al. Toward a definition of asthma for epidemiology. Am Rev Respir Dis 1992;146:633–7.

7. Martinez FD, Wright AL, Taussig LM, et al. Asthma and wheezing in the first six years of life. N Engl J Med 1995;332:133–8.

8. Jenkins MA, Clarke JR, Carlin JB, et al. Validation of questionnaire and bronchial hyperresponsiveness against respiratory physician assessment in the diagnosis of asthma. Int J Epidemiol 1996;25:609–16.

9. The International Study of Asthma and Allergies in Childhood (ISAAC) Steering Committee. Worldwide variation in prevalence of symptoms of asthma, allergic rhinoconjunctivitis, and atopic eczema: ISAAC. Lancet 1998;351:1225–32.

10. Habbick BF, Pizzichini MMM, Taylor B, et al. Prevalence of asthma, hay fever and eczema in children in 2 Canadian cities: the international study of asthma and allergies in childhood. Can Med Assoc J 1999;160:1824–8.

11. Shaw RA, Crane J, Pearce N, et al. Comparison of a video questionnaire with the IUATLD written questionnaire for measuring asthma prevalence. Clin Exp Allergy 1992;22:561–8.

12. Pizzichini MMM, Rennie D, Senthilselvan A, et al. Agreement between the ISAAC written and video asthma symptom questionnaires in two regions of Canada. Pediatr Pulmonol. In press.

13. Chinn S, Burney P, Jarvis D, Luczynska C, on behalf of the European Community Respiratory Health Survey (ECRHS). Variation in bronchial responsiveness in the European Community Respiratory Health Survey (ECRHS). Eur Respir J 1997;10:2495–501.

14. Jones DT, Sears MR, Holdaway MD, et al. Childhood asthma in New Zealand. Br J Dis Chest 1987;81:332–40.

15. Pizzichini MMM, Pizzichini E, Sears MR. Asthma diagnosis and severity of symptoms in Canadian children. Eur Respir J 1996;9 Suppl 23:216s.

16. Burney PGJ, Chinn S, Rona RJ. Has the prevalence of asthma increased in children? Evidence from the national study of health and growth 1973–86. Br Med J 1990;300:1306–10.

17. Rona RJ, Chinn S, Burney PGJ. Trends in the prevalence of asthma in Scottish and English primary school children 1982–92. Thorax 1995;50:992–3.

18. Gergen PJ, Mullaly DI, Evans R. National survey of prevalence of asthma among children in the United States, 1976 to 1980. Pediatrics 1988;81:1–7.

19. Ninan TK, Russell G. Respiratory symptoms and atopy in Aberdeen schoolchildren: evidence from two surveys 25 years apart. Br Med J 1992;304:873–5.

20. Senthilselvan A. Prevalence of physician-diagnosed asthma in Saskatchewan, 1981 to 1990. Chest 1998;114:388–92.

21. Dubois P, Degrave E, Vandenplas O. Asthma and airway hyperresponsiveness among Belgian conscripts, 1978–91. Thorax 1998;53:101–5.

22. Keating G, Mitchell EA, Jackson R, et al. Trends in sales of drugs for asthma in New Zealand, Australia and the United Kingdom, 1975–81. Br Med J 1984;289:348–51.

23. Sinclair BL, Clark DWJ, Sears MR. Use of anti-asthma drugs in New Zealand. Thorax 1987;42:670–5.

24. Klaukka T, Peura S, Martikainen J. Why has the utilization of antiasthmatic patients increased in Finland? J Clin Epidemiol 1991;44:859–63.

25. Sears MR, Taylor DR, Print CG, et al. Regular inhaled beta-agonist treatment in bronchial asthma. Lancet 1990;336:1391–6.

26. Sears MR, Taylor DR. The β_2-agonist controversy. Observations, explanations and relationship to asthma epidemiology. Drug Safety 1994;11:259–83.

27. Sears MR. Epidemiological trends in asthma. Can Respir J 1996;3:261–8.

28. Gerritsen J, Koeter GH, Postma DS, et al. Airway responsiveness in childhood as a predictor of the outcome of asthma in adulthood. Am Rev Respir Dis 1991;143:1468–9.

29. Roorda RJ, Gerritsen J, van Aalderen WMC, et al. Follow-up of asthma from childhood to adulthood: influence of potential childhood risk factors on the outcome of pulmonary function and bronchial responsiveness in adulthood. J Allergy Clin Immunol 1994;93:575–84.

30. Godden DJ, Ross S, Abdalla M, et al. Outcome of wheeze in childhood. Symptoms and pulmonary function 25 years later. Am J Respir Crit Care Med 1994;149:106–12.

31. Williams H, McNicol KN. Prevalence, natural history and relationship of wheezy bronchitis and asthma in children. An epidemiological study. Br Med J 1969;4:321–5.

32. Oswald H, Phelan PD, Lanigan A, et al. Outcome of childhood asthma in mid-adult life. Br Med J 1994;309:95–6.

33. Jenkins MA, Hopper JL, Bowes G, et al. Factors in childhood as predictors of asthma in adult life. Br Med J 1994;309:90–3.

34. Sears MR, Holdaway MD, Flannery EM, et al. Parental and neonatal risk factors for atopy, airway hyper-responsiveness, and asthma. Arch Dis Child 1996;75:392–8.

35. Sears MR, Willan A, Herbison GP, et al. Associations between atopy, hyperresponsiveness and persistence of childhood asthma. Eur Respir J 1997;10 Suppl 25:162s.

36. Sears MR, Flannery EM, Herbison GP, et al. Does smoking worsen asthma or add a new disease? [abstract] Am J Respir Crit Care Med 1997;155:A76.

37. Strachan DP, Butland BK, Anderson HR. Incidence and prognosis of asthma and wheezing illness from early childhood to age 33 in a national British cohort. Br Med J 1996;312:1195–9.

38. Strachan D, Gerritsen J. Long-term outcome of early childhood wheezing: population data. Eur Respir J 1996;9:42–7s.

39. Oswald H, Phelan PD, Lanigan A, et al. Childhood asthma and lung function in mid-adult life. Pediatr Pulmonol 1997;23:14–20.

40. Agertoft L, Pedersen S. Effects of long-term treatment with an inhaled corticosteroid on growth and pulmonary function in asthmatic children. Respir Med 1994;88:373–81.

41. Venables KM, Chan-Yeung M. Occupational asthma. Lancet 1997;349:1465–9.

42. Ronmark E, Jonsson E, Lundback B. Remission of asthma 1986–1996—Report from the Obstructive Lung Disease in Northern Sweden study. Eur Respir J 1997;10 Suppl 25:164s.

43. Panhuysen CIM, Vonk JM, Koeter GH, et al. Adult patients may outgrow their asthma. A 25-year follow-up study. Am J Respir Crit Care Med 1997;155:1267–72.

44. Burrows B, Barbee RA, Cline MG, et al. Characteristics of asthma among elderly adults in a sample of the general population. Chest 1991;100:935–42.

45. Fraser PM, Speizer FE, Waters SDM, et al. The circumstances preceding death from asthma in young people in 1968 to 1969. Br J Dis Chest 1971;65:71–84.

46. Jackson RT, Beaglehole R, Rea HH, Sutherland DC. Mortality from asthma: a new epidemic in New Zealand. Br Med J 1982;285:771–4.

47. Jackson R, Sears MR, Beaglehole R, Rea HH. International trends in asthma mortality: 1970 to 1985. Chest 1988;94:914–8.

48. British Thoracic Association Subcommittee. Accuracy of death certificates in bronchial asthma. Thorax 1984;39:505–9.

49. Sears MR, Rea HH, De Boer G, et al. Accuracy of certification of deaths due to asthma. A national study. Am J Epidemiol 1986;124:1004–11.

50. Rea HH, Sears MR, Beaglehole R, et al. Lessons from the national asthma mortality study: circumstances surrounding death. N Z Med J 1987;100:10–3.

51. Johnson AJ, Nunn AJ, Somner AR, et al. Circumstances of death from asthma. Br Med J 1984;288:1870–2.

52. Tough SC, Green FHY, Paul JE, et al. Sudden death from asthma in 108 children and young adults. J Asthma 1996;33:179–88.

53. Ulrik CS, Frederiksen J. Mortality and markers of risk of asthma death among 1,075 outpatients with asthma. Chest 1995;108:10–5.

54. Crane J, Pearce N, Flatt A, et al. Prescribed fenoterol and death from asthma in New Zealand, 1981–83: case-control study. Lancet 1989;1:918–22.

55. Pearce N, Grainger J, Atkinson M, et al. Case-control study of prescribed fenoterol and death from asthma in New Zealand, 1977–81. Thorax 1990;45:170–5.

56. Grainger J, Woodman K, Pearce N, et al. Prescribed fenoterol and death from asthma in New Zealand, 1981–7: a further case-control study. Thorax 1991;46:105–11.

57. Spitzer WO, Suissa S, Ernst P, et al. The use of β-agonists and the risk of death and near death from asthma. N Engl J Med 1992;326:501–6.

58. Suissa S, Ernst P, Boivin J-F, et al. A cohort analysis of excess mortality in asthma and the use of inhaled beta agonists. Am J Respir Crit Care Med 1994;149:604–10.

59. Cockcroft DW, McPaarland CP, Britto SA, et al. Regular inhaled salbutamol and airway responsiveness to allergen. Lancet 1993;342:833–7.

60. Cockcroft DW, O'Byrne PM, Swystun VA, Bhagat R. Regular use of inhaled albuterol and the allergen-induced late asthmatic response. J Allergy Clin Immunol 1995;96:44–9.

61. Ernst P, Spitzer W, Suissa S, et al. Risk of fatal and near fatal asthma in relation to inhaled corticosteroid use. JAMA 1992;268:3462–4.

62. Sears MR. Role of β₂-agonists in asthma fatalities. In: Sheffer AL, editor. Lung biology in health and disease, Vol. 115: Fatal Asthma. New York: Marcel Dekker; 1998. p. 457–81.

63. Sears MR. Epidemiology. In: Barnes PJ, Rodger IW, Thomson NC, editors. Asthma. Basic mechanisms and clinical management. 3rd ed. San Diego: Academic Press; 1998. p. 1–33

CHAPTER 2

Genetics of Asthma

Andrew J. Sandford, PhD,
Tracey D. Weir, BMLSc,
Peter D. Paré, MD

There is little doubt that genes contribute to the etiology of asthma and allergic diseases. However, the inheritance patterns of asthma and allergy demonstrate that these are "complex genetic disorders" rather than single gene disorders that follow classic mendelian genetics. Another important feature that distinguishes complex genetic disorders from single gene disorders is their prevalence in the population. Asthma occurs in 4 to 8% of the population, whereas the most frequent single gene disorder of the lungs, cystic fibrosis, occurs in only 0.05% of live Caucasian births.

There are several possible reasons that complex genetic disorders are not inherited in a simple mendelian fashion. First, several genes may predispose to the development of the traits—either more than one gene in the same individual (polygenic inheritance) or different combinations of genes in different individuals (genetic heterogeneity). Second, environmental factors are necessary for expression of the disease phenotype.

The symptoms of asthma—wheeze, cough, and breathlessness—are caused by acute and chronic inflammation in the airways of affected individuals. The airway inflammation is most frequently an IgE-mediated inflammatory response to common aeroallergens. Thus, most of this chapter deals with the genetics of the allergic form of asthma. Other mechanisms that produce an asthmatic phenotype may have a different, or no, genetic basis. However, strong evidence also supports a genetic contribution to nonallergic asthma.[1]

It is our aim in this chapter to present the evidence for a genetic contribution to asthma and to summarize the latest evidence for candidate genes.

CONTRIBUTION OF HEREDITY TO ASTHMA AND ALLERGY

Familial Concordance

One classic method of quantifying the hereditary contribution to a complex disorder is to calculate a parameter termed heritability (H). Heritability is defined as the proportion of phenotypic variance in a population that can be attributed to genetic factors. Estimates of heritability as it relates to asthma and allergy can be derived using the prevalence of asthma or other allergic phenotypes in the general population and in first-degree relatives of affected individuals.[2] The results are variable but all suggest a major genetic contribution to the development of asthma and allergic disorders (H = 0.6–1.0).

Estimates of heritability are influenced by shared environments and shared genes. The increased prevalence of a trait in the first-degree relatives of a proband could be due to their shared environment. For example, certain allergens such as house dust mite or cat dander are specific to the microenvironment of a household. Another complicating factor is the presence of phenocopies within the population. Phenocopies are environmentally induced phenotypes that mimick a phenotype of the genetic disorder of interest. Phenocopies can occur for asthma and allergy phenotypes. For example, in infants and children, asthma may be confused with viral bronchiolitis or "wheezy bronchitis." In adults, asthmatic symptoms such as episodic wheeze and dyspnea can also occur in patients who have chronic obstructive pulmonary disease (COPD). In addition, elevated IgE levels characteristic of atopic disease can be mimicked by a helminthic intestinal parasitic infection.

Studies of Twins

Studies of twins are often used to determine the relative contribution of genes and the environment in complex genetic disorders. For quantitative traits, the intrapair correlation coefficient is calculated. A disease phenotype that has a genetic component is expected to have a higher intrapair correlation coefficient in monozygotic (MZ) twins than in dizygotic (DZ) twins. The results of such studies generally support a role for genes in traits such as total serum IgE and skin-test responses.[3]

The study of discrete phenotypes uses a measure of twin concordance. There is general agreement in results from smaller studies of twins that yield heritability estimates similar to those derived from studies of families.[3] However, the concordance rates are lower in studies of large populations in which the determination of phenotype was based either on a mailed questionnaire[4] or hospital and pharmacy records.[5] These methods of phenotyping may be one reason that the concordance rates are lower than in smaller studies for which asthmatic or allergic twins were specifically ascertained.

The concordance and correlation of a trait between twins will also be influenced by the similar environment that they share, and it is likely that MZ twins will share a more similar environment than DZ twins. One way to separate the effect of shared genes and environment in studies of twins is to compare twins reared apart to twins reared together, as was done in a study by Hanson et al.[6] The prevalence of asthma in the subjects was too low to accurately compare concordance. The concordance for seasonal rhinitis and the correlation coefficient for levels of total IgE were not higher in twins reared together than in those reared apart. These unique data suggest that there is a major genetic contribution to twin concordance and that environmental contribution to concordance is small or negligible.

In a recent study of skin-test responses to ryegrass pollen allergens, the investigators found that the concordance level for responses to each allergen among MZ twins was similar to that found in DZ twins.[7] This result suggests that there is less genetic control of IgE responses to specific antigens than there is for total IgE levels.

Mode of Inheritance

Determination of the mode of inheritance of a genetic disease is known as segregation analysis. Early segregation analyses of asthma found autosomal dominant inheritance.[8] Segregation analyses using total IgE as a phenotype have yielded conflicting results. In these studies, autosomal recessive,[9] dominant,[10] co-dominant,[11] polygenic,[10] and two-loci[12] models have all been suggested. Several investigators have proposed that basal IgE levels are controlled separately from specific IgE responses to aeroallergens.[9]

These conflicting results suggest that there is no major gene for asthma or IgE responses. Furthermore, genetic heterogeneity is likely to exist so that different genes and inheritance patterns are involved in different populations. An additional confounding factor is incomplete penetrance, that is, the reduced probability of observing a phenotype given a specific genotype. Finally, the results of several studies indicate the importance of the gender of the parent who transmits the trait. For example, maternal asthma was found to be a stronger predictor of asthma in the child than paternal asthma.[13] Maternal atopic disease is also a stronger predictor of umbilical cord IgE levels than paternal disease.[14] In families with at least one asthmatic family member, a significant maternal, but not paternal, influence on lung function was found.[15] Similar gender-specific inheritance patterns have been demonstrated in other genetic diseases such as bipolar disorder and Huntington's disease. The mechanism responsible for these effects could be "imprinting" (gender-specific modification of gene expression). However, the cause of these effects with regard to asthma could be environmental, not genetic, for example, modulation of the infant's immune responses in utero via maternal antibodies or cytokines.

ASTHMA AND ALLERGY PHENOTYPES

The definition of the asthmatic or allergic phenotype has been difficult and contentious to ascertain. Phenotypes may be either categorical, such as the presence or absence of wheeze, or continuous (quantitative), such as the serum level of IgE.

Total Serum IgE

Total serum IgE demonstrates a unimodal distribution within the population.[16] The fact that a trait is continuous and unimodal as opposed to bimodal suggests that multiple genes may be involved in its expression. A bimodal distribution would indicate that a single mutant gene might be responsible. Total IgE levels are known to be increased by cigarette smoking, and infections with nematodes can inflate IgE levels almost 100-fold. However, even in a population of nematode-infected individuals, logarithm IgE was normally distributed and unimodal, indicating a polygenic and environmental influence.

Skin Tests and Specific IgE

Although total serum IgE levels are unimodally distributed, skin-test responses and serum IgE levels to specific allergens are often bimodally distributed within a population. Among 3,102 unselected individuals, 24% and 9% had positive skin-test responses to Bermuda grass and house dust mite antigen, respectively.[17] While the distribution of skin-test responses peaks at 10 mm for grass and 5 mm for dust mite, the majority of the population forms a second peak at 0 mm. A similar bimodal distribution can be demonstrated for serum levels of specific IgE in a population. The bimodal distribution of skin-test responses and specific IgE serum could be due to the presence of a genetically susceptible group or to heterogeneity of exposure to the allergens. However, the fact that the distribution is bimodal for a ubiquitous aeroallergen (Bermuda grass) supports genetic susceptibility as the important cause of the bimodal distribution.

Bronchial Hyper-responsiveness

Another feature of airway disease that may have a hereditary component is bronchial hyper-responsiveness (BHR).[18] Most population studies have shown a unimodal distribution of measures of bronchial responsiveness with considerable overlap between normal, atopic, asthmatic, and nonasthmatic individuals.[19] However, a bimodal distribution has been demonstrated in nonatopic family members of asthmatic probands[20] and in parents of asthmatic children,[18] suggesting a major genetic component.

Longo et al proposed that BHR is controlled by an autosomal dominant gene with incomplete penetrance.[18] This gene could impart moderate BHR, which could then be enhanced by allergic inflammation. However, others have suggested that BHR is predominantly acquired based on discordance in the degree of airway responsiveness between allergic and nonallergic MZ twins.[21] According to this viewpoint, BHR in atopic individuals who do not have lower respiratory tract symptoms is a reflection of subclinical airway inflammation.

Several studies have demonstrated a strong association between BHR and atopy.[22] However, atopics may not have BHR, and subjects who have BHR may not be atopic, leading to the hypothesis that BHR is a separately inherited phenotypic trait. In support of this theory, a high prevalence of BHR was found in both atopic and nonatopic relatives of children with atopic asthma.[23] Moreover, there was frequent concordance of BHR in MZ twins who were not concordant for atopy or symptomatic asthma.[24] At the present time, there is no consensus among experts as to the independent contribution of heredity to BHR.

End-Organ Response

There is evidence that there is a genetic contribution to the organ-specific manifestations of allergic disease that can be separated from the inherited tendency to generate excessive IgE and develop some form of allergic symptoms. Parents who have asthma are more likely to have offspring who will have asthma rather than allergic rhinitis or eczema, and vice versa.[2] Similarly, MZ and DZ twins who are concordant for an allergic disorder are more likely to be concordant for the same organ involvement.[4] There also may be a separate genetic influence on the symptoms of specific manifestations of asthma. Duffy and Mitchell found that cough and wheeze segregated separately in families who have asthma.[25]

IDENTIFICATION OF ASTHMA AND ATOPY GENES

Several approaches are being used to identify the genes involved in susceptibility to asthma and atopy. The most systematic approach is to search the entire human genome one segment at a time, but this is time consuming and expensive, Such genome screens are performed on families with asthma or atopy, and the genes are detected by co-inheritance (or linkage) of a particular chromosomal region with the trait under consideration.

An alternative approach is to directly target specific genes that are candidates for suscep-tibility on the basis of their function. Association studies of unrelated subjects or family stud-ies can be used in this approach.

The specific genes and chromosomal regions identified by such techniques are summa-rized in Figure 2–1. The strength of the evidence in favor of each region or gene is estimated in Table 2–1. The role of each candidate gene in the pathogenesis of allergy and asthma is summarized in Figure 2–2.

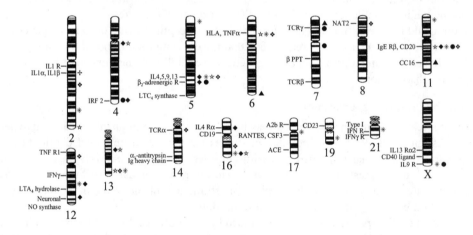

Figure 2–1 Linkages to asthma and related phenotypes. The phenotypes are shown to the right of each chromosome: ✻ = asthma; ◆ = total serum IgE; + = wheeze, ☆ = atopy; ● = bronchial hyper-responsiveness; ❖ = specific IgE; ▲ = eosinophil counts. Chromosomal locations are approximate. Only linkages with p < .01 are shown. Candidate genes from each region are shown to the left of each chromosome. A2b = adenosine 2b; ACE = angiotensin converting enzyme; CC = Clara cell; CD = cluster designation; CSF = colony-stimulating factor; HLA = human leukocyte antigen; IFN = inter-feron; Ig = immunoglobulin; IL = interleukin; IRF = interferon regulatory factor; LT = leukotriene; NAT2 = N-acetyltransferase; NO = nitric oxide; PPT = preprotachykinin; R = receptor; RANTES = regulated on activation, normal T expressed and secreted; TCR = T cell antigen receptor; TNF = tumour necrosis factor.

Genome Screens

The first genome screen for asthma and atopy phenotypes found 6 potential linkages.[26] Four of these linkages were replicated in an additional study group. However, there was little con-sistency in the linked phenotypes in the first group compared with the second, which may reflect pleiotropy of gene action (ie, one gene affecting multiple phenotypes).

The Collaborative Study on the Genetics of Asthma (CSGA) identified linkage of asthma

Table 2–1 *Levels of Evidence for Candidate Genes in Allergy and Asthma Phenotypes*

Evidence Level*	Criteria†	Candidate Genes
1	A and E or B and E	Interleukin-4, β_2-adrenergic receptor, tumour necrosis factor α, interleukin-4 receptor α, HLA, α_1-antitrypsin
2	A or B	β subunit of the high-affinity IgE receptor
3	C and E or D and E	*N*-acetyltransferase, angiotensin converting enzyme
4	C or D	Interleukins -5, -9, and -13, glucocorticoid receptor, CD14, Clara cell protein 16, transporter antigen peptide 1, interleukin-9 receptor, immunoglobulin heavy-chain genes, T cell antigen receptor α, T cell antigen receptor β

*1 = highest; 4 = lowest.

†A. Candidate gene is localized to a linked region of the human genome, and the linkage has been *replicated* in at least two separate populations. B. Candidate gene contains, or is close to, a polymorphism(s) *repeatedly* associated with an allergy or asthma phenotype. C. Candidate gene is localized to a linked region of the human genome. D. Candidate gene contains, or is close to, a polymorphism(s) associated with an allergy or asthma phenotype. E. Candidate gene contains a polymorphism(s) that is proven to increase or decrease the gene product's function or level in a manner that could contribute to the pathogenesis of allergy or asthma.

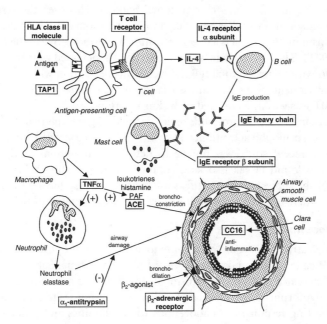

Figure 2–2 Functional roles of candidate genes implicated in the pathogenesis of allergy and asthma. The candidate genes are shown in the boxes: (1) Major histocompatibility complex class II and transporter antigen peptide (TAP) variants may allow allergens to be presented more effectively to T cells. (2) Specific T cell receptor types may allow more effective T cell response to allergens. (3) More (or more active) interleukin-4 (IL-4) or its receptor could cause an exaggerated production of IgE. (4) IgE heavy-chain variants may bind to IgE receptors with greater affinity. (5) More effective high-affinity IgE receptors may cause a greater affinity. (5) More effective high-affinity IgE receptors may cause an exaggerated response to IgE cross-linking by allergen and release of more IL-4. (6) Tumor necrosis factor α (TNFα) variants may increase the degree of airway inflammation. (7) Angiotensin converting enzyme (ACE) variants could promote bronchoconstriction and airway smooth muscle proliferation. (8) The allergic inflammatory response to mediators and cytokines may increase because of decreased antiproteolytic activity of α_1-antitrypsin. (9) The smooth muscle response to contractile agonists released from effector cells could be enhanced due to defective or down-regulated β_2-adrenergic receptors.

to 6 novel regions.[27] The authors confirmed 5 other previously reported linkages, such as those on chromosomes 5q[28] and 12q.[29] However, there was generally a lack of reproducibility between different ethnic groups, which may reflect genetic heterogeneity in different populations.

A third genome screen was performed in a genetically isolated population.[30] The study identified 10 regions showing possible linkage to asthma or related phenotypes. Four regions (including chromosomes 5q and 12q) also showed linkage in a replication sample and had previously been linked in other populations. These results show that even in an isolated population with limited genetic diversity there may be several asthma susceptibility genes.

Finally, the CSGA group performed a search for genes that influence IgE responsiveness to house dust mite allergens.[31] Linkage was demonstrated to the human leukocyte antigens (HLA) region and to 2 other regions identified by the previous genome screens. In addition, 2 novel linked regions were detected. Interestingly, the only linked region in all four genome screens was chromosome 13q. However, there are currently no obvious candidate genes located in this region.

Chromosome 5q

Chromosome 5q contains a wealth of candidate genes for asthma and atopy, such as interleukin-4 (IL-4), IL-5, IL-9, IL-13, the glucocorticoid receptor, cluster designation 14 (CD14), and the β_2-adrenergic receptor (β_2AR). Several groups have found linkage to chromosome 5q31–q33 with total IgE as the phenotype.[28] Linkage of specific IgE responses to common. aeroallergens was also found in this chromosomal region.[32] However, the results of other recent linkage and association studies have failed to confirm some of these findings.[33]

A polymorphism in this region is a C→T transition at position −590 in the IL-4 gene promoter (IL-4 C−590T). The −590T allele was associated with increased gene transcription in a reporter assay and with increased total IgE in vivo.[34] The association with IgE levels was not replicated in a subsequent study, but an association with asthma was found.[35] In another study, IL-4 C−590T was weakly associated with skin-test responses.[36]

An additional candidate gene from this region is the IL-5 gene. Interleukin-5 is the major cytokine controlling eosinophil activation, and eosinophilia is characteristic of airway inflammation; however, a recent study was unable to detect any mutations in the IL-5 gene.[37] Another recent study found a weak association of total serum IgE with a polymorphism from the IL-9 gene after the subjects were stratified for specific IgE responses.[38] Interleukin-9 was suggested as a candidate for asthma by an investigation of the genetics of BHR in mice.[39]

β_2 -Adrenergic Receptor

The theory that defective β_2AR could contribute to asthma was proposed long before markers near the β_2AR gene on chromosome 5q were linked to asthma. Subsequent association studies provided evidence that polymorphisms in the β_2AR gene do not cause asthma.[40–42] However, these polymorphisms are associated with altered responses to exogenous β_2AR agonists, possibly affecting responses to endogenous catecholamines and asthma therapy and modulating the resulting asthma phenotype.

The two most common polymorphisms of the β_2AR occur in the extracellular N-terminus at positions 16 (ARG16GLY) and 27 (GLN27GLU). These polymorphisms may affect β_2AR responses by altering receptor trafficking and insertion into the plasma membrane. Data from in vitro studies suggest that cultured human airway smooth muscle cells that are homozygous for GLY16 display greater downregulation of the receptor in response to agonist than cells that are homozygous for ARG16.[43]

The results of several studies demonstrate that individuals who have the GLY16 allele seem to respond less well to exogenous β_2AR agonists than those who have ARG16. Reihsaus et al found that asthmatic patients who had GLY16 were more likely to be steroid dependent, possibly because they respond less well to β_2AR therapy.[41] In another study, asthmatic patients who had GLY16 showed significantly more desensitization to formoterol than those who had

ARG16.[44] In a larger study of 269 children, the ARG16 allele was associated with increased response to albuterol, regardless of asthma.[42] Results of these last two studies also demonstrated that ARG16GLY heterozygotes had intermediate responses.

GLY16 may affect responses to endogenous as well as exogenous β_2AR agonists. Turki et al showed that GLY16 was more prevalent in asthmatic patients who had nocturnal symptoms than in those who did not.[45] Since β_2AR levels are known to decrease during the night, the less responsive GLY16 receptor may contribute to night-time symptoms.

The results of studies of the GLN27GLU locus showed that the GLN27 allele was associated with BHR in asthmatic patients[46] and with increased asthma in children.[47] Since the GLN27 allele is associated with the GLY16 allele,[40,42] it is not clear whether these disease associations are due to GLN27, GLY16, or the GLY16/GLN27 haplotype (combination of alleles). Results from a haplotype association study showed that GLY16/GLN27 was more prevalent in severe asthmatic patients than in mild asthmatic patients (defined by steroid use and lung function).[40]

A silent mutation that is located close to the GLN27GLU polymorphism was associated with asthma and response to salbutamol in Japanese families.[48] This study and one by Hopes et al[47] are the only ones that find a positive association with asthma. At the present time, it is clear that polymorphisms in the β_2AR gene affect responses to β_2AR agonists and may contribute to the asthmatic phenotype. It is still unclear whether determination of the β_2AR genotype would be sufficiently predictive of responsiveness to β_2-agonists to be of clinical value.

Chromosome 11q

Chromosome 11q13 was the first region to be linked to measures of atopy and asthma,[49] but this linkage proved difficult to replicate.[50] More recently, studies have shown either linkage or association of 11q to asthma,[51] total serum IgE,[52] BHR,[53] and specific IgE responses.[32] However, the importance of chromosome 11q in atopic disease remains a controversial issue.[54]

A candidate from the 11q13 region is the gene for the β subunit of the high-affinity receptor for IgE (FcεRIβ).[55] Mutations in this gene could lead to increased signal transduction after allergen binds to IgE and, consequently, to increased secretion of interleukin-4 (IL-4). One such mutation (LEU181) was associated with atopy[56] and asthma[57] but was not detected in any other population.[58] Another mutation in the FcεRIβ gene causes an amino acid substitution (GLU237GLY) in the cytoplasmic tail of the protein. This mutation was associated with positive skin-test responses[59] and with childhood asthma.[60] Bronchial hyperresponsiveness, but not asthma, has been associated with another polymorphism in the FcεRIβ gene.[61]

An alternative candidate gene from this region is the Clara cell–derived anti-inflammatory molecule CC16. A polymorphism in the untranslated region of CC16 was associated with asthma.[62] However, in other studies, no association of CC16 variants was found with asthma[63] or atopy.[64]

Chromosome 12q

Linkage of asthma and total IgE was found to chromosome 12q in an Afro-Caribbean population and confirmed in Caucasian Amish families.[29] This region of the genome was investigated because it contains candidate genes such as interferon-γ. Linkage of total serum IgE levels to the same region has been reported in an independent study of a German population.[65]

Chromosome 16p

The α subunit of the IL-4 receptor (IL-4Rα) is a candidate for atopy due to the central role of IL-4 in the production of IgE. An amino acid substitution in IL-4Rα (GLN576ARG) was discovered in a group of patients who had hyper-IgE syndrome.[66] Subsequently, 576ARG was found to be associated with atopy. Functional studies have revealed that the 576ARG allele produces a receptor that shows enhanced signal transduction in vitro.

Evidence for the role of the IL-4Rα gene in the genetics of atopy was strengthened by a subsequent linkage study.[67] Another mutation in the IL-4Rα gene (ILE50VAL) was associated with atopy and asthma in a Japanese population.[68] The ILE50 allele was associated with increased in vitro cell growth and IgE gene expression in B cell lines in response to IL-4. An alternative candidate from this region is the CD19 gene. CD19 is a B cell marker that modulates development of this cell type. However, an amino acid substitution (A496H) in CD19 was not found to be associated with IgE levels.[69]

Tumor Necrosis Factor α

Tumor necrosis factor α (TNFα) is a powerful pro-inflammatory cytokine. An A→G transition at position −308 in the promoter of the TNFα gene (TNF A −308G) has been shown to be associated with increased TNFα secretion in vitro.[70] The −308G allele has been associated with both asthma[71] and BHR.[72] The −308 polymorphism has also been associated with COPD in a Korean population.[73]

Human Leukocyte Antigens

Both population and family studies have been used to examine relationships between HLA type, asthma, and atopy. Differences in HLA allele frequencies and HLA disease associations in different ethnic groups complicate comparisons between studies. Furthermore, in earlier studies, serologic methods were used to define HLA phenotypes, whereas, in more recent studies, genotypes have been defined by polymerase chain reaction (PCR)-based methods.

Human leukocyte antigen class II antigens (designated DP, DQ, and DR) play a key role in antigen presentation and therefore influence the specificity of the immune response. Many associations between class II alleles and IgE hyper-responsiveness to specific allergens have been demonstrated. Human leukocyte antigen associations with responsiveness to some common aeroallergens have been reviewed previously.[3] In general, significant associations are found only with highly purified simple allergens and not with more complex common ones. For example, the complex allergens of house dust mite (*Der p* and *Der f*) have not been associated with a specific HLA type. However, specific epitopes of *Der p* have been identified at the amino acid level and have been shown to be presented by specific HLA-DR and -DQ gene products.[74]

Perhaps the strongest HLA class II association is with HLA-DR2/Dw2 found in 95% of IgE responders to the ragweed allergen *Amb a* V.[75] A series of experiments provided convincing evidence that only cells with DRB1/2.2 or DRB1/2.12 could present this allergen, indicating that the DRB1 gene is responsible for restricting T cell responses to *Amb a* V.[76] Human leukocyte antigens have also been linked directly with allergic asthma. In *Amb a* V–allergic subjects, Blumenthal et al found an HLA haplotype that was increased in those who had asthma and rhinitis compared with those who had rhinitis only.[77]

There are other regions of the HLA locus that have been implicated in the pathogenesis of allergy; HLA-B8 has been associated with atopy[78] and atopic asthma.[79] Lymphocytes from B8/DR3 individuals have been shown to produce less interferon-γ and more IL-4 upon stimulation in vitro.[80] The genes for transporter antigen peptides (TAP) are located within the HLA locus. The TAP gene products are involved in antigen presentation, and a polymorphism at amino acid position 637 of the TAP1 gene was associated with a high risk of allergic asthma (relative risk = 22 in the homozygous state).[81]

Researchers have also investigated HLA associations with non-IgE-mediated asthma. Aspirin-induced asthma has been associated with the HLA-DQw2 phenotype[82] and the DPB1*0101 genotype.[83] The pathogenesis of asthma induced by isothiocyanates has been strongly associated with specific alleles in the DQB1 gene.[84]

The presence of a particular HLA allele may be necessary, but not sufficient, for responsiveness to an epitope. In the future, investigators may consider the HLA locus in combination with one or more other candidate genes (in particular, the T cell antigen receptor). Such studies will be needed if HLA typing is to be powerful enough to have a predictive value for the identification of individuals at risk for atopy or asthma.

Interleukin-9 Receptor

The interleukin-9 (IL-9) receptor gene is located on the long arm of the X chromosome. This gene was investigated as a candidate asthma gene due to the involvement of IL-9 in the proliferation and differentiation of mast cells. The results of a recent study have provided evidence of linkage of asthma and BHR to a marker within the IL-9 receptor gene.[85] Several variants of the IL-9 receptor are known to affect IL-9 signaling and are therefore candidates for this linkage.

Immunoglobulin Heavy-Chain Genes

Variants of the immunoglobulin heavy-chain locus have been associated with a variety of atopy-related phenotypes. A large multigene deletion was found in one highly atopic subject.[86] However, no deletions of the IgE heavy-chain locus were found in 31 Japanese atopic patients.[87] Immunoglobin G heavy-chain variants were found to be associated with IgG levels and asthma[88] as well as IgE levels and the number of peripheral blood eosinophils.[89]

T Cell Antigen Receptor Genes

Linkage has been demonstrated between the T cell antigen receptor (TCR) α locus and specific IgE responses.[90] The data suggests a recessive genetic effect, and linkage was detected in two separate population samples. The region also contains the δ chain TCR genes and, therefore, they are also candidates for the linkage. Linkage of specific IgE responses, high total serum IgE levels, and asthma to the TCRβ locus was found in a Japanese population.[91] No linkage was found with the TCRα locus in the same population; this may be due to the different ethnicities of the study populations.

N-Acetyltransferase

The enzyme *N*-acetyltransferase (NAT2) is involved in the regulation of histamine. Atopic individuals have been shown to be slow acetylators. There are several polymorphisms in the NAT2 gene that are known to affect the activity of the enzyme. Genotypes associated with defective acetylation were found in 91% of children who had allergies versus 62% in controls.[92]

Angiotensin Converting Enzyme

A polymorphism within the angiotensin converting enzyme (ACE) gene has been shown to be associated with asthma in a French population.[93] It was hypothesized that this association was due to the action of angiotensin II in promoting bronchoconstriction and proliferation of bronchial smooth muscle. However, a larger study of British and Japanese subjects failed to confirm the association.[94]

α_1-Antitrypsin

The gene for α_1-antitrypsin has long been known to play an important role in the pathogenesis of COPD.[95] However, several studies have provided evidence for the involvement of α_1-antitrypsin deficiency in bronchial asthma[96] and asthma severity.[97] However, the evidence remains controversial, because several groups have described increased prevalence of the α_1-antitrypsin deficiency in asthmatic patients irrespective of severity,[98] whereas other studies have found no association between asthma and α_1-antitrypsin levels.[99] Deficiency in α_1-antichymotrypsin has also been associated with asthma, although the genetic mechanisms have not yet been elucidated.[100]

SUMMARY

In this chapter, we have summarized the evidence for a genetic contribution to asthma. An understanding of the genetic variation that predisposes to asthma and atopic diseases could open a variety of potential diagnostic and therapeutic avenues. First, the identification of the specific mutations that alter the immune response could provide targets for gene therapy. However, the risks and costs associated with gene therapy do not presently justify application to alleviate the relatively nonlethal manifestations of allergic diseases. Second, knowledge of the genes that cause asthma and allergy will be important in the development of specific pharmacologic therapy. For example, if variants of the IL-4 gene with enhanced function are identified as causative factors, drug development effort could be directed toward specific modulators of their effects. However, it is possible that the redundancy in the immune and inflammatory responses, coupled with the likelihood of multiple gene involvement, will make such targeting fruitless or dangerous. A third consequence is the possibility of screening. This is likely the most beneficial outcome of the present search for atopy genes. Recent studies suggest that preventing exposure to cigarette smoke and highly allergenic proteins in the first few years of life can modify the clinical onset of atopic diseases.[101] At present, the power of such studies is limited by the inability to predict those at risk with any certainty. Genetic screening of children born to atopic parents will allow more precise identification of those carrying atopy genes, allowing a focused attempt at environmental modification. In the short term, this will permit the design of more powerful prospective studies of "prophylaxis"; in the long run, screening may prove an effective strategy for asthma prevention.

REFERENCES

1.   Pirson F, Charpin D, Sansonetti M, et al. Is intrinsic asthma a hereditary disease? Allergy 1991;46:367–71.
2.   Dold S, Wjst M, von Mutius E, et al. Genetic risk for asthma, allergic rhinitis, and atopic dermatitis. Arch Dis Child 1992;67:1018–22.
3.   Sandford A, Weir T, Paré P. The genetics of asthma. Am J Respir Crit Care Med 1996;153:1749–65.
4.   Duffy DL, Martin NG, Battistutta D, et al. Genetics of asthma and hay fever in Australian twins. Am Rev Respir Dis 1990;142:1351–8.
5.   Nieminen MM, Kaprio J, Koskenvuo M. A population-based study of bronchial asthma in adult twin pairs. Chest 1991;100:70–5.
6.   Hanson B, McGue M, Roitman-Johnson B, et al. Atopic disease and immunoglobulin E in twins reared apart and together. Am J Hum Genet 1991;48:873–9.
7.   Sluyter R, Tovey ER, Duffy DL, Britton WJ. Limited genetic control of specific IgE responses to rye grass pollen allergens in Australian twins. Clin Exp Allergy 1998;28:322–31.
8.   Cook RA, van der Veer A. Human sensitization. J Immunol 1996;1:201–305.
9.   Meyers DA, Beaty TH, Colyer CR, Marsh DG. Genetics of total serum IgE levels: a regressive model approach to segregation analysis. Genet Epidemiol 1991;8:351–9.
10.   Blumenthal MN, Namboodiri K, Mendell N, et al. Genetic transmission of serum IgE Levels. Am J Med Genet 1981;10:219–28.
11.   Martinez FD, Holberg CJ, Halonen M, et al. Evidence for mendelian inheritance of serum IgE levels in Hispanic and non-Hispanic white families. Am J Hum Genet 1994;55:555–65.
12.   Lawrence S, Beasley R, Doull I, et al. Genetic analysis of atopy and asthma as quantitative traits and ordered polychotomies. Ann Hum Genet 1994;58:359–68.
13.   Litonjua AA, Carey VJ, Burge HA, et al. Parental history and the risk for childhood asthma—does mother confer more risk than father? Am J Respir Crit Care Med 1998;158:176–81.
14.   Johnson CC, Ownby DR, Peterson EL. Parental history of atopic disease and concentration of cord blood IgE. Clin Exp Allergy 1996;26:624–9.
15.   Holberg CJ, Morgan WJ, Wright AL, Martinez FD. Differences in familial segregation of FEV$_1$ between asthmatic and nonasthmatic families—role of a maternal component. Am J Respir Crit Care Med 1998;158:162–9.

16. Barbee RA, Halonen M, Lebowitz M, Burrows B. Distribution of IgE in a community population sample: correlations with age, sex, and allergen skin test reactivity. J Allergy Clin Immunol 1981;68:106–11.

17. Barbee RA, Lebowitz MD, Thompson HC, Burrows B. Immediate skin-test reactivity in a general population sample. Ann Intern Med 1976;84:129–33.

18. Longo G, Strinati R, Poli F, Fumi F. Genetic factors in nonspecific bronchial hyperreactivity. An epidemiologic study. Am J Dis Child 1987;141:331–4.

19. Burrows B, Sears MR, Flannery EM, et al. Relationships of bronchial responsiveness assessed by methacholine to serum IgE, lung function, symptoms, and diagnoses in 11-year-old New Zealand children. J Allergy Clin Immunol 1992;90:376–85.

20. Townley RG, Bewtra AK, Nair NM, et al. Methacholine inhalation challenge studies. J Allergy Clin Immunol 1979;64:569–74.

21. Ericsson CH, Svartengren M, Mossberg B, et al. Bronchial reactivity and allergy-promoting factors in mono-zygotic twins discordant for allergic rhinitis. Ann Allergy 1991;67:53–9.

22. Burrows B, Sears MR, Flannery EM, et al. Relation of the course of bronchial responsiveness from age 9 to age 15 to allergy. Am J Respir Crit Care Med 1995;152:1302–8.

23. Godfrey S, Konig P. Exercise-induced bronchial lability in atopic children and their families. Ann Allergy 1974;33:199–205.

24. Konig P, Godfrey S. Exercise-induced bronchial lability in monozygotic and dizygotic twins. J Allergy Clin Immunol 1974;54:280–7.

25. Duffy DL, Mitchell CA. Lower respiratory tract symptoms in Queensland schoolchildren: risk factors for wheeze, cough and diminished ventilatory function. Thorax 1993;48:1021–4.

26. Daniels SE, Bhattacharrya S, James A, et al. A genome-wide search for quantitative trait loci underlying asthma. Nature 1996;383:247–50.

27. Anonymous. A genome-wide search for asthma susceptibility loci in ethnically diverse populations. The Collaborative Study on the Genetics of Asthma (CSGA). Nat Genet 1997;15:389–92.

28. Marsh DG, Neely JD, Breazeale DR, et al. Linkage analysis of IL4 and other chromosome 5q31.1 markers and total serum immunoglobulin E concentrations. Science 1994;264:1152–6.

29. Barnes KC, Neely JD, Duffy DL, et al. Linkage of asthma and total serum IgE concentration to markers on chromosome 12q: evidence from Afro-Caribbean and Caucasian populations. Genomics 1996;37:41–50.

30. Ober C, Cox NJ, Abney M, et al. Genome-wide search for asthma susceptibility loci in a founder population. Hum Mol Genet 1998;7:1393–8.

31. Hizawa N, Freidhoff LR, Chiu YF, et al. Genetic regulation of *Dermatophagoides pteronyssinus*–specific IgE responsiveness—a genome-wide multipoint linkage analysis in families recruited through 2 asthmatic sibs. J Allergy Clin Immunol 1998;102:436–42.

32. Hizawa N, Freidhoff LR, Ehrlich E, et al. Genetic influences of chromosomes 5q31–q33 and 11q13 on specific IgE responsiveness to common inhaled allergens among African American families. J Allergy Clin Immunol 1998;102:449–53.

33. Laitinen T, Kauppi P, Ignatius J, et al. Genetic control of serum IgE levels and asthma: linkage and linkage dis-equilibrium studies in an isolated population. Hum Mol Genet 1997;6:2069–76.

34. Rosenwasser LJ, Klemm DJ, Dresback JK, et al. Promoter polymorphisms in the chromosome 5 gene cluster in asthma and atopy. Clin Exp Allergy 1995;25:74–8.

35. Noguchi E, Shibasaki M, Arinami T, et al. Association of asthma and the interleukin-4 promoter gene in Japanese. Clin Exp Allergy 1998;28:449–53.

36. Walley AJ, Cookson WOCM. Investigation of an interleukin-4 promoter polymorphism for associations with asthma and atopy. J Med Genet 1996;33:689–92.

37. Pereira E, Goldblatt J, Rye P, et al. Mutation analysis of interleukin-5 in an asthmatic cohort. Hum Mutat 1998;11:51–4.

38. Ulbrecht M, Eisenhut T, Bonisch J, et al. High serum IgE concentrations: association with HLA-DR and mark-ers on chromosome 5q31 and chromosome 11q13. J Allergy Clin Immunol 1997;99:828–36.

39. Nicolaides NC, Holroyd KJ, Ewart SL, et al. Interleukin 9: a candidate gene for asthma. Proc Natl Acad Sci U S A 1997;94:13175–80.

40. Weir TD, Mallek N, Sandford AJ, et al. β₂-adrenergic receptor haplotypes in mild, moderate and fatal/near fatal asthma. Am J Respir Crit Care Med 1998;158:787–91.

41. Reihsaus E, Innis M, MacIntyre N, Liggett SB. Mutations in the gene encoding for the β₂-adrenergic receptor in normal and asthmatic subjects. Am J Respir Cell Mol Biol 1993;8:334–9.

42. Martinez FD, Graves PE, Baldini M, et al. Association between genetic polymorphisms of the β₂-adrenoceptor and response to albuterol in children with and without a history of wheezing. J Clin Invest 1997;100:3184–8.

43. Green SA, Turki J, Bejarano P, et al. Influence of β₂-adrenergic receptor genotypes on signal transduction in human airway smooth muscle cells. Am J Respir Cell Mol Biol 1995;13:25–33.

44. Tan S, Hall IP, Dewar J, et al. Association between β₂-adrenoceptor polymorphism and susceptibility to bronchodilator desensitisation in moderately severe stable asthmatic patients. Lancet 1997;350:995–9.

45. Turki J, Pak J, Green SA, et al. Genetic polymorphisms of the β₂-adrenergic receptor in nocturnal and nonnocturnal asthma. Evidence that Gly16 correlates with the nocturnal phenotype. J Clin Invest 1995;95:1635–41.

46. Hall IP, Wheatley A, Wilding P, Liggett SB. Association of Glu 27 β₂-adrenoceptor polymorphism with lower airway reactivity in asthmatic subjects. Lancet 1995;345:1213–4.

47. Hopes E, McDougall C, Christie G, et al. Association of glutamine 27 polymorphism of β₂ adrenoceptor with reported childhood asthma: population based study. BMJ 1998;316:664.

48. Ohe M, Munakata M, Hizawa N, et al. β₂ adrenergic receptor gene restriction fragment length polymorphism and bronchial asthma. Thorax 1995;50:353–9.

49. Cookson WOCM, Sharp PA, Faux JA, Hopkin JM. Linkage between immunoglobulin E responses underlying asthma and rhinitis and chromosome 11q. Lancet 1989;i:1292–5.

50. Marsh DG, Meyers DA. A major gene for allergy—fact or fancy? Nat Genet 1992;2:252–4.

51. Shirakawa T, Hashimoto T, Furuyama J, et al. Linkage between severe atopy and chromosome 11q13 in Japanese families. Clin Genet 1994;46:228–32.

52. Hizawa N, Yamaguchi E, Furuya K, et al. Association between high serum total IgE levels and D11S97 on chromosome 11q13 in Japanese subjects. J Med Genet 1995;32:363–9.

53. van Herwerden L, Harrap SB, Wong ZY, et al. Linkage of high-affinity IgE receptor gene with bronchial hyper-reactivity, even in absence of atopy. Lancet 1995;346:1262–5.

54. Thomas NS, Holgate ST. Genes for asthma on chromosome 11: an update. Clin Exp Allergy 1998;28:387–91.

55. Sandford AJ, Shirakawa T, Moffatt MF, et al. Localisation of atopy and β subunit of high-affinity IgE receptor (FcεRI) on chromosome 11q. Lancet 1993;341:332–4.

56. Shirakawa T, Li A, Dubowitz M, et al. Association between atopy and variants of the β subunit of the high-affinity immunoglobulin E receptor. Nat Genet 1994;7:125–9.

57. Hijazi Z, Haider MZ, Khan MR, Al-Dowaisan AA. High frequency of IgE receptor FcεRI β variant (Leu181/Leu183) in Kuwaiti Arabs and its association with asthma. Clin Genet 1998;53:149–52.

58. Duffy DL, Healey SC, Chenevix-Trench G, et al. Atopy in Australia. Nat Genet 1995;10:260.

59. Hill MR, Cookson WOCM. A new variant of the β subunit of the high-affinity receptor for immunoglobulin E (FcεRI-β E237G): associations with measures of atopy and bronchial hyper-responsiveness. Hum Mol Genet 1996;5:959–62.

60. Shirakawa T, Mao XQ, Sasaki S, et al. Association between atopic asthma and a coding variant of FcεRI β in a Japanese population. Hum Mol Genet 1996;5:1129–30.

61. Trabetti E, Cusin V, Malerba G, et al. Association of the FcεRI-β gene with bronchial hyper-responsiveness in an Italian population. J Med Genet 1998;35:680–1.

62. Laing IA, Goldblatt J, Eber E, et al. A polymorphism of the CC16 gene is associated with an increased risk of asthma. J Med Genet 1998;35:463–7.

63. Gao PS, Mao XQ, Kawai M, et al. Negative association between asthma and variants of CC16(CC10) on chromosome 11q13 in British and Japanese populations. Hum Genet 1998;103:57–9.

64. Mao XQ, Shirakawa T, Kawai M, et al. Association between asthma and an intragenic variant of CC16 on chromosome 11q13. Clin Genet 1998;53:54–6.

65. Nickel R, Wahn U, Hizawa N, et al. Evidence for linkage of chromosome 12q15–q24.1 markers to high total serum IgE concentrations in children of the German Multicenter Allergy Study. Genomics 1997;46:159–62.

66. Hershey GK, Friedrich MF, Esswein LA, et al. The association of atopy with a gain-of-function mutation in the alpha subunit of the interleukin-4 receptor. N Engl J Med 1997;337:1720–5.

67. Deichmann KA, Heinzmann A, Forster J, et al. Linkage and allelic association of atopy and markers flanking the IL4-receptor gene. Clin Exp Allergy 1998;28:151–5.

68. Mitsuyasu H, Izuhara K, Mao XQ, et al. Ile50Val variant of IL4Rα upregulates IgE synthesis and associates with atopic asthma. Nat Genet 1998;19:119–20.

69. Deichmann KA, Justies N, Kruse S, et al. A common polymorphism in the coding part of the CD19 gene is not associated with atopy. Pediatr Asthma Allergy Immunol 1998;12:123–7.

70. Braun N, Michel U, Ernst BP, et al. Gene polymorphism at position –308 of the tumor-necrosis-factor-α (TNF-α) in multiple sclerosis and its influence on the regulation of TNF-α production. Neurosci Lett 1996;215:75–8.

71. Moffatt MF, Cookson WO. Tumour necrosis factor haplotypes and asthma. Hum Mol Genet 1997;6:551–4.

72. Campbell DA, Li Kam Wa E, Britton J, et al. Polymorphism at the tumour necrosis factor locus and asthma. Monogr Allergy 1996;33:125–37.

73. Huang SL, Su CH, Chang SC. Tumor necrosis factor-alpha gene polymorphism in chronic bronchitis. Am J Respir Crit Care Med 1997;156:1436–9.

74. Verhoef A, Higgins JA, Thorpe CJ, et al. Clonal analysis of the atopic immune response to the group 2 allergen of *Dermatophagoides* spp.: identification of HLA-DR and -DQ restricted T cell epitopes. Int Immunol 1993;5:1589–97.

75. Marsh DG, Huang SK. Molecular genetics of human immune responsiveness to pollen allergens. Clin Exp Allergy 1991;21:168–72.

76. Huang SK, Zwollo P, Marsh DG. Class II major histocompatibility complex restriction of human T cell responses to short ragweed allergen, *Amb a* V. Eur J Immunol 1991;21:1469–73.

77. Blumenthal M, Marcus-Bagley D, Awdeh Z, et al. HLA-DR2, [HLA-B7, SC31, DR2], and [HLA-B8, SC01, DR3] haplotypes distinguish subjects with asthma from those with rhinitis only in ragweed pollen allergy. J Immunol 1992;148:411–6.

78. Turner MW, Brostoff TJ, Wells RS, et al. HLA in eczema and hay fever. Clin Exp Immunol 1977;27:43–7.

79. Ostergaard PA, Eriksen J. Association between HLA-A1,B8 in children with extrinsic asthma and IgA deficiency. Eur J Pediatr 1979;131:263–70.

80. Modica MA, Zambito AM, Candore G, Caruso C. Markers of T lymphocyte activation in HLA-B8, DR3 positive individuals. Immunobiology 1990;181:257–66.

81. Ismail A, Bousaffara R, Kaziz J, et al. Polymorphism in transporter antigen peptides gene (TAP1) associated with atopy in Tunisians. J Allergy Clin Immunol 1997;99:216–23.

82. Mullarkey MF, Thomas PS, Hansen JA, et al. Association of aspirin-sensitive asthma with HLA-DQw2. Am Rev Respir Dis 1986;133:261–3.

83. Lympany PA, Welsh KI, Christie PE, et al. An analysis with sequence-specific oligonucleotide probes of the association between aspirin-induced asthma and antigens of the HLA system. J Allergy Clin Immunol 1993;92:114–23.

84. Bignon JS, Aron Y, Ju LY, et al. HLA class II alleles in isocyanate-induced asthma. Am J Respir Crit Care Med 1994;149:71–5.

85. Holroyd KJ, Martinati LC, Trabetti E, et al. Asthma and bronchial hyperresponsiveness linked to the XY long arm pseudoautosomal region. Genomics 1998;52:233–5.

86. Walter MA, Chambers CA, Zimmerman B, Cox DW. A multigene deletion in the immunoglobulin heavy chain region in a highly atopic individual. Hum Genet 1990;85:643–7.

87. Fujii H, Kondo N, Agata H, et al. Genetic analysis of IgE and the IGHE, IGHEP1 and IGHEP2 genes in atopic families. Int Arch Allergy Immunol 1995;106:62–8.

88. Oxelius VA, Hultquist C, Husby S. Gm allotypes as indicators of non-atopic and atopic bronchial asthma. Int Arch Allergy Immunol 1993;101:66–71.

89. Oxelius VA, Carlsson AM, Aurivillius M. Alternative G1m, G2m and G3m allotypes of IGHG genes correlate with atopic and nonatopic pathways of immune regulation in children with bronchial asthma. Int Arch Allergy Immunol 1998;115:215–9.

90. Moffatt MF, Hill MR, Cornelis F, et al. Genetic linkage of T-cell receptor α/δ complex to specific IgE responses. Lancet 1994;343:1597–600.

91. Noguchi E, Shibasaki M, Arinami T, et al. Evidence for linkage between the development of asthma in childhood and the T-cell receptor beta chain gene in Japanese. Genomics 1998;47:121–4.

92. Zielinska E, Niewiarowski W, Bodalski J, et al. Arylamine N-acetyltransferase (NAT2) gene mutations in children with allergic diseases. Clin Pharmacol Ther 1997;62:635–42.

93. Benessiano J, Crestani B, Mestari F, et al. High frequency of a deletion polymorphism of the angiotensin-converting enzyme gene in asthma. J Allergy Clin Immunol 1997;99:53–7.

94. Gao PS, Mao XQ, Kawai M, et al. Lack of association between ACE gene polymorphisms and atopy and asthma in British and Japanese populations. Clin Genet 1998;54:245–7.

95. Laurell CC, Eriksson S. The electrophorectic α_1-globulin pattern of serum in α_1-antitrypsin deficiency. Scand J Clin Lab Invest 1963;15:132–40.

96. Katz RM, Lieberman J, Siegel SC. α_1 antitrypsin levels and prevalence of Pi variant phenotypes in asthmatic children. J Allergy Clin Immunol 1976;57:41–5.

97. Hyde JS, Werner P, Kumar CM, Moore BS. Protease inhibitor variants in children and young adults with chronic asthma. Ann Allergy 1979;43:8–13.

98. Hoffmann JJ, Kramps JA, Dijkman JH. Intermediate α_1-antitrypsin deficiency in atopic allergy. Clin Allergy 1981;11:555–60.

99. Szczeklik A, Turowska B, Czerniawska-Mysik G, et al. Serum α_1-antitrypsin in bronchial asthma. Am Rev Respir Dis 1974;109:487–90.

100. Lindmark B. Asthma and heterozygous α_1-antichymotrypsin deficiency: a possible association. J Intern Med 1990;227:115–8.

101. Arshad SH, Matthews S, Gant C, Hide DW. Effect of allergen avoidance on development of allergic disorders in infancy. Lancet 1992;339:1493–7.

CHAPTER 3

Cellular and Pathologic Characteristics

Ellinor Ädelroth, MD, PhD

———•••———

Asthma has been considered an inflammatory disease since the nineteenth century. In 1882, Sir William Osler published the medical textbook *The Principles and Practice of Medicine*, in which asthma was said to be "a special form of inflammation of the smaller bronchioles."[1] Subsequent evidence of inflammation in asthma was obtained from autopsy studies of subjects who died from asthma; inflammation was initially thought to be related only to severe fatal attacks of the disease.[2–4] Later, by means of bronchoscopy, particularly fiberoptic bronchoscopy, the airways of subjects with varying degrees of asthma severity were investigated. Features of airway inflammation were found early in the course of asthma, at a stage when subjects often have experienced only mild and intermittent symptoms.[5–29]

Initial fiberoptic bronchoscopy studies used bronchoalveolar lavage (BAL), a washing of the airways, to sample cells and solutes from the surface of the airways.[30] Later, bronchoscopy studies also consisted of bronchial mucosal biopsies for light and electron microscopic examinations of the cellular infiltrate and structural components of the mucosa, together with a number of immunochemical techniques, to investigate the state and level of activation of the inflammatory cells found.[13,16,21–23] The relationship between findings from the BAL and the bronchial biopsies is of particular interest, as it might provide indications of dynamic events in the inflammatory process in asthma.[11,12,18]

Recently, the examination of sputum has gained interest, as standardized methods of sputum induction and specimen handling have been developed and subsequently applied in groups of asthmatic patients with a range of severity of the disease.[31–36]

The safety of an invasive method such as fiberoptic bronchoscopy in subjects with ongoing asthma has been of particular concern, and international guidelines for its use have been developed.[37] The procedure is safe and well tolerated when performed by experienced physicians with proper precautions and monitoring (Level II). The safety of the noninvasive method of sputum induction with hypertonic saline in subjects with asthma, airflow limitation, and hyper-responsive airways has also been of concern. However, carefully standardized methods of pretreatment and monitoring of lung function during the procedure guarantee its safety in asthmatic patients as well as in subjects with other lung conditions.[38]

BRONCHOALVEOLAR LAVAGE

During the last 15 years, numerous bronchoscopy studies have been performed in which the BAL technique to sample cells present on the surface of the airway mucosa has been applied.[7–9,11,13,16,20,23] In the BAL fluid, mediators and proteins released into the airways can be detected and quantified.[7–9,11,14,16,23] In almost all BAL studies, increased proportions of eosinophils, mast cells, and lymphocytes have been found in lavage from asthmatic airways as compared to normals (Level II). There are few eosinophils in the airways of nonallergic, nonasthmatic subjects, but even in asymptomatic asthmatic patients, increased eosinophils can be found.[7–9,11–14,16,19–23] Two studies have found that the intensity of the eosinophilic inflammation is related to the severity of asthma.[14,15] There are relatively low numbers of mast cells and T lymphocytes in the BAL fluid of asthmatic patients, but they are increased compared to normals, and more T lymphocytes are activated in asthma (Level II).[20] Asthmatic patients with current symptoms have shown increased T cell activation compared to patients without ongoing symptoms.[21]

Macrophages are the most abundant cells in BAL in both asthmatic and control subjects and are present both in the central airways and in the alveoli. They have a possible role in the pathogenesis of asthma due to some of their properties and their presence throughout the bronchial tree.[39] For example, following allergen challenge in allergic subjects, the increase in alveolar macrophages exceeds that of eosinophils and other cells. Further, alveolar macrophages express low-affinity surface receptors for immunoglobulin E (IgE) (FcεRII, CD23) and can be activated by the binding of antigen to IgE linked to these receptors. They also release a number of mediators on stimulation (leukotrienes, superoxide anions, and other inflammatory products). There is evidence that alveolar macrophages from asthmatic patients are phenotypically and functionally distinct from those of nonasthmatic control subjects in, for example, their ability to spontaneously release increased amounts of reactive oxygen species (Level II).[39,40]

The role of neutrophils in asthma is less clear. The reports of increased proportions of neutrophils in asthma have been scant and, until recently, mostly noted after challenges with substances such as isocyanates,[41] plicatic acid,[42] or ozone.[43] Some recent studies of severe steroid-dependent asthmatic patients have reported a predominantly neutrophilic inflammation in both central and peripheral airways (Level II).[44,45]

More important than the actual number or proportion of cells is the state of activation of the cells as assessed by immunochemical methods. For example, activated eosinophils in BAL can be identified by the use of an EG2-antibody, which reflects the secreted form of eosinophilic cationic protein (ECP); activated mast cells can be detected by AA1, a monoclonal antibody against tryptase, of which mast cells are the main source.[13,16,20,21,23] The findings made under controlled, nonchallenged conditions are all accentuated if an investigation is repeated following local endobronchial or inhaled allergen challenges.[46,47]

Mediators and Proteins in Bronchoalveolar Lavage

The presence of a number of cytokines has been shown to be of importance in modulating events in the airways of asthmatic patients. Bronchoalveolar lavage cells in asthmatic patients demonstrate a Th2-like phenotype with increased levels or expression of interleukin-4 (IL-4) (involved in local IgE regulation and of IL-5), that promotes differentiation of eosinophil precursors and activates and prolongs the survival of mature eosinophils.[24,27,48] Other cytokines, such as granulocyte-macrophage colony–stimulating factor (GM-CSF), tumor necrosis factor (TNF) α, TNFβ, IL-2, IL-6, IL-8, and RANTES, have been found in increased concentrations in BAL from asthmatic patients under basic conditions.[23,27–29,48,49] Four of these cytokines, TNFα, GM-CSF, IL-2, and IL-6, have been found in higher levels in symptomatic asthmatic patients than in nonsymptomatic asthmatic subjects, indicating a relationship to the severity of asthma (Level II).[50]

Other markers of inflammation, such as eosinophilic proteins (eosinophilic cationic protein [ECP], and major basic protein [MBP]), albumin, and fibrinogen are increased in asthmatic patients as are, for example, histamine, and sulphidopeptide leukotrienes (Level II).[7–9,11,49] The BAL concentration of ECP has been shown to correlate with the severity of asthma,[14] suggesting that the state of activation of eosinophils may be important and contribute to airway pathology.

Special Considerations

Whereas BAL samples the alveolar part of the airway, the peripheral airway, more proximal parts might be of more interest in asthma. Some researchers have tried to limit these difficulties by dividing the instillate into aliquots; the initial aliquot supposedly samples more proximal airways and usually constitutes a less amount, and the subsequent aliquots sample more peripheral airways and make up a larger portion.[51] The rapid exchange of the instilled fluid with the extracellular fluid of the lung complicates the measurements of mediators of inflammation recovered by the BAL. Results have been shown to vary if aliquots of the recovered fluid have been analyzed separately or pooled. Thus, there are limitations to the interpretation that can be made from BAL studies due to difficulties in standardizing the technique for the lavage procedure, the type and amount of instillate, separate or pooled aliquots, and dilution factors.[52,53] The interpretation of soluble mediators in lavage fluid should therefore be done with some caution, and extrapolation to conditions in the bronchial mucosa must not be performed, as events in the airway lumen on the airway mucosal surface do not necessarily reflect the situation in the airway mucosa.

BRONCHIAL MUCOSAL BIOPSIES

Early autopsy studies of subjects who died from acute severe attacks of asthma described airway inflammation: extensive mucus with plugging, enlargement of mucous glands, damage to or loss of epithelium, goblet cell hyperplasia, muscular hypertrophy, edema, and an intense cellular infiltration dominated by eosinophilic granulocytes.[2–4] The first bronchoscopy study performed in live asthmatic patients by Glynn and Michaels in 1960 described a similar picture, with an eosinophilic inflammatory infiltrate in the mucosa.[5] Recent endobronchial biopsy studies elaborate further, describing a loss of surface epithelium, thickening of the reticular layer of the basement membrane, and an increased cellular infiltrate in the bronchial mucosa with predominance of eosinophils, mast cells, and T lymphocytes. Figure 3–1 compares the airway of an atopic asthmatic with that of a healthy control subject. As in BAL, these findings have been present in early stages of asthma shortly after the onset of symptoms and recent diagnosis, at a time when symptoms are mild and occasional, and the lung function is completely normal (Level II).[6,10,12–15,17–19,22,23]

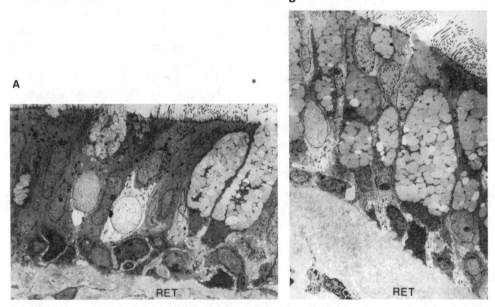

Figure 3–1 Comparison of bronchial surface epithelium and basement membrane reticular collagen (RET) in biopsies from a normal healthy control subject (*A*) and an atopic asthmatic subject (*B*) (×1,950 original magnification). (Reproduced with permission from Jeffrey PK, Godfrey RW, Ädelroth E, et al. Effects of treatment on airway thickening of basement reticular collagen in asthma. A quantitative light and electron microscopic study. Am Rev Respir Dis 1992;145:890–9.)

Epithelium

The loss and shedding of the surface epithelium in asthmatic patients has been debated.[54,55] Is it a true phenomenon or artifactual as a result of the sampling procedure during the bronchoscopy? It is evident that the loss of the epithelium can be patchy, and areas might exist with intact epithelium; however, damage to, or loss of, epithelium is frequently seen in asthmatic patients, both in autopsy material where whole airways can be examined and in the small endobronchial biopsies obtained from living asthmatic patients.[2–5,10,14,18] Thus, there is support for the concept that the epithelium in asthmatic airway mucosa has a special fragility. The epithelial damage could be the result of injury by the toxic cationic proteins such as ECP and MBP, which are found in high concentrations in asthmatic airways. Goblet cell hyperplasia in asthmatic patients is commonly seen and possibly represents a compensatory response to the epithelial damage. As the epithelium acts as a barrier between the airway lumen and underlying target tissues (ie, smooth muscle, vasculature, or inflammatory cells), damage to this barrier by toxic eosinophilic proteins, for example, might facilitate the access of allergens or irritating stimuli to inflammatory cells and nerves deeper in the mucosa. A relationship between epithelial damage and the severity of asthma measured as the degree of airway hyper-responsiveness has been suggested.[10]

Basement Membrane

Thickening of the reticular layer of the basement membrane is present early in asthmatic patients, even in patients who have been diagnosed with asthma for less than 1 year.[19] It is one of the characteristic features of an asthmatic airway described in early autopsy studies (Level II).[2,4] More recent studies, which have applied electron microscopy and immunohistochemical techniques to bronchial mucosal biopsies from subjects with mild to moderate asthma in comparison with controls, have confirmed the thickening of the lamina reticularis of the basement membrane.[10,18] Transmission electron microscopy has demonstrated that the basement membrane consists of three layers: lamina lucida just below the epithelium, lamina densa next, and then the lamina reticularis, composed of collagens and glucoproteins such as fibronectin. The increased thickness of the lamina reticularis in asthmatic airways compared to nonasthmatic airways is due to an increased deposition of collagens III and V and fibronectin. The composition of the basement membrane in asthmatic patients and normals are otherwise the same. Collagens III and V and fibronectin are components of fibrosis, and, therefore, the increased deposition in asthmatic patients has also been called "subepithelial fibrosis."[56]

Cellular Infiltrate in Mild to Moderately Severe Asthma

The most consistent finding in studies in which the cellular infiltrate of bronchial biopsy specimens from asthmatic airways has been compared with that of nonasthmatic control subjects, has been an increase in the number of eosinophils in the asthmatic airway mucosa (Level II).[10,12–15,17–19,21,22] In some studies, a special feature of the eosinophilic inflammation has been identified: the finding of clusters of eosinophil granules lying free in the interstitium.[18,19] This was noticed in the first bronchoscopy study in living asthmatic patients,[5] but did not receive much attention until recently. It is suggested that these clusters are a sign of "the ultimate activation" of eosinophils in vivo and represent either degranulation or lysis of the eosinophil.[57] Free eosinophil granules and intact and degranulating eosinophils are shown in Figures 3–2 and 3–3.

Lymphocytes, mainly T lymphocytes, are the predominant inflammatory cells in the mucosa and are likely to play an important role in the inflammatory response in the airways (Level II).[13,19,22] Lymphocytes have been found in increased numbers in specimens from atopic,[13] nonatopic,[22] or intrinsic asthmatic patients,[22] as well as in specimens from asthmatic patients having died from an attack of asthma.[58] The number of activated T lymphocytes has

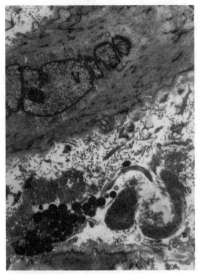

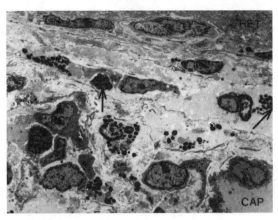

Figure 3–3

Figure 3–2

Figure 3–2 Free eosinophil granules close to a bronchial smooth muscle fiber (M) (×6,450 original magnification). (Reproduced with permission from Jeffrey PK, Godfrey RW, Ädelroth E, et al. Effects of treatment on airway thickening of basement reticular collagen in asthma. A quantitative light and electron microscopic study. Am Rev Respir Dis 1992;145:890–9.)

Figure 3–3 Subepithelial layer from an aspirin-sensitive asthmatic subject receiving inhaled corticosteroid treatment. There was a high number of intact and degranulating eosinophils (*arrows*). Subepithelial reticular collagen (RET), bronchial capillary (CAP), and plasma cell (PC) are shown (×2,700 original magnification). (Reproduced with permission from Jeffrey PK, Godfrey RW, Ädelroth E, et al. Effects of treatment on airway thickening of basement reticular collagen in asthma. A quantitative light and electron microscopic study. Am Rev Respir Dis 1992;145:890–9.)

been shown to correlate with airway obstruction (decreased FEV_1) and with the degree of airway responsiveness.[16] Thus, activated T lymphocytes and their products might be important in the pathogenesis of airway hyper-responsiveness and possibly asthma, regardless of atopy. Increased numbers of mast cells and macrophages[18] have been found in cellular infiltrate, but not universally.[15] Several cytokines, including IL-4, IL-5, IL-8, IL-16, and GM-CSF, have been shown to be upregulated in endobronchial biopsies—in parallel to findings in BAL (Level II).[23–26,29,59] Immunostaining has confirmed the presence of activated cells in the mucosa, also reflecting what has been seen in BAL.[13,21–23]

Smooth Muscle

The smooth muscle mass enlargement in asthmatic airways described in autopsy studies has been further investigated, but it is still not clear if the increase in muscle mass is due to muscle fiber hyperplasia or hypertrophy.[54] It has recently been suggested that the muscle mass increase in larger airways is due to hyperplasia, whereas hypertrophy is present in the smaller airways.[60] Although asthmatic patients have an increased smooth muscle mass, there is no evidence that it behaves abnormally in isolation. It has been shown that the smooth muscle trachea of patients with asthma is more sensitive to histamine compared to normals, but that there is no morphologic difference between smooth muscle from the two groups.[61]

Edema

Autopsy studies have described edema as one of the typical findings in the airway mucosa of asthmatic patients.[2–4] Edema has less often been mentioned as a characteristic feature in the bronchial biopsy specimens from mild asthmatic patients. This is most likely due to the small size of the specimens (2 to 3 mm) or the processing techniques, which make edema difficult to evaluate.

Peripheral Airways

Until very recently, information about airway inflammation has been limited to results from BAL and endobronchial biopsies from proximal airways of mild to moderately severe asthmatic patients. Additional information is now available from peripheral airways of surgically removed asthmatic lungs and from a study in which both endobronchial and transbronchial biopsies have been obtained.[44,45] In these studies, a more intense and severe eosinophilic inflammation was found peripherally in the alveolar tissue. In the study by Kraft and co-workers, the intensity of the peripheral inflammation was further increased when subjects with nocturnal asthma were compared with subjects without nocturnal asthma.[44]

Cellular Infiltrate in Severe Asthmatic patients

Due to the invasive nature of bronchoscopy, there are few studies that include subjects with severe asthma. In a recent study by Wenzel et al, severe glucocorticosteroid-dependent asthmatic patients were investigated with BAL and endobronchial and transbronchial biopsies.[62] The interesting and somewhat surprising results showed an intense neutrophilic inflammation in BAL and both endobronchial and transbronchial biopsies compared with moderately severe asthmatic patients and normal control subjects. These results indicate that severe steroid-dependent asthma may be different from moderate asthma or that the preponderance of neutrophils is due to the steroid treatment or other unknown causes.

Allergen Challenge

According to BAL findings, all features of inflammation in the airway mucosa have been shown to be accentuated after local, and inhaled, allergen challenge, especially when the inflammatory response after a late-phase asthmatic reaction has been investigated (Level II).[63,64]

AIRWAY REMODELING

Airway remodeling is likely important to understand chronic asthma with persistent hyper-responsiveness and sometimes irreversible airway obstruction. It refers to the altered airway structure seen in longstanding asthma and might represent the sequelae of repeated increases in the airway inflammation, such as those following allergen challenge resulting in a late-phase reaction. The thickening of the reticular layer of the basement membrane is a characteristic feature, even in very mild and intermittent asthma, and is also noted soon after the diagnosis of the asthma. As discussed previously, the thickened reticular layer has been shown to be due to increased deposition of subepithelial collagens and glucoproteins, with the presence of fibroblasts that can take on the characteristics of myofibroblasts and possibly be part of the remodeling process.[54,56] In asthmatic patients, it has been suggested that these airway myofibroblasts might participate in the increased production of reticular collagen in the lamina reticularis. In a recent study, increased numbers of myofibroblast-like cells with a contractile phenotype were found in bronchial biopsies obtained 24 hours after allergen challenge resulting in a late-phase reaction.[65] These cells might mature into smooth muscle cells and thus contribute to the increased muscle mass seen in chronic asthma.

Treatment Studies

A number of investigators have used bronchoscopy studies with BAL and biopsies to investigate the effects of anti-inflammatory treatment such as inhaled and oral corticosteroids.[11,17,66-69] These studies have shown that effects of the medication on inflammatory features with fewer inflammatory cells or fewer activated cells can be observed after only a few weeks of treatment (Level IA). There are certain characteristics of the asthmatic airway, such as the thickening of the reticular layer of the basement membrane, which do not seem to be easily affected by short-term or long-term anti-inflammatory treatment (Level II).[11,17,67,69] However, in a recent placebo-controlled parallel group study of inhaled beclomethasone dipropionate for 6 months, the investigators found a significantly reduced thickness of the lamina reticularis in addition to reductions in eosinophils, T lymphocytes, and fibroblasts and improvements in asthma symptoms, lung function, and airway responsiveness measurements.[70] Another recent study indicates that inhaled corticosteroids can reduce the amount of tenascin, a glucoprotein shown to be present in the reticular basement membrane in asthmatic patients and involved in the healing cascade; they are therefore assumed to be involved in the remodeling process.[71] These two studies suggest it may be possible to influence features of the chronic inflammation in asthma, previously thought to be untreatable.[70,71]

Special Considerations

The biopsy specimens obtained through fiberoptic bronchoscopy are 2 to 3 mm in diameter and, even if 5 to 10 specimens are taken during one bronchoscopy, their representation of the whole airway surface area is questionable. There are intrasubject variabilities in findings of inflammatory parameters between anatomic sites.[72] In addition, due to technical factors, most, or perhaps all, biopsies are taken from carinas of lobar or segmental bronchi and, again, their representation of the whole mucosal surface can be questioned. Still, the information gained from bronchoscopy studies has advanced our knowledge about asthma and shown the effects of anti-inflammatory treatments such as corticosteroids on the target organ and overall clinical improvement.

SPUTUM

Bronchoscopy studies of asthmatic patients with mild and intermittent symptoms show signs of airway inflammation early in the course of the condition, a fact that emphasizes the importance of noninvasive methods to detect and follow inflammatory events in the airways. Although sputum eosinophilia has been a well-known feature of asthma for many years, only recently have standardized methods for careful induction with hypertonic saline, specimen handling, and processing been developed.[31,32] The two main methods to induce and process sputum have proved to yield adequate samples for investigation in most cases. They also have a high degree of reproducibility and content validity, that is, sensitivity to change by interventions.[73]

Sputum studies have confirmed the importance of eosinophilic inflammation in asthma (Level II).[31,32,34,35] Increased proportions of sputum eosinophils and metachromatic cells, as well as increased levels of ECP, albumin, and fibrinogen, have been found in stable asthmatic patients compared to nonasthmatic control subjects. The inflammation in the airways as reflected in sputum has been shown to be sensitive to treatment with inhaled and oral corticosteroids (Level I).[36] As the method of induced sputum has been applied to asthmatic patients with more severe disease and ongoing airflow obstruction and to asthmatic patients dependent on oral and inhaled corticosteroids for asthma control, it has been found that some of these patients have a neutrophilic inflammation parallel to that shown by Wenzel et al in their bronchoscopy study (Level II).[62] The reasons for this discrepancy from subjects with mild or moderate asthma are not known, but there are likely subgroups of asthmatics that are not typical of all asthma patients, and further study of these exceptions is needed.

The cellular inflammation found in sputum has been compared to that in bronchial wash or BAL as well as the inflammatory cell infiltrate seen in bronchial mucosal biopsies.[33,74,75] There has been some correlation between sputum and bronchial wash or BAL but much less agreement with results from mucosal biopsies.

SUMMARY

Asthma is an inflammatory condition in which a number of inflammatory cells play important roles. Eosinophilic inflammation is evident in the majority of asthmatic patients investigated so far, but subgroups of severe asthmatic patients have shown a predominantly neutrophilic inflammation. Further studies of this distinction are needed.

Looking to the future, studies are required that are thoroughly designed for well-defined and well-characterized asthmatic patients, with standardized methods for obtaining specimens of sputum, BAL, or biopsies that are of adequate quality for investigation and comprehensive analyses. Agreement among experts on how best to process and handle the obtained material for the evaluation of inflammation is crucial. Additional studies, both bronchoscopy and sputum, are needed to elucidate the effects of various anti-inflammatory treatments on airway inflammation. To achieve these aims, randomized controlled trials of larger groups of asthmatic patients with a range of severity, and trials of sufficient duration to show potential changes, are required, as is collaboration between research groups.

REFERENCES

1.   Osler W. Bronchial asthma. In: Osler W, editor. The principles and practice of medicine. New York: Appelton and Co; 1882. p. 497–501.

2.   Huber HL, Koessler KK. The pathology of bronchial asthma. Arch Intern Med 1922;30:689–760.

3.   Earle BV. Fatal bronchial asthma. Thorax 1953;8:195–206.

4.   Dunnill MS. The pathology of asthma, with special references to changes in the bronchial mucosa. J Clin Pathol 1960;13:27–33.

5.   Glynn AA, Michaels L. Bronchial biopsy in chronic bronchitis and asthma. Thorax 1960;15:142–53.

6.   Laitinen LA, Heino M, Laitinen A, et al. Damage of the airway epithelium and bronchial reactivity in patients with asthma. Am Rev Respir Dis 1985;131:599–606.

7.   De Monchy JGR, Kauffman HF, Venge P, et al. Bronchoalveolar lavage eosinophilia during allergen-induced late asthmatic reactions. Am Rev Respir Dis 1985;131:373–6.

8.   Kirby JG, Hargreave FE, Gleich GJ, O'Byrne PM. Bronchoalveolar cell profiles of asthmatic and non-asthmatic subjects. Am Rev Respir Dis 1987;136:379–83.

9.   Wardlaw AJ, Dunnette S, Gleich GJ, et al. Eosinophils and mast cells in bronchoalveolar lavage in subjects with mild asthma. Relationship to bronchial hyperreactivity. Am Rev Respir Dis 1988;137:62–9.

10.   Jeffery PK, Wardlaw AJ, Nelson FC, et al. Bronchial biopsies in asthma. An ultrastructural quantitative study and correlation with hyperreactivity. Am Rev Respir Dis 1989;149:1745–53.

11.   Ädelroth E, Rosenhall L, Johansson SÅ, et al. Inflammatory cells and eosinophilic activity in asthmatic patients investigated by bronchoalveolar lavage. The effects of antiasthmatic treatment with budesonide or terbutaline. Am Rev Respir Dis 1990;142:91–9.

12.   Djukanovic R, Roche WR, Wilson JW, et al. Mucosal inflammation in asthma. State of the art. Am Rev Respir Dis 1990;142:434–57.

13.   Azzawi M, Bradley B, Jeffery PK, et al. Identification of activated T-lymphocytes and eosinophils in bronchial biopsies in stable atopic asthma. Am Rev Respir Dis 1990;142:1407–13.

14.   Bousquet J, Chanez P, Lacoste JM, et al. Eosinophilic inflammation in asthma. N Engl J Med 1990;323:1016–8.

15.   Bradley BL, Azzawi M, Jacobson M, et al. Eosinophils, T-lymphocytes, mast cells, neutrophils and macrophages in bronchial biopsy specimens from atopic subjects with asthma: comparison with biopsy specimens from atopic subjects without asthma and normal control subjects and relationship to bronchial hyperresponsiveness. J Allergy Clin Immunol 1991;88:664–74.

16.   Walker C, Kaegi MK, Braun P, Blaser K. Activated T cells and eosinophilia in bronchoalveolar lavages from subjects with asthma correlated with disease activity. J Allergy Clin Immunol 1991;88:935–42.

17.   Laitinen LA, Laitinen A, Haahtela T. A comparative study of the effects of an inhaled corticosteroid, budesonide, and a β_2-agonist, terbutaline, on airway inflammation in newly diagnosed asthma. A randomized, double-blind parallel-group controlled trial. J Allergy Clin Immunol 1992;90:32–42.

18. Jeffery PK, Godfrey RW, Ädelroth E, et al. Effects of treatment on airway thickening of basement membrane reticular collagen in asthma. A quantitative light and electron microscopic study. Am Rev Respir Dis 1992;145:890–9.

19. Laitinen LA, Laitinen A, Haahtela T. Airway mucosal inflammation even in patients with newly diagnosed asthma. Am Rev Respir Dis 1993;147:697–704.

20. Robinson DS, Bentley AM, Hartnell A, et al. Activated memory T-helper cells in bronchoalveolar lavage fluid from patients with atopic asthma: relation to asthma symptoms, lung function and bronchial responsiveness. Thorax 1993;48:26–32.

21. Moqbel R, Barkans J, Bradley BL, et al. Application of monoclonal antibodies against major basic protein (BMK-13) and eosinophilic cationic protein (EG1 and EG2) for quantifying eosinophils in bronchial biopsies from atopic asthma. Clin Exp Allergy 1992;22:265–73.

22. Bentley AM, Menz G, Storz C, et al. Identification of T-lymphocytes, macrophages and activated eosinophils in the bronchial mucosa in intrinsic asthma. Am Rev Respir Dis 1992;146:500–6.

23. Woolley KL, Ädelroth E, Woolley MJ, et al. Granulocyte-macrophage colony–stimulating factor, eosinophils and eosinophilic cationic protein in subjects with and without mild, stable atopic asthma. Eur Respir J 1994;7:1576–84.

24. Humbert M, Durham SR, Ying S, et al. IL-4 and IL-5 mRNA and protein in bronchial biopsies from patients with atopic and non-atopic asthma: evidence against "intrinsic" asthma being a distinct immunopathological entity. Am J Respir Crit Care Med 1996;154:1497–504.

25. Berkman N, Krishnan VL, Gilbey T, et al. Expression of RANTES mRNA and protein in airways of patients with mild asthma. Am J Respir Crit Care Med 1996;154:1804–11.

26. Humbert M, Ying S, Corrigan C, et al. Bronchial mucosal expression of genes encoding chemokines RANTES and MCP-3 in symptomatic atopic and nonatopic asthmatic patients: relationship to the eosinophil active cytokine interleukin (IL)-5, granulocyte-macrophage colony–stimulating factor and IL-3. Am J Respir Cell Mol Biol 1997;16:1–8.

27. Tang C, Rolland JM, Ward C, et al. IL-5 production by bronchoalveolar lavage and peripheral blood mononuclear cells in asthma and atopy. Eur Respir J 1997;10:624–32.

28. Redington AE, Madden J, Frew AJ, et al. Transforming growth factor-β in asthma. Measurement in bronchoalveolar lavage fluid. Am J Respir Crit Care Med 1997;156:642–7.

29. Laberge S, Ernst P, Ghaffar O, et al. Increased expression of interleukin-16 in bronchial mucosa of subjects with atopic asthma. Am J Respir Cell Mol Biol 1997;17:193–202.

30. Smith DL, Deshazo RD. Bronchoalveolar lavage in asthma. An update and perspective. Am Rev Respir Dis 1993;148:523–32.

31. Pin I, Gibson PG, Kolendowicz R, et al. Use of induced sputum cell counts to investigate airway inflammation. Thorax 1992;47:25–9.

32. Fahy JV, Liu J, Wong H, Boushey HA. Cellular and biochemical analysis of induced sputum from healthy and asthmatic subjects. Am Rev Respir Dis 1993;147:1126–31.

33. Fahy JV, Kim KW, Liu J, Boushey HA. Prominent neutrophilic inflammation in sputum from subjects with asthma exacerbation. J Allergy Clin Immunol 1995;95:843–52.

34. Pizzichini MMM, Popov TA, Efthimiadis A, et al. Spontaneous and induced sputum to measure indices of airway inflammation in asthma. Am J Respir Crit Care Med 1996;154:866–9.

35. Pizzichini E, Pizzichini MMM, Efthimiadis A, et al. Indices of airway inflammation in induced sputum: reproducibility and validity of cell and fluid phase measurements. Am J Respir Crit Care Med 1996;154:308–17.

36. Pizzichini MMM, Pizzichini E, Clelland L, et al. Sputum in severe exacerbations of asthma: kinetics of inflammatory indices after prednisolone treatment. Am J Respir Crit Care Med 1997;155:1501–8.

37. Workshop summaries and guidelines. Investigative use of bronchoscopy, lavage and bronchial biopsies in asthma and other airway diseases. Clin Exp Allergy 1991;21:533–40.

38. Torodo de la Fuente P, Romagnoli M, Godard P, et al. Safety of inducing sputum in patients with asthma of varying severity. Am J Respir Crit Care Med 1998;157:1127–30.

39. Calhoun WJ, Jarjour NN. Macrophages and macrophage diversity in asthma. In: Busse WW, Holgate ST, editors. Asthma and rhinitis. Boston: Blackwell Scientific Publications; 1995. p. 467–73.

40. Cluzel M, Damon M, Chanez P, et al. Enhanced alveolar cell luminal-dependent chemiluminescence in asthma. J Allergy Clin Immunol 1987;80:195–201.

41. Fabbri LM, Boschetto P, Zocca E, et al. Bronchoalveolar neutrophilia during late asthmatic reactions induced by toluene diisocyanate. Am Rev Respir Dis 1987;136:36–42.

42. Chan-Yeung M, Leriche J, Maclean L, Lam S. Comparison of cellular and protein changes in bronchial lavage fluid of symptomatic and asymptomatic patients with red cedar asthma on follow-up examination. Clin Allergy 1988;18:359–65.

43. Scannell C, Chen L, Aris RA, et al. Greater ozone-induced inflammatory responses in subjects with asthma. Am J Respir Crit Care Med 1996;154:24–9.

44. Kraft M, Djukanovic R, Wilson S, et al. Alveolar tissue inflammation in asthma. Am J Respir Crit Care Med 1996;154:1505–10.

45. Hamid Q, Song Y, Kotsimbos TC, et al. Inflammation of small airways in asthma. J Allergy Clin Immunol 1997;100:44–51.

46. Liu MC, Hubbard WC, Proud D, et al. Immediate and late inflammatory responses to ragweed antigen challenge of the peripheral airways in allergic asthmatic patients. Cellular, mediator and permeability changes. Am Rev Respir Dis 1991;144:51–6.

47. Woolley KL, Ädelroth E, Woolley MJ, et al. Effects of allergen challenge on eosinophils, eosinophil cationic protein, and granulocyte-macrophage colony–stimulating factor in mild asthma. Am J Respir Crit Care Med 1995;151:1915–24.

48. Calhoun WJ, Kelly J. Cytokines in the respiratory tract. In: Chung KF, Barnes PJ, editors. Pharmacology of the respiratory tract. New York: Marcel Dekker Inc; 1993. p. 258–88.

49. Chung KF. Inflammatory mediators in asthma. In: O'Byrne PM, editor. Asthma as an inflammatory disease. New York: Marcel Dekker Inc; 1990. p. 150–83.

50. Broide DH, Lotz M, Cuomo AJ, et al. Cytokines in symptomatic asthma airways. J Allergy Clin Immunol 1992;89:958–67.

51. Rennard SI, Ghafouri M, Thompson AB, et al. Fractional processing of sequential bronchoalveolar lavage to separate bronchial and alveolar samples. Am Rev Respir Dis 1990;141:208–17.

52. Kelly CA, Fenwick JD, Corris PA, et al. Fluid dynamics during bronchoalveolar lavage. Am Rev Respir Dis 1988;138:81–4.

53. Ward C, Duddridge M, Fenwick J, et al. The origin of water and urea sampled at bronchoalveolar lavage in asthmatic patients and control subjects. Am Rev Respir Dis 1992;146:444–7.

54. Jeffery PK. Pathology of asthma. In: Kay AB, editor. Allergy and allergic diseases. Vol. 2. Oxford: Blackwell Science; 1997. p. 1412–28.

55. Söderberg M, Hellström S, Sandström T, et al. Structural characterization of bronchial mucosal biopsies from healthy volunteers. Eur Respir J 1990;3:261–6.

56. Brewster CE, Howarth PH, Djukanovic R, et al. Myofibroblast and subepithelial fibrosis in bronchial asthma. Am J Respir Cell Mol Biol 1990;3:507–11.

57. Persson CAG, Erjefält JS. "Ultimate activation" of eosinophils in vivo: lysis and release of clusters of free eosinophil granules (Cfegs). Thorax 1997;52:569–74.

58. Azzawi M, Johnstone PW, Majumdar S, et al. T-lymphocytes and activated eosinophils in airway mucosa in fatal asthma and cystic fibrosis. Am Rev Respir Dis 1992;145:1477–82.

59. Shute JK, Wrugt B, Lindley IJ, et al. Free and complexed interleukin-8 in blood and bronchial mucosa in asthma. Am J Respir Crit Care Med 1997;155:1877–83.

60. Ebina M, Takahashi T, Chiba T, Motomiya M. Cellular hypertrophy and hyperplasia of airway smooth muscles underlying bronchial asthma. Am Rev Respir Dis 1993;148:720–6.

61. Bai TR. Abnormalities in airway smooth muscle in fatal asthma. Am Rev Respir Dis 1991;143:441–3.

62. Wenzel SE, Szefler SJ, Leung SY, et al. Bronchoscopic evaluation of severe asthma: persistent neutrophilic inflammation associated with high dose glucocorticoids. Am J Respir Crit Care Med 1997;156:737–43.

63. Aalbers R, de Monchy JGR, Kauffman HF, et al. Dynamics of eosinophil infilatration in the bronchial mucosa before and after the late asthmatic reaction. Eur Respir J 1993;6:840–7.

64. Frew AJ, St. Pierre J, Teran LM, et al. Cellular and mediator responses twenty-four hours after local endobronchial allergen challenge of asthmatic airways. J Allergy Clin Immunol 1996;98:133–43.

65. Gizycki MJ, Ädelroth E, Rogers AV, et al. Myofibroblast involvement in the allergen-induced late response in mild atopic asthma. Am J Respir Cell Mol Biol 1997;16:664–73.

66. Wang JH, Trigg CJ, Devalia JL, et al. Effect of inhaled beclomethasone dipropionate on expression of pro-inflammatory cytokines and activated eosinophils in the bronchial epithelium of patients with mild asthma. J Allergy Clin Immunol 1994;90:1025–34.

67. Booth H, Richmond I, Ward C, et al. Effects of high dose inhaled fluticasone propionate on airway inflammation in asthma. Am J Respir Crit Care Med 1995;152:45–52.

68. Robinson D, Hamid Q, Ying S, et al. Prednisolone treatment in asthma is associated with modulation of broncho-alveolar lavage cell interleukin-4, interleukin-5 and interferon-γ cytokine gene expression. Am Rev Respir Dis 1993;148:401–6.

69. Djukanovic R, Homeyard S, Gratziou C, et al. The effect of treatment with oral corticosteroids on asthma symptoms and airway inflammation. Am J Respir Crit Care Med 1997;155:826–32.

70. Hoshino M, Naramura Y, Sim J, et al. Inhaled corticosteroid reduced lamina reticularis of the basement membrane by modulation of insulin-like growth factor (IGF)-I expression in bronchial asthma. Clin Exp Allergy 1998;28:568–77.

71. Laitinen A, Altraja A, Kämpe M, et al. Tenascin is increased in airway basement membrane of asthmatic patients and decreased by an inhaled steroid. Am J Respir Crit Care Med 1997;156:951–8.

72. Richmond I, Booth H, Ward C, Walters EH. Intrasubject variability in airway inflammation in biopsies in mild to moderate stable asthma. Am J Respir Crit Care Med 1996;153:899–903.

73. O'Byrne PM, Inman MD. Induced sputum to assess airway inflammation in asthma. Eur Respir J 1996;9:2435–6.

74. Maestrelli P, Saetta M, Di Stefano A, et al. Comparison of leukocyte counts in sputum, bronchial biopsies, and bronchoalveolar lavage. Am J Respir Crit Care Med 1995;152:1926–31.

75. Grootendorst DC, Sont JK, Willems LNA, et al. Comparison of inflammatory cell counts in asthma: induced sputum vs bronchoalveolar lavage and bronchial biopsies. Clin Exp Allergy 1997;27:769–79.

CHAPTER 4

Diagnosis

D. Robin Taylor, MD, MRCP, FRCPC

The diagnosis and assessment of bronchial asthma is now a "bread-and-butter" issue for clinicians in general medicine, pediatrics, and family practice. Epidemiologic data indicate that over the last two decades, the prevalence of asthma in western countries has increased, particularly among children [see Chapter 1]. In addition, among older adults, the need to diagnose and distinguish asthma from chronic obstructive pulmonary disease (COPD) is becoming increasingly important, given the diverging emphases that there are for treatment of the two conditions. However, although most clinicians are familiar with asthma in its common presentations, in a significant number of cases, a more painstaking approach is called for, either because the clinical picture overlaps with that of other respiratory pathologies, or because the presentation is atypical.

The fundamental principles of therapeutics include establishing the diagnosis, assessing disease severity, and identifying precipitating and aggravating factors. These basics are important in asthma, given its variable natural history. For most diagnoses, the first of these criteria requires identifying and confirming an underlying pathology. Over the past decade, our knowledge of airway pathology in asthma has been an evolving one: the goalposts have been moving. This is reflected in a broadening of, rather than a fundamental change in, the consensus definitions of asthma.

It is now generally accepted that airway inflammation, usually characterized by eosinophilia, is the pathologic hallmark of asthma (Level I).[1] However, diagnosing airway inflammation remains difficult, because the airways are relatively inaccessible—either experimentally or in the clinical setting—for easy observation or sampling. Thus, when a clinical diagnosis remains in doubt, supporting evidence is usually indirect rather than direct. Unfortunately, no single diagnostic test is currently available.[2]

In this chapter, our current approach to the diagnosis of asthma will be reviewed, giving particular attention to the role of the more commonly used diagnostic tests in assessing individual patients.

DEFINITIONS OR DESCRIPTIONS

Definitions of a disease ought to be useful in distinguishing affected from unaffected individuals. To that extent, no satisfactory definition of asthma exists. Rather, consensus statements are *descriptions* of clinical and pathologic scenarios in which asthma is likely to be the diagnosis. The lack of a concrete definition does not necessarily detract from the usefulness of the descriptions; the majority are pragmatic attempts to satisfy the needs of clinicians, epidemiologists, physiologists, cell biologists, and pathologists.

There are several key elements in the historic range of descriptions of asthma: variable airway caliber, responses to drug therapy, bronchial hyper-responsiveness, and airway inflammation. Early definitions of asthma emphasized variable airway obstruction as the primary marker of disease as well as the cause of symptoms (Level III).[3,4] However, airways obstruction in asthma may indeed be irreversible.[5] Likewise, "asthmatic" airway inflammation may give rise to clinical problems other than those of variable airways obstruction,[6] notably cough[7] (Table 4–1).

Table 4–1 *Pathophysiologic Factors Giving Rise to Symptoms in Asthma*

Abnormality of Function	Possible Symptoms
Smooth muscle spasm with airway narrowing	Dyspnea, wheeze, chest tightness
Dynamic hyperinflation, increased work of breathing on inspiration	Chest tightness, dyspnea
Airway hyper-responsiveness	Chest tightness, cough, chest pain, notably on exposure to cold air, dry air, exercise, and other exogenous stimuli
Mucus plugging	Cough, sputum production, chest tightness

Early definitions also included references to the response of the airways to bronchodilator and/or steroid therapy (Level III),[4,8] and all subsequent definitions have included this component. Later attempts to define asthma sought to include bronchial hyper-responsiveness (BHR) to nonspecific bronchoconstrictors. This has been a particular emphasis in definitions of asthma being used for epidemiologic studies (Level II).[9] However, even the inclusion of objectively measured hyper-responsiveness to methacholine or histamine is neither sensitive nor specific enough to be entirely helpful.[10]

For this reason, most current definitions embrace each of these concepts and also include descriptions of underlying airway inflammation (Level III). [1,11–13] They are best summed up by the International Consensus Report.[1]

> Asthma is a chronic inflammatory disorder of the airways in which many cells play a role. In susceptible individuals this inflammation causes symptoms which are usually associated with widespread but variable airflow obstruction that is often reversible either spontaneously or with treatment, and it also causes an associated increase in airway responses to a variety of stimuli.

The major components in that definition are: susceptibility (atopy); airway inflammation; variable airflow obstruction; symptoms; responses to treatment; and responsiveness to exogenous stimuli. Paradoxically, in clinical practice, most of these are assessed or measured *except* for airway inflammation. However, although the presence of one or more of these features may identify an individual's asthma phenotype, their importance will ultimately be determined by whether they predict persisting symptoms, the need for regular treatment, adverse changes in lung function over time, or the risk of mortality.

OTHER DIAGNOSTIC LABELS

Late-Onset or Intrinsic Asthma

This term is used to describe asthma that usually occurs in older adult patients who have no background history of atopy. Skin-prick testing is usually negative and total serum IgE is within normal limits. They may be characterized by sensitivity to aspirin or other nonsteroidal drugs, and they may have coexisting nasal polyposis. There is considerable debate about the differences in underlying pathologic mechanisms between this and the classic form of asthma.[14]

Reactive Airways Dysfunction Syndrome

Reactive airways dysfunction syndrome, or "RADS," is a term first used in 1985 to describe an asthma-like syndrome occurring in previously healthy individuals following acute massive exposure, usually in the workplace, to irritant fumes or gases.[15] Symptoms usually occur within 24 hours and continue for a minimum of 3 months and are associated with persistent nonspecific bronchial hyper-responsiveness. The underlying pathology is not yet clear, and uncertainties remain as to whether RADS is a distinct clinical entity.[16]

EVALUATING SYMPTOMS AND SIGNS

The classic presentation of asthma in adults usually includes symptoms of chest tightness, shortness of breath, and wheeze. Less commonly, the presenting complaint is chest pain or isolated cough. The frequency of symptoms reported in a recent survey is shown in Table 4–2.[17] Of these, wheeze and/or nocturnal symptoms are the best predictors of current asthma.

Table 4–2 *Frequency Distribution of Respiratory Symptoms**

Symptom/Symptom Combination	Frequency (%)
Isolated wheeze	75
Wheeze with dyspnea	65
Exercise dyspnea	66
Wheezing in the absence of a cold	60
Nocturnal chest tightness	48
Nocturnal cough	46
Nocturnal dyspnea	43
Chronic phlegm production	22
Chronic cough	19

* In a population of 204 asthmatic patients with current asthma.
Reprinted with permission from Sistek D, Tschopp JM, Schindler C, et al. Predictive symptoms to diagnose current asthma. Eur Respir J 1998;440 Suppl 28:2851.

As in children with asthma, and despite a broader differential diagnosis, these symptoms usually occur against a background of a positive family history or a personal history of atopy.[18]

Tracing the time course of events is important in confirming a diagnosis of asthma and in distinguishing asthma from other respiratory disorders. Symptoms are usually, but not always, episodic. However, "attacks" occur only in the minority. Nocturnal symptoms are common, occurring in 74% of patients with current asthma in one large survey,[19] a feature that also suggests that the patient is less likely to have COPD. Associations between the onset or worsening of symptoms and trigger factors, such as allergen exposure, exercise, inhalation of cold air or irritating fumes and gases, ingestion of certain foods or metabisulfite, or viral respiratory tract infections, should be established. Often a diagnosis of asthma is made when a precipitating event is reported but against a background of mild symptoms which may have been present but undiagnosed for many years.[20] Occupational exposures should be actively borne in mind [see Chapter 9]. A drug history to include nonsteroidal anti-inflammatories, angiotensin converting enzyme (ACE) inhibitors, and β-blockers (including ophthalmic) is important: each may cause or exacerbate asthma-like symptoms.[11]

Diagnostic difficulties may arise because patients use different words to describe uncomfortable respiratory sensations. Their understanding of symptom terminology may differ from the clinician's, for example, in using the term "wheeze." Likewise, individual thresholds for symptom perception are variable.[21] In one study, 20% of patients underestimated the degree of control and/or severity of their asthma,[22] stressing the need for objective measures of assessment. Many asthmatic patients complain only when their spirometric values are less than 50% predicted. In addition, it appears the symptoms experienced by patients may differ depending on the provoking stimulus, at least in experimental situations. Stimuli causing direct smooth muscle contraction appear to give rise to less severe symptoms than those causing bronchospasm by indirect pathways.[23]

Cough and Cough-Variant Asthma

Cough precipitated by cold-air exposure, exercise, or inhalation of aerosols may represent "cough-variant asthma" (CVA), although these symptoms are not specific. In one large series, 24% of 102 consecutive patients presenting with chronic cough had asthma.[7] The diagnosis of asthma when cough is the sole presenting symptom requires the demonstration of BHR (by methacholine or histamine challenge) and a positive response to inhaled drug therapy. Spirometry and peak-flow monitoring are less helpful (Level I).[24] Long-term follow-up indicates that approximately 50% of patients diagnosed with CVA will require chronic therapy and will go on to demonstrate other symptoms of asthma. In the remainder, there is complete resolution, raising questions about the initial diagnosis.[25]

Asthma in the Elderly

A new diagnosis of asthma in an elderly subject is not at all uncommon.[26] However, making the diagnosis may be problematic, especially because comorbidity giving rise to asthma-like symptoms, notably cardiac disease, is more likely to be present.[27] Compared to young subjects with asthma, the elderly may develop significant airflow obstruction, yet symptoms may be understated.[28] Thus, the diagnosis may either be ignored by the patient or missed by the clinician.

Physical Examination

Although, most patients with asthma will have variable airflow obstruction, its absence does not exclude the diagnosis. The role of physical examination to diagnose airflow obstruction (not necessarily asthma) is very limited. The combined findings of several studies indicate that airflow obstruction is best predicted by the presence of audible wheezing, a forced expiratory time of longer than 9 seconds,[29] and the finding of reduced breath sounds on auscultation.[30] Even in high-probability situations, suggestive symptoms together with peak-flow recordings are much more sensitive in identifying airflow obstruction than any examination findings (Level III).

Given that most patients will have mild disease, these results indicate that physical examination is likely to be unrewarding except in chronic moderate or severe disease or during an acute severe episode. The importance of physical examination lies in identifying pathophysiological processes *other than* airways obstruction.

Examination of the upper airway is often neglected but may yield important clues as to underlying causes of a patient's symptoms. Important findings include mucosal inflammation and hypertrophy, nasal polyposis, and maxillofrontal tenderness. Identifying and controlling chronic rhinitis may be important in relieving lower respiratory tract symptoms.[11,13]

DIFFERENTIAL DIAGNOSIS

The differential diagnosis for asthma is extensive because respiratory symptoms are nonspecific (Table 4–3). The clinician's principal task is to consider and exclude other possible diagnoses. This is particularly important if the response to a trial of therapy, for example, bronchodilator or corticosteroid, has been negative. It is also important to recognize that other clinical problems such as gastroesophageal reflux disease (GERD) may coexist alongside asthma, and that a single diagnosis to explain a patient's symptoms may be inadequate.

Chronic Obstructive Pulmonary Disease

Although considerable overlap may occur between the presenting features of asthma and

Table 4–3 *Differential Diagnosis for Patients Presenting with Respiratory Symptoms Suggestive of Asthma*

Localized pathology	Inhaled foreign body
	Endobronchial tumour
	Vocal cord dysfunction
Pathology in the majority of airways	Chronic obstructive pulmonary disease (COPD)
	Reactive airways dysfunction syndrome (RADS)
	Postinfectious bronchial hyper-responsiveness
	Cystic fibrosis
	Bronchiectasis
	Left ventricular failure
Other pathologies	Gastroesophageal reflux
	Pulmonary embolism
	Pulmonary eosinophilia
	Drug-induced BHR, eg, β-blockers, ACE inhibitors, nonsteroidal anti-inflammatories

BHR = bronchial hyper-responsiveness; ACE = angiotensin converting enzyme.

COPD, the two ought to be distinguished from each other if possible. The long-term prognosis for COPD includes progressive decline in lung function, and although this may occur in asthma, it is much less likely.[31,32] In addition, current approaches to the treatment of COPD are increasingly distinct from asthma, particularly with regard to inhaled drug therapy. This has been highlighted in the results of a large, long-term, prospective, controlled study of inhaled bronchodilator and corticosteroid treatment for nonspecific airways obstruction, in which patients with both COPD and asthma were included. Benefits were obtained predominantly in patients who were nonsmokers, who had a symptom-based diagnosis of asthma, and who demonstrated greater degrees of bronchodilator reversibility and BHR, that is, whose clinical profile was "asthmatic."[33] The clinical features that distinguish asthma from COPD are listed in Table 4–4.

Vocal Cord Dysfunction Syndrome and Other Abnormalities of the Upper Airway

There is evidence that abnormal function of the upper airway may give rise to the classic symptoms of asthma. The current literature suggests two scenarios: vocal cord dysfunction syndrome and, perhaps more controversially, extrathoracic airway responsiveness.

Vocal cord dysfunction syndrome is characterized by incomplete adduction of the vocal cords. Unfortunately, approximately half of such patients will have coexisting asthma, making the diagnosis difficult.[34] In the remainder, a misdiagnosis of asthma is often made, often leading to prolonged inappropriate therapy.[34]

Apart from asthma symptoms, patients may also complain of throat tightness and loss of voice. Stridor is not necessarily a feature. Episodes are usually of rapid onset and may subside just as quickly. They occur mostly by day. Confusingly, they may be precipitated by exercise.[35] Neither inhaled β$_2$-agonists nor corticosteroids are effective in their management, although sometimes patients will be receiving very high doses of both.[34] The diagnosis is suspected if the *inspiratory* limb of the flow-volume loop is flattened but is best confirmed by fiberoptic rhinolaryngoscopy, at which, despite cord adduction, an open glottic "chink" is maintained, distinguishing the syndrome from laryngospasm.[36]

Extrathoracic airway responsiveness has been described as a separate entity but appears to give rise to a similar range of asthma-like symptoms, particularly chronic cough. The

Table 4–4 *Clinical Features Distinguishing Asthma from Chronic Obstructive Pulmonary Disease*

Asthma	Chronic Obstructive Pulmonary Disease
Onset at any time in life	Onset in mid to late adult life
Usually nonsmokers	Almost invariably smokers
Cough and phlegm production less common	Cough and phlegm production common in "bronchitic" type
Dyspnea on effort variable	Dyspnea on effort predictable and progressive over months/years
Nocturnal symptoms relatively common	Nocturnal symptoms uncommon
Diurnal variation in airflow obstruction	Little variation in objective measurements of airflow
Good response to bronchodilator and corticosteroid	Response to bronchodilator and corticosteroid in 15–25% of patients
Bronchial hyper-responsiveness to nonspecific agents in the majority of patients with currently active disease	Bronchial hyper-responsiveness in only a minority of patients

majority of affected subjects have chronic nasal inflammation. The diagnostic hallmark appears to be dose-related changes in the inspiratory limb of the flow-volume loop during a histamine or methacholine challenge (Level II), although this diagnostic approach has not been adequately validated.[37]

Gastroesophageal Reflux Disease

The clinical presentations of GERD are said to include adult-onset asthma and intractable asthma.[38] Certainly, the respiratory symptoms associated with gastroesophageal reflux include atypical chest pain, cough, and wheeze, often occurring at night. In one study, cough occurred three times more frequently than wheeze.[39]

Distinguishing GERD from asthma may be difficult. The two conditions often coexist and dynamic interactions rather than simple cause-effect relationships are thought to occur between them.[40] There is evidence that GERD is more common in patients with asthma than in control groups, ranging from 30 to 89%, and "silent" GERD (presumably meaning free of upper gastrointestinal symptoms) is said to occur in 25 to 30% of asthmatic patients.[41]

Postinfective Airways Obstruction

Otherwise healthy individuals may demonstrate airways obstruction for a period of days or even weeks following a lower respiratory tract infection.[42] Symptoms typical of asthma may be present. In a large study including 395 adults with no other history of airways obstruction, spontaneous improvement in the forced expiratory volume in 1 second (FEV_1) of greater than 15% was recorded within 4 to 5 weeks of the acute illness in 23%.[43] Although for some atopic subjects with confirmed asthma the only trigger factor for symptoms is a "cold," caution should be exercised in diagnosing asthma in the immediate aftermath of respiratory tract infection (Level IIB).

CONFIRMING THE DIAGNOSIS: USE OF DIAGNOSTIC TESTS

Spirometry

Spirometry is becoming increasingly accessible to most clinicians and should always be used to confirm the diagnosis of airflow obstruction (Level IIIA).[11,44] Peak-flow recordings are insufficient for this purpose.[45] The most sensitive and reproducible indicator of airways obstruction is the FEV_1:VC (vital capacity) ratio (Level IIA),[45,46] even allowing for the possibility that airways obstruction is likely to be variable and may therefore be absent at the time of testing. In addition, despite the presence of obstruction, the FEV_1 may be in the normal range with respect to predicted values. Although the ratio falls with age, it is almost always abnormal if it is less than 70% (Level II).[47] Changes in the FEV_1:VC ratio with treatment should not be used to assess reversibility (Level III).[47]

Thereafter, the severity of airflow obstruction is best assessed using the *postbronchodilator* FEV_1 (Level III).[45] This value reflects obstruction due to mucosal edema, mucus plugging, and possibly long-term airway remodeling, rather than reactive smooth muscle spasm. Because of larger intraindividual variability, other parameters such as forced expiratory flow ($FEF_{25/75}$) are considered less useful.[47]

A summary of recommendations for spirometry is presented in Table 4–5.

Table 4–5 *Notes on the Use of Spirometry in Assessing Airflow Obstruction and Bronchodilator Response*

Airway obstruction	FEV_1:VC ratio most important parameter in distinguishing the presence of obstruction (Level IIA)
	$FEF_{25/75}$ (% predicted) and instantaneous flow rates should not be used to diagnose airways obstruction (Level IIA)
	Low FEV_1:VC ratio may occur in healthy subjects if the VC is abnormally high
	Severity assessment should be based on FEV_1 not FEV_1:VC; postbronchodilator values should be used (Level III)
Bronchodilator response	12% increase in FEV_1, calculated from the prebronchodilator value AND a 200 mL increase in either FEV_1 or VC are reasonable criteria for a positive response (Level IIB)
	FEV_1:VC ratio should not be used to judge response (Level III)
	Patients may still respond to bronchodilator even though the test is negative in the laboratory

Adapted from American Thoracic Society statement. Lung function testing: selection of reference values and interpretive strategies. Am Rev Respir Dis 1991;144:1202–18, and Enright P, Lebowitz M, Cockcroft D. Asthma outcome. Physiologic measures: pulmonary function tests. Am J Respir Crit Care Med 1994;149:S9–18.

Peak-Flow Monitoring

Peak-flow meters are portable, easy to use, and relatively inexpensive. However, they have limitations including: (1) they require adequate co-ordination and effort; (2) some models are inaccurate at their extremes of range; (3) they do not always identify small airway obstruction; and (4) their coefficients of variation are almost twice that of FEV_1.[48]

Although the relationship between peak-flow rates and asthma symptoms is variable,[49] serial measurements provide the opportunity to monitor *changes* in airway caliber *over time*. This may be critical in the diagnosis of asthma (Level IIIB).[50] One-time measurements have no diagnostic value but may be used to assess asthma severity as long as comparisons against "best peak-flow" (rather than predicted) values can be made.[49]

Twice-daily peak-flow measurements over 14 or more days should be obtained (Level IIIB).[49] Diurnal variation in peak flow is significantly greater in asthmatic patients and is a good predictor of diagnosed asthma and the severity of symptoms.[51,52] It is roughly related to

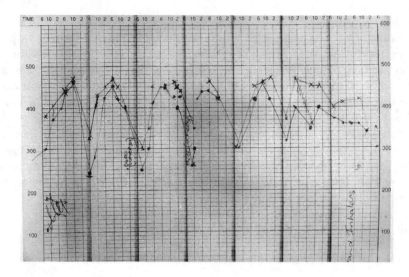

Figure 4–1A Serial peak-flow recordings obtained in a patient who presented with unstable asthma. At the time of diagnosis, the patient was experiencing severe nocturnal symptoms. There is significant diurnal variation with the amplitude % mean on the first day measuring 64.8%. The response to oral corticosteroid therapy shows a steady increase in prebronchodilator morning peak flow and a reduction in diurnal variation.

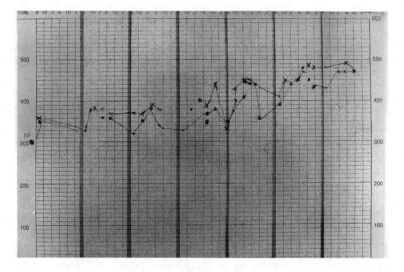

Figure 4–1B Serial peak-flow recordings obtained in a patient with a childhood history of asthma but who allegedly had been free of symptoms for many years. He had smoked for most of his adult life and presented with shortness of breath. There is minimal diurnal variability (amplitude % mean on the first day measures 18.2%). However, a trial of oral prednisone resulted in significant reversal of airflow obstruction, confirming the diagnosis of asthma.

the magnitude of BHR.[45] It is best expressed by calculating the amplitude (evening peak expiratory flow-rate [PEF] minus morning PEF) as % of the mean (evening PEF plus morning PEF/2).[53] In normal individuals, the median measurement is 4.9%.[52] Values greater than 19% have been shown to discriminate between asthmatic and nonasthmatic individuals.[54] Other indices derived from peak-flow data have been evaluated but are not frequently used. In one study, the "two lowest % mean," that is, the mean, of the two lowest PEF values as % of the period mean, was found to be the most sensitive index for diagnosed asthma (Level IIC).[55]

Visual assessment of graphically recorded twice-daily measurements of peak flow often reveals patterns that are characteristic of asthma,[56] particularly if a trial of corticosteroids is being used (Figures 4–1*A* and *B*). However, more frequent recordings are more likely to yield a positive result,[57] especially if occupational asthma is being considered.

Responses to Drug Therapy Trials

Inhaled Bronchodilator

The demonstration of an improvement in airflow following either bronchodilator or corticosteroid is an accepted criterion in support of the diagnosis of asthma (Level III).[44,45] Bronchodilator response is measured 15 minutes after inhaling a standard dose of a short-acting β-agonist, given either via a metered-dose inhaler and spacer, or by nebulizer. Reversibility is calculated as the percentage improvement in FEV_1 compared to the baseline measurement,[58] although this method of calculation tends to exaggerate the apparent response if the baseline FEV_1 is particularly low. For this reason, results may better be expressed with reference to predicted values, although this is not yet common practice.[59] Likewise, it is also recommended that the absolute change in FEV_1 from baseline should be greater than 200 mL.[47]

There is no agreement as to what constitutes a diagnostic response. In a large normal population sample, 95% of subjects showed reversibility in the range 0 to 9%.[60] An improvement of 12% or greater is the minimum criterion to confirm reversibility,[47] and greater than 15% is the usually accepted figure (Level IIC).Unfortunately, the demonstration of significant reversibility is usually not helpful in distinguishing asthma from COPD. In one study comprising 395 patients, reversibility averaged 10.6% for COPD and 16.4% for asthmatic patients, respectively.[61] Significant overlap precluded the test being used to discriminate between the two.

Oral Corticosteroid

Numerous factors affect the acute response to an inhaled bronchodilator (Table 4–6), and some patients may not demonstrate any improvement: the test is often falsely negative.[58] This does not exclude asthma. In such patients, a subsequent trial of oral corticosteroid, usually prednisone 30 to 50 mg daily for a minimum of 14 days, is recommended.[62] In response to corticosteroid, serial peak-flow measurements may demonstrate attenuation of diurnal variation as well as a rise in the mean values,[56] and are diagnostically more sensitive than before/after spirometry (Level II)[63] (see Figure 4–1*A*). This approach is more likely to be helpful in dealing with patients whose asthma is of longer duration and of greater severity,[64] and with current or ex-smokers in whom the differential diagnosis includes COPD (see Figure 4–1*B*). Steroid responsiveness almost certainly identifies those who have asthma (Level III).[65]

Measuring Nonspecific Bronchial Hyper-responsiveness

Increased airway responsiveness to nonspecific agents such as histamine or methacholine is a characteristic of asthma but does not define it, and the relationships between nonspecific BHR and clinical patterns of asthma are poorly understood. Bronchial challenge testing is based on obtaining a dose-response curve from which the provocative dose/concentration of

Table 4–6 *Factors that May Result in a Falsely Negative Bronchodilator Response Test*

Chronicity of airflow obstruction

Severity of airflow obstruction

Presence of respiratory infection

Timing of testing (response less likely late pm)

Adequacy of withdrawal of prescribed bronchodilator therapy before test

Adequacy of drug delivery of test dose, notably inhaler technique in a patient who may not have had
   previous experience with inhalers

Timing of spirometric measurement after taking bronchodilator

Adapted from Shim C. Response to bronchodilators. Clin Chest Med 1989;10:155–63.

methacoline or histamine resulting in a 20% fall in FEV_1 (PC_{20}/PD_{20}) is calculated.
Measuring the slope of the dose-response curve (DRC) is an alternative method of evaluating the result when making between-patient comparisons.[66] The test is reproducible by comparison with exercise or allergen challenge testing.[45]

   Bronchial hyper-responsiveness correlates with the cellular component of   airway
inflammation,[67] and the majority of patients with currently symptomatic asthma have measurable BHR, which correlates with variation in airway caliber,[68] susceptibility to triggers,[69]
symptoms,[70,71] and clinical severity (Level II).[72,73] However, despite this apparent advantage,
the use of these challenge tests to aid diagnosis is limited. In population studies, BHR is normally rather than bimodally distributed.[74] The cutoff between hyper-responsive and nonhy-
per-responsive individuals has been arbitrarily set at 8 mg/mL or 8 μmol/L.[10] Individuals with
diagnosed asthma may still have a negative test, and those with a positive test may be either
asymptomatic or have a respiratory complaint other than asthma (Figure 4–2) (Level II).

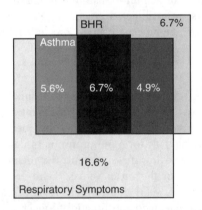

Figure 4–2 Venn diagram showing the overlap relationship between bronchial hyper-responsiveness,
diagnosed asthma, and respiratory symptoms in a population of 2,363 Australian schoolchildren aged
8 to 11 years. Of the schoolchildren, 45.5% with diagnosed asthma failed to demonstrate BHR, and
36.6% with BHR were asymptomatic. (Reproduced with permission from Salome CM, Peat JK,
Britton WJ, Woolcock AJ. Bronchial hyper-responsiveness in two populations of Australian schoolchildren. Relation to respiratory symptoms and diagnosed asthma. Clin Allergy 1987;17:271–81.)

The sensitivities and specificities of bronchial challenge testing recorded in a number of studies has been summarized in a recent review (Level II).[10] They average approximately 60% and 90%, respectively. In the clinical setting, in which the pretest probability of asthma is likely to be high, for example, 50%, the positive predictive value has been calculated to be about 85% (moderately good at predicting asthma), but the negative predictive value was 70% (unhelpful in excluding it) (Level II).[10] However, this judgment is not a consistent one, and opinion appears to have shifted over the years. Earlier it was suggested that because of its allegedly high sensitivity, testing for BHR might be used to exclude asthma [45,75]

What, then, is the role for BHR testing? The issue remains a controversial one.[2,76] In epidemiology, it is used together with symptoms over a specified time period and/or doctor-diagnosed asthma to describe the asthma phenotype.[9] In clinical practice, demonstrating BHR is recommended as a second- or third-line investigation where symptoms are atypical, or where airflow obstruction cannot be demonstrated either by spirometry or by serial peak-flow measurements (Level IIIC).[13] Although the latter may, in fact, be less sensitive, they represent a more practical approach to confirming the diagnosis of asthma.[77,78] More recently, the predictive values of combining two tests has been investigated. In one study, peak-flow measurements and BHR testing together identified nearly 90% of symptomatic asthmatic patients.[79] Finally, BHR testing is recommended as part of a diagnostic algorithm for the management of chronic cough, even though false-positives may occur (Level IIB).[7,80] More recently it has been used as a guide to adjustment of inhaled corticosteroid therapy. The clinical applicability of this approach remains to be determined.[81]

Exercise

The frequency of exercise-induced bronchospasm (EIB) among asthmatic subjects is reported to range from 40 to 90%,[82] and evidence of EIB may be found on testing subjects who deny exercise-related symptoms. Provocative exercise testing has a role in establishing a diagnosis of asthma in patients with exercise-related dyspnea, in whom wheeze is absent and for whom resting spirometry and serial peak-flow measurements are unremarkable.[45] The differential diagnosis includes lack of fitness; glottic dysfunction; occult cardiac or other pulmonary disease, for example, multiple pulmonary emboli; and abnormal muscle substrate use, such as McArdle's disease.[82]

Standardizing exercise tests is important.[83] The key elements are sustained exercise (for at least 5 minutes) breathing dry air at a work rate of 50 to 60% of V_{O_2}max or to 90% of the maximum predicted heart rate. Free running has been used in children. Changes in airway caliber occur at the *end* of exercise and are maximal 5 to 10 minutes thereafter. Lung function is measured for up to 30 minutes, by which time spontaneous recovery has usually begun. A fall in FEV_1 of 10% minimum, but preferably 15% or greater, is diagnostic. Changes in peak flow are less sensitive.[84] The repeatability of the test is rather poor with coefficients of variation ranging from 19 to 25%.

The sensitivity of exercise testing for diagnosed asthma in epidemiologic studies is reported to be 70 to 80%.[85] As for nonspecific BHR, these figures depend on pretest probabilities. However, the specificity of exercise testing is high, ranging from 87 to 97%, that is, a positive test is more likely to occur in asthma than in other lung diseases (Level II).[85,86] A positive test in asymptomatic individuals is also predictive of the later development of symptomatic asthma.[87] Although the magnitude of EIB is greater in patients with greater degrees of nonspecific BHR, correlations between EIB and methacholine/histamine reactivity are poor, suggesting that the tests evaluate different pathophysiologic aspects of the asthma syndrome.[88] A summary of recommendations for commonly used diagnostic tests is contained in Table 4–7.

Table 4–7 *Key Recommendations for Using Diagnostic Investigations in the Diagnosis of Asthma*

Recommendation	Levels of Evidence
Spirometry to confirm airways obstruction	IIIA
FEV$_1$:VC ratio to be used for diagnosis of airflow obstruction (abnormally low); response to bronchodilator should be measured simultaneously (greater than 15% improvement = positive test)	IIA, IIC
Serial peak-flow measurements twice daily over 2–6 weeks to be used diagnostically if spirometry is normal, or in any case to assess initial severity; also used to evaluate response to treatment which may include a diagnostic trial of corticosteroid	IIIB
Nonspecific BHR may be measured if spirometry or peak flow measurements are diagnostically unhelpful; recommended in a diagnostic approach to chronic cough	IIIC, IIB
Exercise testing to help to distinguish asthma from other respiratory pathologies or if exercise symptoms predominate	IIC

Other Investigations

Sputum Examination

The analysis of sputum induced after inhaling nebulized hypertonic saline has been developed in recent years as a useful means of assessing airway inflammation. The technique requires considerable resources and expertise, but in experienced hands it is repeatable and valid. The methodology is not yet widely used in clinical practice as a diagnostic tool.[89]

Nonisotonic Airway Challenge

Nonisotonic aerosols have been shown to induce bronchoconstriction and may be used to evaluate airway hyper-responsiveness, particularly if associated with exercise-related symptoms.[90] Techniques using hypertonic saline or mannitol have been described[91–93] and are similar to those for histamine or methacholine. Hypertonic saline challenge has been used in large epidemiologic studies of asthma,[91] but its role in clinical practice has not been adequately studied.

Other Tests

A list of other potentially helpful investigations appears in Table 4–8.

SEVERITY AND CONTROL

Confirming the periodicity of symptoms is helpful in establishing the diagnosis of asthma but has also been included in guidelines for assessing disease severity (Table 4–9).[50] However, although intermittent symptoms usually imply less severe disease than do persistent ones, this approach requires some caution. Of critical importance is the identification of a small number of patients with either brittle or potentially fatal asthma, whose general control may be satisfactory but who are subject to acute life-threatening attacks.[94]

At the time of diagnosis, objective measures of severity usually help in assessing initial treatment requirements and may be used as a baseline against which response to treatment is measured. The stratification of mild, moderate, and severe asthma is, for the most part, arbi-

Table 4–8 *Supplementary Investigations Used in the Diagnosis and Assessment of Asthma Symptoms, and Evaluation of Diagnosed Asthma**

Investigation	Comment
Chest radiography	Useful only in excluding other causes of wheezy dyspnea, eg, tumor, foreign body, cardiac disease
Fiberoptic laryngoscopy / bronchoscopy	Should be used with caution; helpful in visualizing the larynx to confirm vocal cord dysfunction; bronchoscopy indicated to investigate monophonic wheeze, particularly in a smoker
CT scan of sinuses	The most useful investigation of the upper airway if coexisting sinusitis or nasal polyposis has not been firmly established by clinical or endoscopic examination
Total serum IgE	Often elevated in asthma; very high levels may point to allergic bronchopulmonary aspergillosis
Skin-prick testing	Helpful to confirm allergic basis for asthma

*Level III evidence.
CT = computed tomography; Ig = immunoglobulin.
Reprinted with permission from American Academy of Allergy, Asthma and Immunology. Practical parameters for treatment of asthma. J Allergy Clin Immunol 1995;96:746–8.

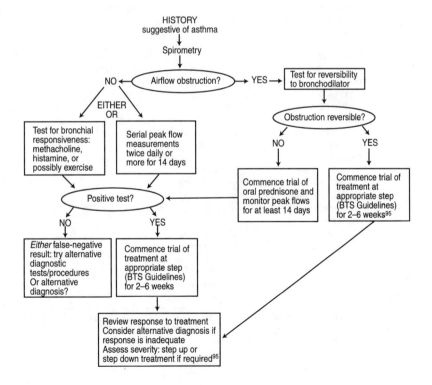

Figure 4–3 Algorithm for the diagnosis of asthma (Level IIIC). The algorithm does not easily allow for a diagnosis of asthma in patients with moderate or severe, long-standing, and poorly treated asthma, in which airflow obstruction remains largely irreversible even after an intensive trial of corticosteroid treatment (with or without other therapy). This outcome needs to be borne in mind. (Adapted from National Institutes of Health. Guidelines for the diagnosis and management of asthma. Expert panel report. NIH; 1991 Publication No.: 91-3042A.)

Table 4-9 *Indicators of Asthma Severity*

Severity	Clinical Features*	Treatment Requirements*†	Lung Function	Bronchial Hyper-responsiveness‡
Chronic mild asthma	Intermittent brief symptoms, less than 1–2 times per week Minimal nocturnal symptoms: < 2 times per month Few exacerbations and asymptomatic in between Good exercise tolerance, although occasional exercise symptoms No emergency medical requirements	Occasional use of relief bronchodilator, usually a short acting β-agonist (step 1)	Spirometry normal or abnormal: FEV_1 70–100% predicted§ PEFR greater than 80% predicted* PEFR variability 10–20%	PC20 2-8 mg/ml
Moderate	Symptoms > 1–2 times per week Nocturnal symptoms > 2 times per month Impaired exercise tolerance Occasional acute episodes, maybe lasting several days	Regular use of inhaled anti-inflammatory agents (step 2)	Spirometry usually abnormal, with FEV_1 50–69% predicted§ PEFR 60–80% predicted* PEFR variability 20–30%	PC_{20} 0.25–2 mg/mL
Severe	Daily persistent symptoms Frequent nocturnal symptoms Physical activities limited School or work absences Frequent exacerbations: sometimes requiring emergency treatment or hospital admission	Progressive increase in therapy depending on response Step 3: High-dose inhaled steroids or low-dose plus long-acting β-agonist Step 4: Additional measures eg, inhaled long-acting β-agonist, oral theophylline, inhaled anti-cholinergic, or inhaled nedocromil Step 5: Addition of oral steroid	FEV_1 less than 50% predicted§ PEFR less than 60% predicted* PEFR variability > 30%	PC_{20} < 0.25 mg/mL

Data adapted from: *National Institutes of Health[11]; †British Thoracic Society[95]; ‡Juniper et al.[72]; §American Thoracic Society statement[47].

trary. Thus, for spirometry there are some discrepancies between consensus statements regarding thresholds of severity. These are unlikely to be of practical significance in managing individual patients.

Thereafter, the goal posts shift. Severity is likely to be modified by treatment interventions. For this reason, severity may also be defined by the amount of treatment patients require in order to *maintain control.*[11,50,95] This is the basis for the symptom-based, step-wise approach to managing chronic asthma advocated in current guidelines (Level III).[50,95] However, severity and control are not synonymous: mild asthma may be poorly controlled and severe asthma may be well controlled.[96]

CONCLUSION

The diagnosis of asthma is usually straightforward and depends on a history of variable symptoms, supported by objective evidence of variable airflow obstruction that responds promptly to treatment. A diagnostic algorithm is presented in Figure 4–3.The absence of one or more of these features suggests an alternative explanation for symptoms of dyspnea with wheeze or cough, and depends on age and smoking status. Chronic obstructive pulmonary disorder and cardiac disease, as well as vocal cord dysfunction and gastroesophageal reflux, are important alternative or coexisting diagnoses. Although bronchial hyper-responsiveness underlies the clinical presentation of asthma, its objective measurement is recommended only if the diagnosis of asthma remains unconfirmed.

REFERENCES

1. US Department of Health and Human Services. International consensus report on the diagnosis and treatment of asthma. NIH Publication No.:92-3091. Eur Respir J 1992;5:601–41.

2. Britton J, Lewis S. Objective measures and the diagnosis of asthma. BMJ 1998;317:227–8.

3. Fletcher CM, Gibson JG, Hugh-Jones P, Scadding JG. Terminology, definitions and classification of chronic pulmonary emphysema and related conditions. Thorax 1959;14:286–99.

4. Meneely GR, Renzetti AD, Steele JD, et al. Chronic bronchitis, asthma and pulmonary emphysema. A statement by the committee on diagnostic standards for non-tuberculous respiratory disease. Am Rev Respir Dis 1962;85:762–8.

5. Brown PJ, Greville HW, Finucane KE. Asthma and irreversible airflow obstruction. Thorax 1984;39:131–6.

6. Woolcock AJ. How does inflammation cause symptoms? Am J Respir Crit Care Med 1996;153:S21–2.

7. Irwin RS, Curley FJ, French CL. Chronic cough: the spectrum and frequency of causes and key components of the diagnostic evaluation. Am Rev Respir Dis 1990;141:640–7.

8. Godfrey S. What is asthma? Arch Dis Child 1985;60:97–100.

9. Toelle BG, Peat JK, Salome CM, et al. Towards a definition of asthma for epidemiology. Am Rev Respir Dis 1992;146:633–7.

10. James A, Ryan G. Testing airway responsiveness using inhaled methacholine or histamine. Respirology 1997;2:97–105.

11. National Institutes of Health. Guidelines for the diagnosis and management of asthma. Expert panel report. NIH; 1991 Publication No.:91-3042A.

12. British Thoracic Society, British Paediatric Association, Royal College of Physicians of London, et al. Guidelines on the management of asthma. Thorax 1993;48:S1–24.

13. American Academy of Allergy Asthma and Immunology. Practice parameters for the diagnosis and treatment of asthma. J Allergy Clin Immunol 1995;96:707–48.

14. Kroegel C, Jager L, Walker C. Is there a place for intrinsic asthma as a distinct immunopathological entity? Eur Respir J 1997;10:513–5.

15. Brooks SM, Weiss MA, Bernstein IL. Reactive airways dysfunction syndrome (RADS); persistent asthma syndrome after high level irritant exposures. Chest 1985;88:376–84.

16. Alberts WM, Brooks SM. Reactive airways dysfunction syndrome. Curr Opin Pulm Med 1996;2:104–10.

17. Sistek D, Tschopp JM, Schindler C, et al. Predictive symptoms to diagnose current asthma. Eur Respir J 1998;440 Suppl (28):2851.

18. Sherman CB. Late-onset asthma: making the diagnosis, choosing drug therapy. Geriatrics 1995;50:24–33.

19. Turner-Warwick M. Epidemiology of nocturnal asthma. Am J Med 1988;85 Suppl:6–8.

20. Dodge R, Cline MG, Lebowitz MD, Burrows B. Findings before the diagnosis of asthma in young adults. J Allergy Clin Immunol 1994;94:831–5.

21. Rubinfield AR, Pain MCF. Perception of asthma. Lancet 1976;24:882–4.

22. Nguyen BP, Wilson SR, German DF. Patients' perceptions compared with objective ratings of asthma severity. Ann Allergy Asthma Immunol 1996;77:209–15.

23. Marks GB, Yates DH, Sist M, et al. Respiratory sensation during bronchial challenge testing with methacholine, sodium metabisulphite, and adenosine monophosphate. Thorax 1996;51:793–8.

24. Irwin RS, French CT, Smyrnios NA, Curley FJ. Interpretation of positive results of a methacholine challenge and 1 week inhaled bronchodilator use in diagnosing and treating cough variant asthma. Arch Intern Med 1997;157:1981–7.

25. Braman S, Pordy W, Corrao W, et al. Cough variant asthma: a 3–5 year follow-up. Am Rev Respir Dis 1982;125 Suppl 4(2):133.

26. Burrows B, Barbee RA, Cline MG, et al. Characteristics of asthma among elderly adults in a sample of the general population. Chest 1991;100:935–42.

27. Braman SS. Asthma in the elderly patient. Clin Chest Med 1993;14:413–22.

28. Connolly MJ, Crowley JJ, Charan NB, et al. Reduced subjective awareness of bronchoconstriction provoked by methacholine in elderly asthmatic and normal subjects as measured on a simple awareness scale. Thorax 1992;47:410–3.

29. Holleman DR, Simel DL. Does the clinical examination predict airflow limitation? JAMA 1995;273:313–9.

30. Badgett RG, Tanaka DJ, Hunt DK, et al. The clinical evaluation for diagnosing obstructive airways disease in high-risk patients. Chest 1994;106:1427–31.

31. Lange P, Parner J, Vestbo J, et al. A 15-year follow-up study of ventilatory function in adults with asthma. N Engl J Med 1998;339:1194–200.

32. Silverstein M, Reed C, O'Connell E. Long-term survival of a cohort of community residents with asthma. N Engl J Med 1994;331:1537–41.

33. Kerstjens HAM, Overbeek SE, Schouten JP, et al and the Dutch Non-Specific Lung Disease Group. Airways hyperresponsiveness, bronchodilator response, allergy and smoking predict improvement in FEV_1 during long-term inhaled corticosteroid treatment. Eur Respir J 1993;6:868–76.

34. Newman KB, Mason UG, Schmaling KB. Clinical features of vocal cord dysfunction. Am J Respir Crit Care Med 1995;152:1382–6.

35. McFadden ER, Zawadski DK. Vocal cord dysfunction masquerading as exercise-induced asthma. Am J Respir Crit Care Med 1996;153:942–7.

36. Wood RP, Milgrom H. Vocal cord dysfunction. J Allergy Clin Immunol 1996;98:481–5.

37. Bucca C, Rolla G, Brussino L, et al. Are asthma-like symptoms due to bronchial or extrathoracic airway obstruction? Lancet 1995;346:791–5.

38. Interiano B, Guntupalli KK. Clinical aspects of asthma. Curr Opin Pulm Med 1996;2:60–5.

39. Johnson WE, Hagen JA, DeMeester TR, et al. Outcome of respiratory symptoms after anti-reflux surgery on patients with gastroesophageal reflux disease. Arch Surg 1996;131:489–92.

40. Ayres JG, Miles JF. Oesophageal reflux and asthma. Eur Respir J 1996;9:1073–8.

41. Simpson WG. Gastro-oesophageal reflux disease and asthma: diagnosis and management. Arch Intern Med 1995;155:798–804.

42. O'Connor SA, Jones DP, Collins JV, et al. Changes in pulmonary function after naturally acquired respiratory infection in normal persons. Am Rev Respir Dis 1979;120:1087–93.

43. Melbye H, Kongerud J, Vorland L. Reversible airflow limitation in adults with respiratory infection. Eur Respir J 1994;7:1239–45.

44. National Institutes of Health. Guidelines for the diagnosis and management of asthma. National asthma education program. Expert panel report. NIH; 1992 Publication No.:92-3091.

45. Enright P, Lebowitz M, Cockcroft D. Asthma outcome. Physiologic measures: pulmonary function tests. Am J Respir Crit Care Med 1994;149:S9–18.

46. Gardner RM, Hankinson JL, Clausen JL, et al. Standardization of spirometry—1987 update. Official statement of the American Thoracic Society. Am Rev Respir Dis 1987;136:1285–98.

47. American Thoracic Society statement. Lung function testing: selection of reference values and interpretative strategies. Am Rev Respir Dis 1991;144:1202–18.

48. Cross D, Nelson HS. The role of the peak flow meter in the diagnosis and management of asthma. J Allergy Clin Immunol 1991;87:120–8.

49. Quanjer PH, Lebowitz MD, Gregg I, et al. Peak expiratory flow: conclusions and recommendations of a working party of the European Respiratory Society. Eur Respir J 1997;10: Suppl 24:2–8S.

50. National Institutes of Health, Lung and Blood Institute. Global Initiative for Asthma: global strategy for asthma management and prevention. NHLBI/WHO workshop report, March 1993. Bethesda (MD): NIH; 1995 Publication No.:95-3659.

51. Hetzel MR, Clark TJH. Comparison of normal and asthmatic circadian rhythms in peak expiratory flow. Thorax 1980;35:732–8.

52. Quackenboss JJ, Lebowitz M, Krzyzanowski M. The normal range of diurnal changes in peak expiratory flows. Am Rev Respir Dis 1991;143:323–30.

53. Higgins BG, Britton JR, Chinn S, et al. The distribution of peak flow variability in a population sample. Am Rev Respir Dis 1989;140:1368–72.

54. Jamison JP, McKinley RK. Validity of peak expiratory flow variability for the diagnosis of asthma. Clin Sci (Colch) 1993;85:367–71.

55. Siersted HC, Hansen HS, Hansen NG, et al. Evaluation of peak expiratory flow variability in an adolescent population sample. Am J Respir Crit Care Med 1994;149:598–603.

56. Turner-Warwick M. On observing patterns of airflow obstruction in chronic asthma. Br J Dis Chest 1977;71:73–86.

57. D'Alonzo GE, Steinijans VW, Keller A. Measurements of morning and evening airflow grossly underestimate the circadian variability of FEV_1 and peak expiratory flow in asthma. Am J Respir Crit Care Med 1995;152:1097–9.

58. Shim C. Response to bronchodilators. Clin Chest Med 1989;10:155–63.

59. Brand PLP, Quanjer PH, Postma DS, et al. Interpretation of bronchodilator response in patients with obstructive airways disease. Thorax 1992;47:429–37.

60. Dales RE, Spitzer WO, Tousignant P, et al. Clinical interpretation of airway response to bronchodilator: epidemiologic considerations. Am Rev Respir Dis 1988;138:317–20.

61. Kesten S, Rebuck AS. Is the short-term response to inhaled beta-adrenergic agonist sensitive or specific for distinguishing between asthma and COPD? Chest 1994;105:1042–5.

62. Weir DC, Robertson AS, Gove RI, Burge PS. Time course of response to oral and inhaled corticosteroids in non-asthmatic chronic airflow obstruction. Thorax 1990;45:118–21.

63. Mitchell DM, Gildeh P, Dimond AH, Collins JV. Value of serial peak expiratory flow measurements in assessing treatment response in chronic airflow limitation. Thorax 1986;41:606–10.

64. Hudon C, Tircotte H, Laviolette M, et al. Characteristics of bronchial asthma with incomplete reversibility of airflow obstruction. Ann Allergy Asthma Immunol 1997;78:185–202.

65. Chanez P, Vignola AM, O'Shaughnessy T, et al. Corticosteroid reversibility in COPD is related to features of asthma. Am J Respir Crit Care Med 1997;155:1529–34.

66. O'Connor G, Sparrow D, Taylor D, et al. Analysis of dose response curves to methacholine. Am Rev Respir Dis 1987;136:1412–7.

67. Chetta A, Foresi A, Del Donno M. Bronchial responsiveness to distilled water and methacholine and its relationship to inflammation and remodelling of the airways in asthma. Am J Respir Crit Care Med 1996;153:910–7.

68. Gibson PG, Mattoli S, Sears MR, et al. Variable airflow obstruction in asymptomatic children with methacholine airway hyper-responsiveness. Clin Invest Med 1988;11:105.

69. Woolcock AJ, Reddel H, Trevillion L. Assessment of airway responsiveness as a guide to diagnosis, prognosis and therapy in asthma. Allergy Proc 1995;16:23–6.

70. Pattemore PK, Asher MI, Harrison AC, et al. The interrelationship among bronchial hyperresponsiveness, the diagnosis of asthma, and asthma symptoms. Am Rev Respir Dis 1990;142:549–54.

71. Clough JB, Williams JD, Holgate ST. Effect of atopy on the natural history of symptoms, peak expiratory flow, and bronchial responsiveness in 7 and 8 year old children with cough and wheeze. Am Rev Respir Dis 1991;143:755–60.

72. Juniper EF, Frith PA, Hargreave FE. Airway responsiveness to histamine and methacholine: relationship to minimum treatment to control symptoms of asthma. Thorax 1981;36:575–9.

73. Ryan G, Latimer KM, Dolovich J, Hargreave FE. Bronchial responsiveness to histamine: relationship to diurnal variation of peak flow rate, improvement after bronchodilator and airway calibre. Thorax 1982;37:423–9.

74. Salome CM, Peat JK, Britton WJ, Woolcock AJ. Bronchial hyperresponsiveness in two populations of Australian schoolchildren. Relation to respiratory symptoms and diagnosed asthma. Clin Allergy 1987;17:271–81.

75. Cockcroft DW, Hargreave FE. Airway hyper-responsiveness: relevance of random population data to clinical usefulness. Am Rev Respir Dis 1990;142:497–500.

76. Taylor DR. Making the diagnosis of asthma. BMJ 1997;315:4–5.

77. DenOtter JJ, Reijnen GMW, Van den Bosch WJHM, et al. Testing bronchial hyper-responsiveness: provocation or peak flow variability? Br J Gen Pract 1997;47:487–92.

78. Higgins BG, Britton JR, Chinn S, et al. Comparison of bronchial reactivity and peak flow variability measurements for epidemiologic studies. Am Rev Respir Dis 1992;145:588–93.

79. Siersted HC, Mostgaard G, Hyldebrandt N, et al. Inter-relationships between diagnosed asthma, asthma-like symptoms and abnormal airway behaviour in adolescence: the Odense Schoolchild study. Thorax 1996;51:503–9.

80. McGarvey LPA, Heaney LG, Lawson JT, et al. Evaluation and outcome of patients with chronic nonproductive cough using a comprehensive diagnostic protocol. Thorax 1998;53:738–43.

81. Sont JK, Willems LN, Bel H, et al. Clinical control and histopathological outcome of asthma when using airway hyperresponsiveness as an additional guide to long term treatment. Am J Respir Crit Care Med 1999;159:1043–51.

82. McFadden ER. Exercise-induced airway obstruction. Clin Chest Med 1995;16:671–81.

83. Anderson SD, Schoeffel RE. The importance of standardizing exercise tests in the evaluation of asthmatic children. In: Oseid S, Edwards AM, editors. The asthmatic child in play and sport. Kent, England: Pitman Medical; 1982. p. 21–5.

84. Custovic A, Arifhodzic N, Robinson A, Woolcock A. Exercise testing revisited. The response to exercise in normal and atopic children. Chest 1994;105:1127–32.

85. West JV, Robertson CF, Roberts R, Olinsky A. Evaluation of bronchial responsiveness to exercise in children as an objective measure of asthma in epidemiological surveys. Thorax 1996;51:590–5.

86. Godfrey S, Springer C, Noviski N, et al. Exercise but not methacholine differentiates asthma from chronic lung disease in children. Thorax 1991;46:488–92.

87. Jones A, Bowen M. Screening for childhood asthma using an exercise test. Br J Gen Pract 1994;44:127–31.

88. Haby MM, Anderson SD, Peat JK, et al. An exercise challenge protocol for epidemiological studies of asthma in children: comparison with histamine challenge. Eur Respir J 1994;7:43–9.

89. O'Byrne PM, Inman MD. Induced sputum to assess airway inflammation in asthma. Eur Respir J 1996;9:2435–6.

90. Makker HK, Holgate ST. Relation of hypertonic saline responsiveness of the airways to exercise induced asthma symptom severity and to histamine or methacholine reactivity. Thorax 1993;48:142–7.

91. Anderson SD, Smith CM, Rodwell LT, duToit JI. The use of non-isotonic aerosols for evaluating bronchial hyper-responsiveness. In: Spector SL, editor. Provocation testing in clinical practice. New York: Marcel Dekker; 1994. p. 249–77.

92. American Academy of Allergy, Asthma and Immunology Practical Parameters for the diagnosis and treatment of asthma. J Allergy Clin Immunol 1995;96:746.

93. Anderson SD, Brannan J, Spring J, et al. A new method for bronchial provocation testing in asthmatic subjects using a dry powder of mannitol. Am J Respir Crit Care Med 1997;156:758–65.

94. Ayres JG, Miles JF, Barnes PJ. Brittle asthma. Thorax 1998;53:315–21.

95. British Thoracic Society. The British guidelines on asthma management: 1995 review and position statement. Thorax 1997;52 Suppl.

96. Cockcroft DW, Swystun VA. Asthma control versus asthma severity. J Allergy Clin Immunol 1996;98:1016–8.

CHAPTER 5

Diagnosis in Children

Alexander C. Ferguson, MB, ChB, FRCPC

Asthma is a disease of respiration, often with paroxysms of difficult breathing; the word is derived from the Greek "asthma-matos" (breath hard).[1] The term has come to be used in different ways: (1) a general description of any reversible airway obstruction; (2) specifically to imply symptomatic airway inflammation; (3) a term describing a particular episode of airway obstruction; (4) a term describing a tendency to recurring episodes of airway obstruction; and (5) as combinations of all of these. In children, the word has been applied as an umbrella term to cover a variety of "wheezy" illnesses;[2] whereas, in adults, it is used more specifically to indicate recurring and, at least partly, reversible airway obstruction associated with chronic eosinophilic inflammation and bronchial hyper-responsiveness.[3] From a clinical point of view, a precise diagnostic definition based on symptoms and signs indicative of well-defined pathophysiology is important in leading to appropriate therapy and accurate predictions of initial outcome and long-term prognosis. Unfortunately, unlike diagnosis in adults, this degree of diagnostic precision is not yet possible in children. Indeed, the application of adult treatment principles to wheezing children based on bronchial biopsy findings of T lymphocyte–orchestrated airway inflammation mediated by eosinophils and other inflammatory cells has resulted in calls for the early and aggressive introduction of inhaled corticosteroid therapy,[4,5] which may be quite inappropriate (Level III).[6,7]

DIAGNOSIS BASED ON PATTERNS OF WHEEZY ILLNESS

Wheezy illness in young children is common. Community studies[8–13] have shown that 15 to 48% of children will have one or more episodes of wheeze, in the first 6 years of life, with most episodes clearly associated with viral infection, and prolonged symptom-free periods between.[4] Many infants have only one or two episodes, whereas others have monthly episodes during the winters of their first 2 or 3 years. The prevalence of cough or wheeze at night and on crying, exercise, or emotional upset between viral "colds" increases from age 3 years onwards but can be present after 1 year of age. Intercurrent symptoms, more characteristic of older children with asthma, increase with age as the number of infants who have only acute episodes decreases. Many children who later develop chronic symptoms and atopy begin with episodic wheezing related to recurrent viral infections and are initially indistinguishable from those whose wheezing episodes decrease and disappear by school age.

Park et al[10] found that 80% of children who wheezed in the first 5 years of life were wheeze free by age 10 years, but there was a wide range of duration of symptoms. The age of onset of wheezing was unhelpful in predicting outcome. Children developing atopic asthma may have early onset symptoms suggesting a high degree of airway sensitization for intrinsic or environmental reasons and a poor prognosis, whereas those who wheeze as a result of reduced airway caliber in infancy will improve as their lungs grow with age. Although a greater percentage of children who wheezed during their first year of life than those who commenced at an older age were symptom free by age 10 years, because 45% of early wheeze (≤ 5 years) starts in the first year, twice as many of this early onset group were still wheezing at age 10 years. Only 20% of those with wheeze beginning after the second year were still hav-

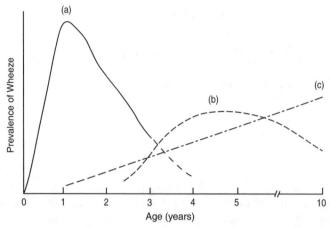

Figure 5–1 Three proposed patterns of wheeze in early childhood, with differing risk factors and time course: (*a*) recurrent lower respiratory illness with wheezing related to abnormal airway mechanics, maternal smoking, and genetic factors; (*b*) episodic viral wheeze; and (*c*) atopic asthma. (Reproduced with permission from Wilson NM. The significance of early wheezing. Clin Exp Allergy 1994;24:522–90.)

ing wheezing at age 10 years. Prognostic differences between different patterns of wheeze are therefore not clearly identifiable. As well, 50% of children with intercurrent symptoms (rather than with only viral-induced episodes) were wheeze free by 10 years of age. In another study, over 20% of nonatopic children were still wheezing at age 7 years.[11] It is probable, therefore, that there are at least three different populations of young children with wheeze, each with a different prognosis and, for the clinician, no clear-cut way to identify the category into which an individual child will fit (Level II).[15,16] Figure 5–1 illustrates the three proposed patterns of wheeze in childhood. The picture is further complicated by apparently continual switching which can occur between wheezing and not-wheezing sets in the population over periods of years.[17]

DIAGNOSIS BASED ON RISK FACTORS

Community studies of large cohorts of children extending over many years and in a variety of countries are required to clearly identify the relative risk of different factors in the development of asthma, as described in adults. Several studies are underway, and preliminary information is becoming available. It is clear that events occurring before birth are important. Genetic inheritance and familial factors have been linked to asthma development, and recent studies[18] have confirmed susceptibility genes on chromosomes 5q, 6p, 11p, 12q, 13q, and 14q and suggested other regions on 2q, 5p, 11p, 17p, 19p, and 21q. Parental tobacco smoking and maternal atopy are also important. Studies of infants in the first 3 months of life, using a squeeze technique to measure forced expiratory flow at functional residual capacity, have shown reduced airflow and bronchial hyper-responsiveness on histamine challenge in infants whose parents were smokers, atopic, or both.[19,20] Infants who wheeze with viral infections in the first 3 years of life have been shown to have abnormal lung function prior to the onset of wheezing (Level II).[13,19,21] This is thought to be related to the small caliber of the conducting airways, with resolution of wheezing episodes as lung growth continues. Follow-up studies to the age of 6 years have shown that this group of children continue to have abnormal lung function.[13]

In a community-based cohort of 826 children studied at 3 and 6 years of age (Level II),[13] over 50% of children had never wheezed, but about 20% had at least 1 episode of wheeze during the first year of life with no further episodes by age 6 years. Fifteen percent had no wheezing before 3 years of age but had developed wheezing by age 6 years, and about 13% had wheezing both before 3 years of age and at 6 years. Those who wheezed only in the first 3 years of life continued to have diminished lung function, had mothers who smoked but not mothers with asthma, and did not have elevated serum immunoglobulin E (IgE) at 9 months of age or atopy identified by allergen skin tests. Those who wheezed both before 3 years and at 6 years were significantly more likely to have mothers with asthma, increased serum IgE at 9 months and 6 years, normal lung function in the first year of life, and diminished lung function at 6 years. Those with persistent wheezing had the lowest levels of lung function. Sixty percent of infants with wheezing had stopped wheezing by age 6 years, but there was a significant risk of persistent wheezing at age 6 years in those with an increased serum IgE at 9 months of age but not at birth (as tested in cord blood). It is possible, therefore, that allergen exposure and sensitization may be an important risk factor in young children (Level II).

Respiratory viral infection is important in provoking episodes of wheeze, and infection with respiratory syncytial virus has been associated with persistent bronchial hyper-responsiveness in some children.[22] As well, rhinovirus infection has been associated with an eosinophilic inflammatory response in the airways of subjects with wheezing.[23–25] Whether this occurs in the majority of children who grow out of their wheezy illness is unknown. Atopy (positive skin tests to common environmental allergens) in children age 3 years and older is strongly associated with recurring wheezing,[26] as is total serum IgE,[27] and with more severe and persistent asthma (Level II).[17,28–30] In a large cohort of children aged 11 years who had been followed prospectively for wheezing illness, assessment of bronchial responsiveness to methacholine, peak-flow variability and atopy identified three groups.[31] Those with wheezing that occurred only in the first 3 years of life had no bronchial hyper-responsiveness or atopy; those with wheezing only in midchildhood had peak-flow variability but no response to methacholine and no atopy; whereas those who had persistent wheezing at any age had atopy, peak-flow variability, and methacholine hyper-responsiveness. Boys are at greater risk of recurring wheeze during childhood, and women are at greater risk than men in adulthood. In early adulthood, more men than women may move to a group with more severe symptoms,[32] but this is not predictable. Fourteen studies have been published from 1952 to 1997 describing the natural history of wheezing in childhood (summarized by Barbee and Murphy[33]). These include several large community cohorts followed up for up to 35 years. Overall, about 50% of adults who had wheezy illness in childhood no longer have symptoms, and about 40% have persisting wheeze in early middle age (Level II). Airway responsiveness in childhood tends to predict airway responsiveness in adulthood and is greater in those with persistent symptoms among whom it does not improve over time (Level II).

It is evident that from a diagnostic point of view there is no risk factor which, when identified in conjunction with wheezing in childhood, clearly indicates recurring and/or persistent wheezing symptoms (Level II). It is probably more helpful to consider factors that may operate over different time periods and to which individual children may be more or less susceptible. Silverman and Wilson[34] have illustrated this approach in Figure 5–2, pointing out that clinical phenotypes are not static so that, for example, transient viral-induced wheezing of early infancy can occur in those who later develop wheeze associated with atopy. At present, combinations of factors, such as a history of asthma in a first-degree relative together with atopy in the child who has recurring episodes of wheezy illness, may weigh more toward a decision to intervene with "preventive" asthma therapy and a more guarded prognosis than in a child with wheezy illness alone, but a definitive diagnosis of asthma on this basis remains elusive.

DIAGNOSIS BASED ON PATHOLOGY

There is little information linking pathologic changes in the airways of children to symptoms, nor has the underlying pathophysiology associated with different clinical patterns of wheezy illness been clearly identified. Studies using fiberoptic bronchoscopy and bronchoalveolar lavage[35,36] to assess the bronchial inflammatory response in atopic school-aged children (aged

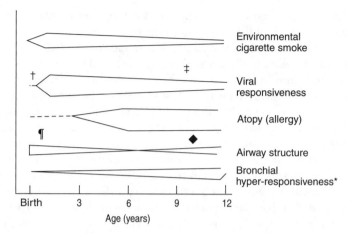

Figure 5–2 Risk factors for childhood wheeze and asthma and the ages at which they appear to operate:* = primary (hereditary) and secondary (to atopic inflammation); = viral wheeze related to suboptimal airway function; = viral exacerbations of atopic asthma; = fetal lung development; = remodeling consequent on chronic inflammation. (Reproduced with permission from Silverman M, Wilson N. Wheezing phenotypes in childhood. Thorax 1997;52:936-7.)

6 to 18 years) with mild recurring wheeze found similar percentages of lymphocytes in lavage fluid as in adults but with increased proportions of neutrophils and eosinophils. Basophils and mastocytes were present but not in sufficient numbers to quantify. Eosinophil cationic protein (ECP) and mast cell tryptase (MCT), markers of cell activation, were present, as in adults, and concentrations of MCT but not ECP were associated with bronchial responsiveness to methacholine. These findings are consistent with the pathologic changes described in the airways of adults with mild asthma (Level II). From a diagnostic point of view, bronchoalveolar lavage studies in children with asthma are limited by the ethical difficulty of using investigative procedures that involve some degree of discomfort and risk (Level III).

Bronchoalveolar lavage has also been performed in asthmatic children who were receiving general anesthetics for unrelated reasons.[37] Three groups of children, aged 1 to 15 years, were examined: 52 with atopic asthma (median age, 8 years); 23 with atopic disease but not asthma (median age, 8.3 years); and 20 with only viral-associated wheeze (median age, 3.1 years). The numbers of eosinophils and mast cells were significantly increased in the airways of those with atopic asthma but not in those of the other groups. This is consistent with a different mechanism of wheezy illness in nonatopic preschool children. The possibility of differentiating atopic wheezing (eosinophilic) from nonatopic wheezing (episodic viral associated) is complicated by the observation that viruses that commonly act as provocative agents for wheeze are associated with activation of bronchial epithelial cells, secretion of eosinophil attractant factors, and the development of eosinophilic inflammation.[23,24,38] Other evidence suggests that viral bronchiolitis provoking a primary episode of wheezing in previously healthy infants is associated with persistent blood eosinophilia, persistent activation of T helper lymphocytes, and a Th2 lymphocyte phenotypic response (atopic) in those who develop persistent wheezing.[39] Whether these children are genetically susceptible to this outcome and are inherently atopic is unknown, but the results are consistent with a similar group of infants who, after having bronchiolitis, had recurring wheeze and increased levels of ECP in their nasopharyngeal secretions, whereas those without recurring wheeze did not.[40] Respiratory viral infection may, however, provoke bronchial hyper-responsiveness and wheezing by stimulating release of interleukin-11 from epithelial cells,[41] which may explain, in part, episodic viral-induced wheezing in nonatopic infants without evidence of eosinophilic inflammation. As well, some infants with bronchiolitis may have pre-existing impairment of respiratory function and a propensity to lower respiratory symptoms.[19]

Recurring respiratory viral infection is therefore an important provocative factor for wheezing illness at all ages, but recurring wheezing thus caused may not be indicative of asthma especially in young children (Level II).

The use of serum ECP as a diagnostic marker of atopic asthma and as a measure of response to therapy has been proposed, especially in children in whom current symptoms are minimal or absent.[42–44] In a study of 24 children with symptomatic asthma, 10 with asymptomatic asthma, and 16 with allergic rhinitis alone, there was no difference in serum ECP levels between any of the groups, and most values were within the normal range (Level II).[45] Serum ECP correlated with blood eosinophil counts but not symptom score, forced expiratory volume in 1 second (FEV_1), forced expiratory flow at mid-expiration ($FEF_{25/75}$), or the provocative concentration of methacholine/histamine causing a 20% fall in FEV_1 (PC_{20}). Other tests for asthma based on pathogenetic mechanisms including sputum eosinophilia, quantification of blood eosinophils, and serum IgE have not been shown to be sufficiently sensitive or specific to be of practical value in diagnosing asthma in individual children.

Diagnosis Based on Symptoms

Asthma is primarily a clinical diagnosis based on recurring symptoms including cough, wheeze, and, often, shortness of breath. "Doctor-diagnosed" asthma, a commonly used term especially in epidemiologic studies, is based on responses of subjects to simple questions and is dependant on accurate recall by the patient. It is often associated with recurrent cough in the absence of wheeze and can be of little practical value (Level II). In the preschool population, the proportion of children with doctor-diagnosed asthma among those with current cough, and even more so among those with current wheeze, increases with age, suggesting that the diagnosis also depends on the duration of symptoms.[11]

Noises generated in the upper respiratory tract can be mistaken for wheezing, and it is often difficult to separate noise related to secretions from wheeze related to airway narrowing. There is often no clear demarcation from lower respiratory illness not considered asthma, or between mild asthma and normal respiratory function. Many children are treated for recurring chest infections or pneumonia before a diagnosis of asthma is made,[46] and a diagnosis of asthma increases the probability of the child receiving antiasthma therapy rather than antibiotics.[47]

In a survey of general practitioners in the United Kingdom and New Zealand,[48] the symptoms regarded as most important in diagnosing asthma in children less than 5 years of age were night cough and cough provoked by emotional upsets (UK physicians) and cough provoked by temperature change and recurrence of similar episodes (New Zealand physicians). New Zealand physicians were more likely to initiate treatment with anti-inflammatory therapy. In older children, the presence of cough alone has also been deemed sufficient to make a diagnosis of asthma,[49] and in adolescents, cough, rather than wheeze or shortness of breath, has been the symptom most associated with undiagnosed asthma based on concurrent evidence of airflow obstruction (FEV_1) or bronchial hyper-responsiveness (methacholine or exercise challenge, peak expiratory flow [PEF] variability).[50]

Other studies do not support the use of cough alone as a diagnostic feature of asthma in children; the significance of nocturnal cough is especially poorly understood (Level II). A community-based cohort of 100 young children with previously documented recurring wheeze was restudied[51] when the children reached school age to examine the relationship of nocturnal cough to current symptoms. Fifty-nine children were asymptomatic and 41 had current wheezing. Nocturnal coughing was more common, and episodes of coughing were more frequent among current wheezers (39% vs 19%). However, nocturnal cough was not associated with bronchial responsiveness, PEF variability, degree of morning dip in PEF, mean overnight arterial O_2 saturation, ventilatory function, maternal smoking, or treatment of asthma. Cough at night was associated with lower overnight air temperature, and there was poor agreement between recorded and reported night cough. In another community-based study,[52] the determinants of recurrent cough, defined as two or more episodes unrelated to upper respiratory infection in the previous year, was investigated in 987 children. Those with recurring cough but no wheeze (154) did not differ from those with neither cough nor wheeze (610) as regards serum IgE level, allergen skin-test response, FEV_1 (percentage of predicted value), and bronchial responsiveness to cold-air challenge. Those with recurring cough and wheezing (116), in contrast, had more respiratory illness, more atopy, more airflow obstruction, and more bronchial responsiveness to cold-air challenge. Coughing without wheeze was associated with parental smoking, whereas cough with wheeze was associated with male sex, maternal atopy, wheezing in infancy, and increased serum IgE, all markers of asthma. As well, cough occurring alone usually resolved by age 11 years, in contrast to cough with wheeze, all of which suggests that the pathogenesis of recurring cough in the absence of wheeze is different from asthma.

The relationship of cough, wheeze, and breathlessness, alone and in combination, has been assessed in the context of "doctor-diagnosed asthma."[53] Two cross-sectional community surveys of children aged 5 to 11 years were performed 2 years apart. The rate of participation was excellent; 92% of 2,035 subjects and 87% of 4,288, respectively (Level II). The proportion of children in the first and second surveys with no symptoms were 70% and 69.5%; with cough alone, 8.9% and 9.2%; and with cough, wheeze, and breathlessness, 8.3% and 7.3%, respectively. In contrast, "doctor-diagnosed asthma" increased from 17.4% in the first survey to 27.1% in the second. Cough alone was associated with the level of local air pollution, whereas the triad of symptoms was associated with atopy, family history of atopy, and prematurity. The diagnosis of asthma in those with cough alone increased from 1 in 8 to 1 in 4, suggesting that the increase in "doctor-diagnosed asthma" was due to diagnostic transfer. In a randomized placebo-controlled trial[54] of inhaled salbutamol and beclomethasone for recurrent cough in 43 school-aged children, neither drug had any effect on cough frequency or score, irrespective of the presence of bronchial hyper-responsiveness (Level II). Cough by itself, therefore, does not appear to be related to the risk factors associated with asthma in school-aged children.

Wheezing as a symptom is neither very sensitive nor specific for the diagnosis of asthma. It may be present in a variety of respiratory conditions (Table 5–1) and may be absent even when airway obstruction and inflammation are present. The results of a large prospective community survey[55] of children up to age 11 years found that, in subjects under 1 year of age, neither cough nor wheeze occurring only with colds increased the risk of subsequent asthma (Level II). From age 1 to 2 years, children who had wheezing with or without shortness of breath, with colds, but not cough alone, were more likely to be later diagnosed with asthma (odds ratio [OR] 2.1, $p < .05$). From age 3 to 4 years, the risk increased for wheeze with short-

Table 5–1 *Diagnoses to Be Considered for Wheezy Illness in Children*

Infancy	Childhood	Both
Tracheo-/bronchial malacia	Acquired tracheo-/bronchial stenosis	Lobar emphysema
Congenital tracheo-/bronchial stenosis	Tuberculosis	Bronchogenic cyst
Left ventricular failure	Granulomas	Vascular ring
Bronchiolitis	Vocal cord paralysis	Pulmonary abscess
Bronchopulmonary dysplasia	Acquired vocal cord dysfunction	Lymphadenopathy
Tracheal web		Mediastinal masses
Immune deficiency		Hemangiomas
Laryngeal papillomata		Cystic fibrosis
		Ciliary dyskinesia
		Tumors
		Aspiration

ness of breath (OR 7.2, $p < .0001$). Wheezing beginning at or persisting from 3 to 4 years of age is therefore clearly associated with future asthma (Level II). Wheezing recognized by parents may be a useful tool for monitoring established asthma in children and deciding on the need to increase drug therapy or seek urgent medical care.[56] This requires training in the detection of wheezing by listening over the chest and mouth, and must then be correlated with PEF and wheezing heard by physicians.

Children with asthma defined as "wheezing in the past year and airway hyper-responsiveness," which identifies school-aged children with more severe abnormalities compared to those with either feature alone, have been studied in parallel with children whose asthma was defined as "recent wheeze" and "doctor diagnosed" to determine the predictive value of each definition.[57] At the beginning and end of the 10-year study period, 407 children (aged 8 to 10 years at the start) were assessed for the presence of wheezing and other symptoms, medication use, bronchial responsiveness, and atopy. Classification was consistent for about 70% of all three groups over the 10-year period, with those who had "wheezing in the past year and airway hyper-responsiveness" having more severe illness and a poorer outcome (Level II).

DIAGNOSIS BY LABORATORY INVESTIGATION

A diagnosis of asthma is generally made in the context of recurring wheezy symptoms and evidence of reversible airway obstruction on evaluation of spirometry and/or bronchial hyper-responsiveness on exercise, histamine, methacholine, or eucapnic cold-air challenge in children old enough to perform these maneuvers. Bronchial hyper-responsiveness is not, in itself, diagnostic of asthma, as it can be present, if less severe, in other conditions such as cystic fibrosis and allergic rhinitis. The role of bronchial challenge with cold air or methacholine in predicting a future diagnosis of asthma with recurring episodes of wheeze is inconclusive (Level III). In one study, it has been evaluated in 281 children ages 5 to 9 years, followed up prospectively over a 6-year period.[58] Those free of wheeze at a given visit, but with evidence of bronchial hyper-responsiveness, were more likely to have developed wheezing by the next visit (OR 3.91, 95% confidence interval [CI] 1.21 to 12.66) after controlling for other risk factors. The occurrence of successive tests demonstrating airway hyper-responsiveness was independently associated with a higher probability of recurring episodes of wheezing. In a study[59] of the cumulative incidence of newly diagnosed asthma (recurrent wheezing) between 6 and 11 years of age, 360 children were tested for responsiveness to cold dry air at age 6 years. The cumulative incidence of asthma was 12%. After adjustment for confounding factors, only mild wheeze at age 6 years (OR 7.5, 95% CI 3.6 to 15.9, $p < .001$) and allergen skin-test positivity (OR 3.6, 95% CI 1.5 to 8.5, $p < .01$) were significant predictors of asthma; responsiveness to cold air was not. Thus, assessment of airway responsiveness may play a role in predicting the development and persistence of asthmatic symptoms, but this needs to be confirmed by other studies (Level II).

Some older children, and all children under the age of 6 years, have difficulty performing spirometric tests. Attempts have therefore been made to assess whether changes in breath sounds, recorded by tape from electronic auscultation over the trachea, can be used to detect significant changes in airflow. Wheeze, cough, increased respiratory rate, and prolonged expiration were found not to correlate with bronchial responsiveness to methacholine[60] or reduced peak expiratory flow in diagnosing or evaluating the severity of asthma.[61] Assessment of breath sounds in children who are unable to perform pulmonary function maneuvers is of no value in diagnosing asthma (Level II).

Serologic markers of asthma have also been assessed. Elevated serum IgE and the presence of allergen-specific skin tests for IgE antibody are risk factors for the development of asthma, as identified in large cohorts of children, but for individuals, the predictive value is less clear. As well, studies of IgG and IgG subclasses, secretory IgA, immune complex formation, eosinophil basic proteins, intercellular adhesion molecules, leukotrienes, and myeloperoxidase in serum, and of interleukins in bronchoalveolar lavage fluid and leukotrienes in urine have not, thus far, clearly differentiated wheezing phenotypes in young children (Level II).[62–64] In one study[65] of infants having a first episode of wheeze, those with a serum ECP level greater than 20 µg/L were more likely to have recurring episodes (three or more) over the next year than those who did not (OR 12.4, 95% CI 4.6 to 33.5), suggesting that it might be possible to identify a subgroup of infant wheezers who have persistent asthma later in childhood.

DIAGNOSIS BY RESPONSE TO DRUG THERAPY

School-aged children with recurring wheezing, in whom diagnoses other than asthma have been eliminated, are often given a trial of inhaled or oral corticosteroids, and, if they respond, are diagnosed with asthma. This approach remains controversial. In younger children, the role of a therapeutic trial of antiasthma drugs is even less clear, but the use of moderately high doses of inhaled corticosteroids (ICS) for a 6- to-8 week period has been recommended.[4,66] Is using a response to ICS as a diagnostic indicator of asthma appropriate? Several randomized controlled trials[67–71] of oral salbutamol and/or ICS therapy in infants from 2 months to 4 years of age show that these drugs can control recurring symptoms of wheeze related to viral infections and bronchiolitis (Level II). In three of the studies,[69–71] high doses of nebulized budesonide were used, and the infants were not selected as to risk factors; indeed, the presence of a family history of asthma or of personal atopy usually was not recorded. There was also selection of those with the most severe symptoms, who may not be representative of the general population of infant wheezers. In one study,[72] lower doses of budesonide and sodium cromoglycate were equally effective in reducing recurring episodes of wheeze and hospital admissions, compared to those in placebo group, but children in whom atopy was identified had significantly more wheezing episodes and admissions than those without. Other randomized controlled studies did not demonstrate beneficial effects in either infants[73,74] or school-aged children (Level II).[75]

Children with no genetic predisposition for asthma as expressed by absence of atopy, chronic airway inflammation, and bronchial hyper-responsiveness may respond to bronchodilator and inhaled corticosteroid therapy because of viral-induced changes in airway function, airway hyper-responsiveness unrelated to atopy, or other poorly understood anatomic and physiologic factors leading to airway obstruction.[76] Viral infection may also result in airway obstruction that persists for several weeks because of the small size of infants' airways, decreased mucociliary transport, ineffective clearing of secretions by coughing, and transient bronchial hyper-responsiveness. As well, a lack of response to therapy does not exclude a diagnosis of asthma in atopic infants with a family history of asthma, as airway obstruction may occur from excessive mucus, cellular debris, and mucosal edema caused by viral infection or other provoking factors; this is consistent with the concept of overlapping clinical patterns of wheezy illness during early childhood, as previously discussed (Level III). A diagnosis of asthma cannot therefore be made based solely on response to therapy.

SUMMARY

Recurring wheezy illness in children is clearly heterogeneous in origin, and the proportion who have asthma as defined by airway inflammation and heightened airway responsiveness[77] is unknown. The clinician should therefore be cautious about labeling wheezy illness in a child as asthma for therapeutic, social, psychological, and financial reasons, and, especially in younger children, the implied need for long-term antiasthma medications. The phenotypes of wheezy illness need to be more precisely defined to facilitate an understanding of pathogenesis, and the implementation of preventive and therapeutic strategies. When faced with a child who has recurring wheezy illness, other specific diagnoses should be ruled out by a careful clinical history, physical examination, and appropriate investigations (see Table 5–1). The great majority of children with wheeze will remain uncategorized, and a diagnosis of asthma will be considered. Several possible ways of defining asthma have been suggested.[2] These include severity of symptoms; number of attacks; wheeze persisting to, or occurring for the first time at, a particular age; wheeze with atopy; and wheeze with bronchial hyper-responsiveness. All have important limitations, as previously discussed, and none are well founded scientifically.

The most practical approach is to consider recurring wheezing in the context of provoking factors (exercise, allergens, viral infections, respiratory irritants), persistent and prolonged wheezing after viral infection, evidence of asthma in first-degree relatives, and atopy in the child. In the atopic school-aged child with wheezing and evidence of reversible airway obstruction on spirometry or peak-flow measurements, the diagnosis is reasonably defined and treatment can be commenced. For others, a trial of antiasthma therapy (inhaled corticosteroid) is the best approach in all except those with the mildest symptoms and no evidence of airway obstruction. In the preschool child, only those with moderate or severe wheezing should receive a trial of drug therapy.[78] Children at all ages should be carefully monitored for beneficial and adverse effects of therapy, with linear growth measured and plotted on a growth chart. If therapy using adequate drug doses delivered efficiently to the airway is not effective within 2 to 3 months, it should be withdrawn and the diagnosis reconsidered. Those who respond should continue to be monitored and have therapy adjusted according to published guidelines.

REFERENCES

1. The Concise Oxford Dictionary. 6th ed. Oxford: Oxford University Press; 1976. p. 57.
2. Silverman M, Wilson N. Asthma—time for a change in name? Arch Dis Child 1997;77:62–5.
3. Woolcock AJ. Treatment of asthma. In: Busse WW, Holgate ST, editors. Asthma and rhinitis. Boston: Blackwell Scientific Publications; 1995. p. 1364.
4. The British guidelines on asthma management: 1995 review and position statement. Thorax 1997;52 Suppl 1:S1–21.
5. Pedersen S. Early use of inhaled corticosteroids in children with asthma. Clin Exp Allergy 1997;27:995–1006.
6. Hogg C, Bush A. Childhood asthma—all that wheezes is not inflammation. Clin Exp Allergy 1997;27:991–4.
7. Warner JO. The down-side of early intervention with inhaled corticosteroids. Clin Exp Allergy 1997;27:999–1001.
8. Strachan DP. The prevalence and natural history of wheezing in early childhood. J R Coll Gen Pract 1985;35:182–4.
9. Ogston SA, Florey CD, Walker CH. The Tayside infant morbidity and mortality study: effect on health of using gas for cooking. Br Med J 1985;290:957–60.
10. Park ES, Golding J, Carswell F, Stewart-Brown S. Pre-school wheezing and prognosis at 10. Arch Dis Child 1986;61:642–6.
11. Luyt DK, Burton PR, Simpson H. Epidemiological study of wheeze, doctor diagnosed asthma and cough in preschool children in Leicester. Br Med J 1993;306:1386–90.
12. Martinez FD, Wright AL, Taussig LM, et al. Asthma and wheezing in the first six months of life. The Group Health Medical Associates. N Engl J Med 1995;332:133–8.
13. Martinez FD, Morgan WJ, Wright AL, et al. Diminished lung function as a predisposing factor for wheezing respiratory illness in infants. N Engl J Med 1988;319:1112–7.
14. Johnston SL, Pattemore PK, Sanderson G, et al. Community study of the role of viral infections in exacerbations of asthma in 9–11 year old children. Br Med J 1995;310:1225–9.
15. Wilson NM. The significance of early wheezing. Clin Exp Allergy 1994;24:522–9.
16. Burr ML, Limb ES, Maguire MJ, et al. Infant feeding, wheezing and allergy: a prospective study. Arch Dis Child 1993;68:724–8.
17. Strachan DP, Butland BK, Anderson RH. Incidence and prognosis of asthma and wheezing illness from early childhood to age 33 in a national British cohort. Br Med J 1996;312:1606–7.
18. The Collaborative Study on the Genetics of Asthma (CSGA). A genome wide search for asthma susceptibility loci in ethnically diverse populations. Nat Genet 1997;15:389–92.

19. Young S, O'Keeffe PT, Arnott J, Landau LI. Lung function, airway responsiveness, and respiratory symptoms before and after bronchiolitis. Arch Dis Child 1995;2:16–24.

20. Stick SM, Burton PR, Gurrin L, et al. Effects of maternal smoking during pregnancy and a family history of asthma on respiratory function of newborn infants. Lancet 1996;348:1060–4.

21. Tager IB, Hanrahan JP, Tosteson TD, et al. Lung function: pre- and post-natal smoke exposure and wheezing in the first year of life. Am Rev Respir Dis 1993;147:811–7.

22. Weiss ST, Tager IB, Munoz A, Speizer FE. The relationship of respiratory infections in early childhood to the occurrence of increased levels of bronchial responsiveness and atopy. Am Rev Respir Dis 1985;131:573–8.

23. Grunberg K, Smits HH, Timmeo MC, et al. Experimental rhinovirus 16 infection. Effects on cell differentials and soluble markers in sputum in asthmatic subjects. Am J Respir Crit Care Med 1997;156:609–16.

24. Geru JE, Calhoun W, Swenson C, et al. Rhinovirus infection preferentially increases lower airway responsiveness in allergic subjects. Am J Respir Crit Care Med 1997;155:1872–6.

25. Terajima MN, Yamaya M, Sekizawa K, et al. Rhinovirus injection of primary cultures of human tracheal epithelium: role of ICAM-1 and IL-beta. Am J Physiol 1997;273:749–59.

26. Burrows B, Halonen M, Lebowitz MD, et al. The relationship of serum immunoglobulin E, allergy skin tests, and smoking to respiratory disorders. J Allergy Clin Immunol 1982;70:199–204.

27. Burrows B, Martinez FD, Halonen M, et al. Association of asthma with serum IgE levels and skin-test reactivity to allergens. N Engl J Med 1989;320:271–7.

28. Buffum WP, Settipane GA. Prognosis of asthma in childhood. Am J Dis Child 1996;112:214–7.

29. Blair H. Natural history of childhood asthma. Arch Dis Child 1997;52:613–9.

30. Sporik R, Holgate ST, Platts-Mills TAE, Cogswell JJ. Exposure to house-dust mite allergen (der P1) and the development of asthma in childhood. N Engl J Med 1990;323:502–7.

31. Stein RT, Holberg CJ, Morgan WJ, et al. Peak flow variability, methacholine responsiveness and atopy as markers for detecting different wheezing phenotypes in childhood. Thorax 1997;52:946–52.

32. McNicol KN, Williams HB. Spectrum of asthma in children—1, clinical and physiological components. Br Med J 1973;4:7–11.

33. Barbee RA, Murphy S. The natural history of asthma. J Allergy Clin Immunol 1998;102:S65–72.

34. Silverman M, Wilson N. Wheezing phenotypes in childhood. Thorax 1997;52:936–7.

35. Ferguson AC, Wong FWM. Bronchial hyper-responsiveness in asthmatic children: correlation with macrophages and eosinophils in broncholavage fluid. Chest 1989;96:988–91.

36. Ferguson AC, Whitelaw M, Brown H. Correlation of bronchial eosinophil and mast cell activation with bronchial hyper-responsiveness in children with asthma. J Allergy Clin Immunol 1992;90:609–13.

37. Stevenson EC, Turner G, Heaney LG, et al. Bronchoalveolar lavage findings suggest two different forms of childhood asthma. Clin Exp Allergy 1997;27:1027–35.

38. Ragar KJ, Langland JO, Jacobi BL, et al. Activation of antiviral protein kinase leads to immunoglobulin E class switching in human B cells. J Viral 1998;72:1171–6.

39. Renzi PM, Turgeon JP, Yang JP, et al. Cellular immunity is activated and a TH-2 response is associated with early wheezing in infants after bronchiolitis. J Pediatr 1997;130:584–93.

40. Reijonen RM, Korppi M, Kleemola M, et al. Nasopharyngeal eosinophil cationic protein in bronchiolitis: relation to viral findings and subsequent wheezing. Pediatr Pulmonol 1997;24:35–41.

41. Einarrson O, Geba GP, Zhu Z, et al. Interleukin-11: stimulation in vivo and in vitro by respiratory viruses and induction of airways hyper-responsiveness. J Clin Invest 1996;97:915–24.

42. Bisgaard H, Gronborg H, Mygind N, et al. Allergen induced increase of eosinophil cationic protein in nasal lavage fluid: effect of the glucocorticoid budesonide. J Allergy Clin Immunol 1990;85:891–5.

43. Venge P, Henriksen J, Dahl R. Eosinophils in exercise induced-asthma. J Allergy Clin Immunol 1991;88:699–704.

44. Hedlin G, Ahlstedt S, Hakansson L, Venge P. Levels in serum of eosinophilic cationic protein (ECP), eosinophil chemotactic activity (ECA) and tryptase before and during bronchial challenge in cat allergic children with asthma. Pediatr Allergy Immunol 1992;3:144–9.

45. Ferguson AC, Vaughan R, Brown H, Curtis C. Evaluation of serum eosinophilic cationic protein as a marker of disease activity in chronic asthma. J Allergy Clin Immunol 1995;95:23–8.

46. Levy M, Bell L. General practice audit of asthma in childhood. Br Med J 1984;289:1115–6.

47. Anderson HR, Cooper JS, Bailey PA, Palmer JC. Influence of morbidity, illness label and social family and health service factors on drug treatment of childhood asthma. Lancet 1981;2:1030–2.

48. Reid J, Walker S, Penrose A, Charlton R. The diagnosis and initial treatment of asthma in young children in New Zealand and the United Kingdom. N Z Med J 1998;111:248–51.

49. Canadian Asthma Consensus Group. Summary of recommendations from the Canadian asthma consensus report, 1999. Can Med Assoc J 1999;161 Suppl 11:S6–7.

50. Siersted HC, Boldsen J, Hansen HS, et al. Population based study of risk factors for underdiagnosis of asthma in adolescence: Odense schoolchild study. Br Med J 1998;316:651–5.

51. Brooke AM, Lambert PC, Burton PR, et al. Night cough in a population-based sample of children: characteristics, relation to symptoms and associations with measures of asthma severity. Eur Respir J 1996;9:65–71.

52. Wright AL, Holberg CJ, Morgan WJ, et al. Recurrent cough in childhood and its relation to asthma. Am J Respir Crit Care Med 1996;153:1259-65.

53. Kelly YJ, Brabin BJ, Milligan PJ, et al. Clinical significance of cough and wheeze in the diagnosis of asthma. Arch Dis Child 1996;75:489–93.

54. Chang AB, Phelan PD, Carlin JB, et al. A randomized placebo controlled trial of inhaled salbutamol and beclomethasone for recurrent cough. Arch Dis Child 1998;79:6–11.

55. Dodge R, Martinez FD, Cline MG, et al. Early childhood respiratory symptoms and the subsequent diagnosis of asthma. J Allergy Clin Immunol 1996;98:48–54.

56. Lee H, Arroyo A, Rosenfield W. Parents' evaluations of wheezing in their children with asthma. Chest 1996;109:91–3.

57. Toelle BG, Peat JK, Vanden Berg RH, et al. Comparison of three definitions of asthma: a longitudinal perspective. J Asthma 1997;34:161–7.

58. Carey VJ, Weiss ST, Tager IB, et al. Airways responsiveness, wheeze onset, and recurrent asthma episodes in young adolescents. The East Boston Childhood Respiratory Disease Cohort. Am J Respir Crit Care Med 1996;153:356–61.

59. Lombardi E, Morgan WJ, Wright AL, et al. Cold air challenge at age 6 and subsequent incidence of asthma. A longitudinal study. Am J Respir Crit Care Med 1997;156:1863–9.

60. Sprikkelman AB, Grol MH, Lourens MS, et al. Use of tracheal auscultation for the assessment of bronchial responsiveness in asthmatic children. Thorax 1996;51:317–9.

61. Rietveld S, Rijssenbeek-Nouvens LH. Diagnosis of spontaneous cough in childhood asthma: results of continuous tracheal sound recording in the homes of children. Chest 1998;113:50–4.

62. Bjorksten B. Immunological outcome measures. Eur Respir J Suppl 1996;21:22–7S.

63. Grigg J, Venge P. Inflammatory markers of outcome. Eur Respir J Suppl 1996;21:16–21S.

64. Carlsen KH. Markers of airway inflammation in preschool wheezers. Monaldi Arch Chest Dis 1997;52:455–60.

65. Koller DY, Wojnerowski C, Herkner KR, et al. High levels of eosinophil cationic protein in wheezing infants predict the development of asthma. J Allergy Clin Immunol 1997;99:752–6.

66. Cochran D. Diagnosing and treating chesty infants. BMJ 1998;316:1546–7.

67. Fox GF, March MJ, Milner AD. Treatment of recurrent acute wheezing episodes in infancy with oral salbutamol and prednisolone. Eur J Pediatr 1996;155:512–6.

68. Kraemer R, Graf Bigler U, Casaulta Aebischer C, et al. Clinical and physiological improvement after inhalation of low-dose beclomethasone diprprionate and salbutamol in wheezy infants. Respiration 1997;64:342–9.

69. Wennergren G, Nordvall SL, Hedlin G, et al. Nebulized budesonide for the treatment of moderate to severe asthma in infants and toddlers. Acta Paediatr 1996;85:183–9.

70. de Blic J, Delacourt C, Le Bourgeois M, et al. Efficacy of nebulized budesonide in treatment of severe infantile asthma: a double blind study. J Allergy Clin Immunol 1996;98:14–20.

71. Volvovitz B, Soferman R, Blau H, et al. Rapid induction of clinical response with a short-term high-dose starting schedule of budesonide nebulizing suspension in young children with recurring wheezing episodes. J Allergy Clin Immunol 1998;101:464–9.

72. Reijonen T, Korppi M, Kuikka L, Remes K. Anti-inflammatory therapy reduces wheezing after bronchiolitis. Arch Pediatr Adolesc Med 1996;150:512–7.

73. Stick SM, Burton PR, Clough JB, et al. The effects of inhaled beclomethasone dipropionate on lung function and histamine responsiveness in recurrently wheezy infants. Arch Dis Child 1995;73:327–32.

74. Richter H, Seddon P. Early nebulized budesonide in the treatment of bronchiolitis and the prevention of post bronchiolitic wheezing. J Pediatr 1998;132:849–53.

75. Doull IJ, Lampe FC, Smith S, et al. Effect of inhaled corticostereoids on episodes of wheezing associated with viral infection in school age children: randomized double blind placebo controlled trial. BMJ 1997;315:858–62.

76. Taussig LM. Wheezing in infancy: when is it asthma? Pediatr Pulmonol Suppl 1997;16:90–1.

77. National Institutes of Health, Lung and Blood Institute. Global strategy for asthma management and prevention. NHLBI/WHO workshop report, March 1993. Bethesda (MD): National Institutes of Health: 1995 Publication No.: 95-3659.

78. Price JF. The early use of inhaled corticosteroids: concluding comments. Clin Exp Allergy 1997;27;10104–6.

CHAPTER 6

Role of the Outdoor Environment

Sverre Vedal, MD, MSc

It seems a reasonable notion that contaminants or allergens in the outdoor air that we breathe can aggravate asthma in those who already have it, and possibly cause new cases of asthma. As asthma is one airways disease that is likely determined by an interplay of environmental exposures and inherent susceptibility factors, it should be affected by contaminants or allergens in the outdoor air that come into contact with airways. The purpose of this chapter is to review and evaluate the evidence that addresses whether this hypothesis is valid.

Because evidence-based approaches generally have been applied in clinical settings, a formal evidence-based approach has not been used to assess the effects of the ambient environment on asthma. Relevant evidence comes largely from only two general types of studies: (1) experimental exposure chamber studies using subjects with asthma and (2) observational (nonexperimental) epidemiologic studies involving asthmatic patients. By definition, the observational studies can provide no better than Level II evidence. Although there exists a considerable body of work on the effects of both air pollution and allergens using animal models of asthma, since the value of such work to asthma in humans from the perspective of "levels of evidence" is low, findings based on animal models will not be discussed here.

Two general questions will be addressed: (1) Do exposures to the ambient environment cause asthma? and (2) Do exposures to the ambient environment aggravate asthma? The ambient environment will be taken to include outdoor air pollution and allergens, and meteorology.

Do Exposures to the Ambient Environment Cause Asthma?

A number of study designs could be used to address the question of whether exposure to ambient air pollution or allergens causes asthma. It is not readily apparent how experimental studies or clinical trials involving humans could realistically address this question. However, observational studies could address it. For example, cohort studies, in which population samples with different ambient air pollution or allergen exposures are followed over time to assess the development of asthma could be relevant. One obvious difficulty with this cohort design is the assignment of the diagnosis "asthma" to individuals at some point in time. A related problem is that an exposure might bring a subject with "subclinical" asthma to clinical attention and therefore make it appear that the exposure was causally related to asthma, when, in this instance, one could argue that the role of the exposure was to aggravate pre-existing asthma. Another type of longitudinal design that might be useful is one in which long-term temporal changes in asthma prevalence in a region are correlated with temporal changes in air pollution concentrations. Alternatively, asthma prevalence could be compared in population samples with different exposures. These studies could range from typical cross-sectional studies, in which the investigator has data on each subject in the study, to so-called ecologic cross-sectional studies, in which data on asthma prevalence and estimated exposure are only available at the population level.

In all of these observational studies, the investigator has no role in "assigning" the exposure. Great care must therefore be taken in interpreting the findings to avoid inferring an observed association as causal, when in fact it might be a spurious association due to other causal factors related to exposure. For example, factors associated with low socioeconomic status, other than air pollution, could be causally associated with asthma and associated with high air pollution exposure. In such a situation, an investigator would find an association between air pollution and asthma that would be a spurious association due to these other factors linked with low socioeconomic status. This is an example of bias due to confounding. It can also be difficult, if not impossible, in such studies to disentangle the effects of air pollution, allergens, and meteorology.

Level I Evidence

There are no human experimental data available that directly address the question of whether ambient exposures cause asthma.

Level II Evidence

The best evidence to date that air pollution exposure causes asthma is provided by a cohort study of Seventh Day Adventists in California.[1] In this study of over 3,000 nonsmoking adults followed up over a 15-year period, the risk of men developing doctor-diagnosed asthma was associated with average ambient ozone concentration. Because data were available on individuals, it was possible to attempt to control for other potential risk factors for the development of asthma. Interestingly, no such association with air pollution was observed in women.

Whereas there are prospective data linking infant exposure to indoor allergens and subsequent asthma,[2] there are no good observational studies that directly support a causal role for exposure to ambient outdoor allergens in asthma. In fact, evidence to the contrary is provided by a birth cohort study from New Zealand in which skin-test sensitivity to indoor allergens was associated with development of asthma but grass sensitivity was not.[3]

Level III Evidence

There is marked geographic heterogeneity in estimates of asthma prevalence.[4] At issue here is whether any of this heterogeneity is due to differences in population exposures to the outdoor environment. A large number of cross-sectional studies relating asthma prevalence to some average measures of the outdoor environment have been reported. Because of the significant potential for uncontrolled confounding in these studies, the level of evidence that they provide is generally low. Apart from the few studies reviewed below, these studies will not be reviewed here.

Studies comparing respiratory symptoms, illness prevalence, and atopic status in children in the former East and West Germany are intriguing in that they demonstrate a higher prevalence of atopic disease in West Germany but more cough and sputum production in East Germany.[5] It was speculated that allergy was related to modern "Western" environments where indoor allergen exposures were higher due to more tightly sealed homes, and where ambient pollution was largely created by automobile combustion and resultant oxidant pollution."Bronchitic" symptoms were related to an "old-style" type of air pollution due, for example, to coal burning with resultant high ambient concentrations of sulfur dioxide and particles. On the basis of these studies, it is unlikely that combustion-related pollution of the type that contains a mix of sulfur dioxide and particulate matter causes asthma (Level IIID).

Given estimates of recently increased asthma prevalence and morbidity (see Chapter 1), it is reasonable to postulate that exposure to oxidant-type air pollution (nitrogen dioxide and ozone) generated largely from automobile combustion might be one factor contributing to this increase in prevalence of asthma. Evidence that this is not the case is provided by the observation that these increases in asthma have occurred in settings where there have been no concurrent increases in oxidant pollution concentrations.[6] One component of the air pollution mix whose concentrations are apparently increasing is the ultrafine fraction (particles < 0.1 μm) of inhalable particles. Newer (and cleaner) diesel engines paradoxically emit many times more ultrafine particles than older engines.[7] There are no data that directly address the role of ultrafine particles in asthma causation. However, several studies have observed increases in asthma prevalence in people residing near major roadways.

Evidence for a causal role for outdoor allergens or meteorology in asthma is weak. The interesting observations on increased birch sensitization in infants born shortly before the birch pollen season suggests that exposure to outdoor pollen at a critical period of life is important in producing related allergy and possibly asthma.[8] An intriguing, but speculative, hypothesis that spans the distinction between airborne particle pollution and aeroallergens is that latex antigens on inhalable ambient particles might contribute to the increase in asthma prevalence.[9]

DO EXPOSURES TO THE AMBIENT ENVIRONMENT AGGRAVATE ASTHMA?

In general, the evidence supporting a role for the ambient environment in aggravating asthma is far stronger than that supporting its role in causing asthma. The number of study designs that can be used to address the question of asthma aggravation is potentially greater than that addressing the question of a causal relationship. In this setting, experimental designs can be used effectively and are the only source of Level I evidence. While the findings from these experimental studies should generally be considered more valid than findings from observational studies, as discussed above, they are often plagued by concerns as to their relevance or generalizability. For example, whereas it is true that the ability to define and control the exposure of subjects in experimental studies is an advantage, exposures in the "real world" are complex and typically include mixtures of pollutants from several sources. Furthermore, it is generally only possible to recruit asthmatic patients with relatively mild asthma for these experimental studies. It may be difficult to extrapolate the findings of such studies to asthmatic patients with more severe disease.

Typically, observational study designs used to address whether outdoor environmental factors can aggravate asthma are those in which short-term changes in these factors are correlated with changes in an asthma outcome measure, such as hospitalizations, medication use, symptom reporting, and level of lung function. Studies using short-term (usually daily) counts of events such as hospitalizations or emergency department visits are referred to as time-series studies. In these studies, the investigator must attempt to ensure that the short-term temporal association that might be observed in such a study is not confounded by factors that change over time in concert with air pollution concentrations and that also affect asthma. For example, meteorologic factors would be prime examples of factors potentially confounding the air pollution associations in such time-series studies. Panel studies refer to studies in which a group of subjects (eg, asthmatic patients) provides individual-level outcome data (eg, reports of symptoms or level of lung function) repeatedly over the study period.

Asthma "epidemics," in which relatively dramatic increases in adverse asthma events are observed, such as dramatically increased hospitalization rates, can also provide insight into outdoor environmental factors that adversely affect asthma. Identification of soybean unloading in Barcelona harbor as the critical factor in the repeated epidemics in Barcelona is perhaps the best example of the use of such data.[10] Interpretation of epidemic data can be complicated by the same difficulties, such as confounding, that plague the other types of observational data on asthma.

It is well appreciated that air pollution is composed of many individual pollutants whose contributions to the air pollution mix can vary markedly across geographic regions. One approach to countering this complexity is to restrict the study as much as possible to single components of this mix, such as in experimental exposure studies, at the expense of being able to investigate effects of any real-world air pollution atmosphere. Another approach is to study effects of individual sources, as exemplified by studies relating effects of a single source's emissions on asthma, or those relating effects of proximity to a source (eg, a major roadway) on asthma. We may not learn much about the specific components responsible for any observed effects from such studies, but they are potentially of great public health significance. Finally, one can study real-world pollution settings and attempt to identify the component or components of the mix, when these individual components are measured, that might be responsible for any observed effects. Because the individual components of the pollutant mix are often highly correlated, it may not be possible in these studies to confidently identify which pollutant is having an effect. The individual pollutants that have most commonly been investigated in studies on asthma include tropospheric ozone, particles and the acidic component of particles (acid aerosol), sulfur dioxide, and nitrogen dioxide.

Level I Evidence

A large body of experimental data derived from exposure chamber studies has addressed the role of air pollution in aggravating asthma. Exposure to ozone causes respiratory symptoms, reduction in level of lung function, increased bronchial responsiveness, and airways inflammation in subjects with asthma (Level IA)[11,12] as well as in those without asthma. The effect on lung function is not affected by treatment with β-agonists. Interestingly, in those with exercise-induced bronchospasm, ozone does not worsen the degree of airflow obstruction after exercise (Level IA).[13] The effects on lung function and bronchial responsiveness may not differ in subjects with asthma and those without asthma,[14] although this observation is controversial.[15] However, the inflammatory effects of ozone exposure in the lung, in particular, the neutrophilic inflammatory component, seem to be more pronounced in asthmatic subjects (Level IB).[16,17] Whether ozone produces an increased eosinophilic inflammatory component in asthmatic patients is controversial, with some studies showing no increased eosinophils in bronchoalveolar lavage[16] and others showing increased eosinophils.[11]

It is not known whether treatment with anti-inflammatory agents can prevent these experimental effects of ozone in asthma. In a recent randomized, crossover study reported only in preliminary form, 1 month of inhaled budesonide decreased baseline percentage of induced sputum neutrophils. In addition, the increase in sputum neutrophils following ozone exposure was not statistically significant on budesonide, but it did significantly increase off budesonide.[18] The mean increase in percent neutrophils following ozone nevertheless appeared similar with and without budesonide, suggesting that the inhaled steroid had little effect.

The adverse effects of ozone in asthma need not necessarily be direct effects. Experimental studies have documented enhanced lung function responses to allergen exposure following exposure to relatively low concentrations of ozone,[19-21] although this is not a universal finding (Level IB).[22]

For nitrogen dioxide, the experimental studies have been remarkably inconsistent in demonstrating effects on lung function and bronchial responsiveness in asthmatic patients (Level IC).[23,24] However, allergen responsiveness to ozone also seems to increase following exposure to nitrogen dioxide (Level IB),[25,26] although in one study, effects of nitrogen dioxide on allergen responsiveness required the presence of sulfur dioxide.[27]

Exposure to sulfur dioxide can produce bronchoconstriction and respiratory symptoms in asthmatic patients at much lower concentrations than in those without asthma.[28] Many pharmacologic agents, especially β-agonists, abolish or attenuate the adverse effects of sulfur dioxide in asthmatic patients. Inhaled corticosteroids do not influence the effects of sulfur dioxide.

Most experimental studies of particle exposure in asthmatic patients have been carried out only with specific components of the ambient particle mix, with most having assessed only the effect of acid aerosol exposure in asthma. As for nitrogen dioxide, the results across studies have been inconsistent.[29,30] Recently, preliminary data using concentrated ambient particles in exposure chamber studies of mild asthmatic patients have been reported.[31] No adverse effects on symptoms, level of lung function, or markers of nasal or airway inflammation were observed. Recent in vivo studies using diesel exhaust particles have demonstrated that diesel particles can enhance immunoglobulin E (IgE) responses in the nose following pollen exposure in pollen-sensitive subjects.[32] The relevance of this finding to the clinical or population setting is not known.

In summary, the strongest experimental support for adverse effects due to air pollution exposure in asthmatic patients is for sulfur dioxide and ozone directly, and for ozone and nitrogen dioxide in enhancing lung function responses to inhaled allergen.

The role of allergen in aggravating asthma also has been investigated experimentally. Exposure to aeroallergen in the laboratory[33] and in a natural setting[34] reduces levels of lung function and increases bronchial responsiveness (Level IA).

Exercise-induced bronchospasm in asthmatic patients is aggravated by inhalation of dry, cold air and ameliorated by inhalation of humidified, warm air (Level IA).[35]

Level II Evidence

Air Pollution

A very large and rapidly expanding body of observational work addresses the role of ambient air pollution in aggravating asthma. The grade of evidence from these types of studies can, by definition, be no greater than Level II, although rarely one might argue that a "natural experiment" could occur in an observational setting that might be considered Level I evidence. Most of the relevant observational studies are time-series studies, although panel studies of groups of subjects with asthma are also common. Asthma outcomes investigated have included hospitalizations, emergency department visits, asthma-medication use, reported respiratory symptoms, and level of lung function. Summary of findings from observational studies will be organized by type of study and by outcome. Although observed effects (or absence of effects) will be summarized for specific pollutants, it should be emphasized that it is often difficult or impossible in these studies to disentangle the effects of one pollutant from another.

Time-series studies assessing the association between short-term variation in air pollution concentrations and daily asthma hospitalizations and emergency department visits have been performed in many settings with various air pollutant mixtures. In many, but by no means all, of the published time-series studies, associations between short-term changes in ambient ozone concentrations and adverse asthma outcomes were observed. Therefore, although the weight of evidence would support the presence of an association, the studies are not consistent in this regard. For example, whereas associations between short-term increases in ozone concentrations and asthma hospitalizations were reported in studies from New York City,[36] Buffalo,[36] Toronto,[37] Seattle,[38] and Helsinki,[39] no associations were observed in studies from Paris,[40] Amsterdam,[41] London,[42] or Sydney.[43] Effects of ozone on emergency department visits due to asthma were observed in New Jersey,[44] New Brunswick,[45] and Mexico City,[46] but not in Seattle,[47] Santa Clara County, California,[48] Israel,[49] or Vancouver, Canada.[50] Ozone was not associated with increased asthma visits to primary care physicians in London.[51]

For effects of nitrogen dioxide, the evidence is also inconsistent. No significant associations between short-term changes in ambient nitrogen dioxide concentrations and hospitalizations for asthma were observed in Toronto,[37] Helsinki,[39] or Amsterdam,[41] but significant associations were observed in Paris[40] and Sydney.[43] For emergency department visits, an association was seen in California,[48] Barcelona,[52] Finland,[53] and Israel[49] but not in Vancouver.[50] No association with nitrogen dioxide was observed for adult visits to primary care physicians in London, but a strong association was present for child visits.[51]

The evidence is also inconsistent for sulfur dioxide. No significant associations between short-term changes in ambient sulfur dioxide concentrations and hospitalizations for asthma were observed in Toronto,[37] Seattle,[38] or Amsterdam,[41] but they were seen in Paris[40] and Helsinki.[39] For emergency department visits, an association was seen in Vancouver,[50] Mexico City,[46] and Israel[49] but not in Seattle[47] or Valencia.[54]

For particulate matter (PM), the most studied of these pollutants, associations between short-term changes in ambient PM concentrations and adverse asthma outcomes were observed in many, but by no means all, of the published studies. Therefore, although the weight of evidence might support the presence of an association, the studies are not entirely consistent in this regard. For example, whereas associations between short-term increases in PM concentrations and asthma hospitalizations were reported in studies from New York City,[36] Buffalo,[36] Toronto,[37] and Birmingham, United Kingdom,[55] no associations were observed in studies from Paris,[40] Helsinki,[39] Amsterdam,[41] or Sydney.[43] Effects of PM on asthma emergency department visits were observed in Seattle,[47,56] Santa Clara County,[48] and Valencia, Spain,[54] but not in Mexico City.[46,57] Increased asthma visits to primary care physicians in London were associated with PM in adults but not in children.[51] For the acid aerosol component of PM, associations were observed with hospital visits in Toronto.[37]

Interestingly, increases in carbon monoxide have also been associated with asthma hospitalizations for adults[38] and emergency department visits for children[56] in Seattle, and for visits to primary care physicians in London.[51] Interpretation of these observed effects for carbon monoxide is problematic given our understanding of carbon monoxide toxicity, although viewing carbon monoxide as a marker for automobile exhaust has some appeal.

Panel studies of asthmatic patients have been relatively consistent in observing adverse effects of short-term changes in air pollution concentrations on symptom reporting, level of lung function, and medication use. Increased symptom reporting was seen in association with short-term increases in PM (British Columbia,[58] Denver,[59] southern California,[60] the Netherlands,[61,62] and three cities in Eastern Europe[63]), in ozone,[60] in sulfur dioxide (the Netherlands,[62] three cities in Eastern Europe[63]), and in nitrogen dioxide (the Netherlands,[62] Sweden[64]). However, no effect on symptom reporting also has been reported for PM[60,65] and sulfur dioxide.[64]

Effects on reducing level of lung function were seen for PM (British Columbia,[58] the Netherlands,[62] three cities in Eastern Europe[63]), for sulfur dioxide (three cities in Eastern Europe,[63] Denmark[66]), and for nitrogen dioxide (Denmark[66]). No effect on lung function also has been observed for PM,[61] sulfur dioxide,[61,64] and nitrogen dioxide.[61,64] Association between reported increased asthma-medication use and increased particle sulfate concentrations in Czechoslovakia,[67] and increased ozone and PM concentrations in the Netherlands[61] also have been reported.

In the time-series and panel studies, an effect of at least one component of the air pollution mix is almost invariably observed. As seen, however, there is no impressive consistency with respect to any single pollutant. The findings for carbon monoxide suggest that the findings for any of the air pollutants in these longitudinal observational studies may not, in fact, increase our understanding of the effects of each specific pollutant on asthma. Any of the pollutants may well be reflections of the sources of various pollutant mixtures in a given setting, in which case, better understanding of health effects may be gained by taking a source-based approach to exposure rather than the traditional air concentration approach.

Allergens

There seems little doubt that exposure to outdoor allergens can cause exacerbations of asthma, sometimes dramatically, as demonstrated by the strong association between soybean unloading in the Barcelona harbor and "epidemic" days of asthma (Level IIA).[10] There is also suggestive evidence that exposure to outdoor mold spores, at least in the case of Alternaria, can cause severe asthma exacerbations[68] and that outdoor molds may be associated with asthma deaths.[69] In an older study, asthmatic students at the University of Minnesota experienced more symptoms during periods of high ambient dust, especially when the wind direction was favorable with respect to the grain mills.[70] The association was only present in the students with grain dust skin sensitivity. Based on specific serum IgE levels in asthmatic patients presenting emergently, ryegrass pollen was strongly implicated in the dramatic seasonal peak in asthma emergency department visits in northern California.[71]

It is less certain that outdoor allergens play a significant role in contributing to the less dramatic asthma exacerbations that are commonplace. Again, panel studies of asthmatic subjects as well as time-series studies have been used to address this issue. No consistent effect of pollens on asthma hospitalizations was observed in London.[6] Similarly, no effect of pollens or mold spores was observed for children's asthma emergency visits in Israel[49] or for pollens in Finland.[53] However, both grass pollen and mold spores were associated with asthma emergency visits in Mexico City.[57] In a panel study of asthmatic patients in southern California, fungal spores, but not pollen, were associated with increased symptoms, decreased level of lung function, and increased medication use.[60] Inconsistencies in the above findings on aeroallergens may be due to different effects of ambient aeroallergens in different settings.

Meteorology

Reported effects of meteorology on asthma outcomes also have been inconsistent. The most dramatic effects of meteorology have been those on asthma "epidemics" following thunderstorms, such as those described in London[72] and Melbourne.[73] The Melbourne epidemics may have been due to the inhalation of starch granules released from pollen during the rapid meteorologic changes that occur during thunderstorms.[74] Use of a time-series design also has allowed investigators to observe an effect of thunderstorms in England on asthma hospitalizations, an effect that was increased with increases in pollen.[75] More typically, the approach to assessing the effects of meteorology employs daily records of temperature, humidity, and sometimes barometric pressure. Using such an approach, no effects of meteorology on emergency visits were observed in Valencia.[54] In Israel, increased visits were associated with increased barometric pressure and with temperature but not with humidity,[49] whereas temperature was associated with increased visits in Finland.[53] In Sweden, whereas changes in temperature were not associated with increased symptoms or decreased level of lung function in asthmatic patients, on-demand use of asthma medications increased with lower temperature.[64] In Denmark, temperature and humidity were both associated with reduction in level of lung function in adult asthmatic patients.[66] As for the effects of ambient aeroallergens, the lack of consistency of effect of the meteorologic factors across studies may be due to true differences in settings with different climates.

Level III Evidence

A large number of cross-sectional studies relating asthma prevalence to some averaged measures of outdoor environmental factors have been reported. Because of the significant potential for uncontrolled confounding in these studies, the level of evidence that they provide is generally low. These studies will therefore not be reviewed here. An interesting example, however, is provided by the group of studies examining asthma prevalence and severity and proximity to roadways. Residential proximity to high traffic flow in San Diego was associated with more frequent medical visits due to asthma, but it did not increase the risk of asthma.[76] In general, the relationship between asthma prevalence and proximity to roadways has not been consistent.[77,78]

CONCLUSION

Table 6–1 summarizes the levels of evidence for several claims regarding the adverse effects of outdoor environmental factors on asthma. In general, the evidence at this time supporting roles for ambient environmental factors in causing asthma is weak. It seems unlikely, barring new understanding of the effects of pollutant components that are not decreasing, such as ultrafine particles, that these factors play a significant role in explaining recent increases in asthma prevalence. On the other hand, evidence supporting roles for ambient environmental factors in aggravating asthma is relatively strong. Experimental studies convincingly demonstrate adverse effects of air pollutants, aeroallergens, and inspired air conditions on

Table 6–1 *Levels of Evidence for Claims about the Adverse Effects of Outdoor Environmental Factors on Asthma*

Environmental Factor	Claims	Levels of Evidence
Air pollution	Air pollution, in general, causes asthma	IIIE
	Ozone causes asthma	IIB
	Air pollution, in general, aggravates asthma	IIB
	Sulfur dioxide and ozone can aggravate asthma	IA
	Ozone and nitrogen dioxide enhance the effect of allergen on lung function	IB
Allergen	Aeroallergens cause asthma	IID and IIIB
	Aeroallergens aggravate asthma	IA and IIB
Meteorology	Inspired-air conditions affect exercise-induced bronchospasm	IA
	Meteorologic factors aggravate asthma	IIA

asthma. It is still very much an open question to what extent these demonstrated effects contribute to the day-to-day variability of the disease in most people with asthma.

REFERENCES

1. McDonnell WF, Abbey DE, Nishino N, Lebowitz MD. Long-term ambient ozone concentration and the incidence of asthma in nonsmoking adults: the AHSMOG Study. Environ Res 1999;80:110–21.
2. Sporik R, Holgate T, Platts-Mills T, et al. Exposure to house-dust mite allergen (Der p I) and the development of asthma in childhood. N Engl J Med 1990;323:502–7.
3. Sears MR, Herbison GP, Holdaway MD, et al. The relative risks of sensitivity to grass pollen, house dust mite and cat dander in the development of childhood asthma. Clin Exp Allergy 1989;19:419–24.
4. International Study of Asthma and Allergies in Childhood (ISAAC) Steering Committee. Worldwide variation in prevalence of symptoms of asthma, allergic rhinoconjunctivitis and atopic eczema: ISAAC. Lancet 1998;351:1225–32.
5. von Mutius E, Martinez FD, Fritzsch C, et al. Prevalence of asthma and atopy in two areas of West and East Germany. Am J Respir Crit Care Med 1994;149:358–64.
6. Anderson HR. Air pollution and trends in asthma. In: Ciba Foundation, editor. The rising trends in asthma [symposium 206]. Chichester: Wiley; 1997. p. 190–207.
7. Finlayson-Pitts BJ, Pitts JN. Tropospheric air pollution: ozone, airborne toxics, polycyclic aromatic hydrocarbons, and particles. Science 1997;276:1045–51.
8. Bjorksten F, Suoiemi I, Koski V. Neonatal birch pollen contact and subsequent allergy to birch pollen. Clin Allergy 1980;10:585–91.
9. Williams PB, Buhr MP, Weber RW, et al. Latex allergen in respirable particulate air pollution. J Allergy Clin Immunol 1995;95:88–95.
10. Anto JM, Sunyer J, Rodriguez-Roison R, Vazques L. Community outbreak of asthma associated with inhalation of soya bean. N Engl J Med 1989;320:1097–102.
11. Peden DB, Boehlecke B, Horstman D, Devlin R. Prolonged, acute exposure to 0.16 ppm ozone induces eosinophilic airway inflammation in allergic asthmatic patients. J Allergy Clin Immunol 1997;100:802–8.
12. Aris RM, Christian D, Hearne PQ, et al. Ozone-induced airway inflammation in human subjects as determined by airway lavage and biopsy. Am Rev Respir Dis 1993;148:1363–72.

13. Wyemer AR, Gong H, Lyness A, et al. Pre-exposure to ozone does not enhance or produce exercise-induced asthma. Am J Respir Crit Care Med 1994;149:1414–9.

14. Silverman F. Asthma and respiratory irritants (ozone). Environ Health Perspect 1979;29:131–6.

15. Horstman DH, Ball BA, Brown J, et al. Comparison of pulmonary responses of asthmatic and non-asthmatic subjects performing light exercise while exposed to a low level of ozone. Toxicol Ind Health 1995;11:369–85.

16. Scannell C, Chen LL, Aris R, et al. Greater ozone-induced inflammatory responses in subjects with asthma. Am J Respir Crit Care Med 1996;154:24–9.

17. Frampton MW, Balmes JR, Cox C, et al. Mediators of inflammation in bronchoalveolar lavage fluid from non-smokers, smokers and asthmatic subjects exposed to ozone—a collaborative study. Health Effects Inst Res Rep 1997;78:73–9.

18. Vagaggini B, Taccola M, Conti I, et al. Effect of one month treatment with budesonide on functional and bio-logical response to ozone in mild asthmatic subjects. Am J Respir Crit Care Med 1999;159:A493.

19. Molfino NA, Wright SC, Katz I, et al. Effect of low concentrations of ozone on inhaled allergen responses in asthmatic subjects. Lancet 1991;338:199–203.

20. Jorres R, Nowak K, Magnussen H. Effects of ozone exposure on airway responsiveness to inhaled allergens in subjects with allergic asthma or rhinitis. Am J Respir Crit Care Med 1996;153:56–64.

21. Kehrl HR, Peden DB, Ball B, et al. Increased specific airway reactivity of persons with mild allergic asthma after 7.6 hours of exposure to 0.16 ppm ozone. J Allergy Clin Immunol 1999;104:1198–204.

22. Ball BA, Folinsbee LJ, Peden DB, Kehrl HR. Allergen bronchoprovocation of patients with mild allergic asthma after ozone exposure. J Allergy Clin Immunol 1996;98:563–72.

23. Bylin G, Lindvall T, Rehn T, Sundin B. Effects of short-term exposure to ambient nitrogen dioxide concentra-tions on human bronchial reactivity and lung function. Eur J Respir Dis 1985;66:205–17.

24. Jorres R, Magnussen H. Effect of 0.25 ppm nitrogen dioxide on the airway response to methacholine in asymp-tomatic asthmatic patients. Lung 1991;169:77–85.

25. Tunnicliffe W, Burge P, Ayres J. Effect of domestic concentrations of nitrogen dioxide on airway responses to inhaled allergen in asthmatic patients. Lancet 1994;344:1733–6.

26. Strand V, Rak S, Svartengren M, Bylin G. Nitrogen dioxide exposure enhances asthmatic reaction to inhaled allergen in subjects with asthma. Am J Respir Crit Care Med 1997;155:881–7.

27. Devalia J, Rusznak C, Herdman M, et al. Effect of nitrogen dioxide and sulphur dioxide on airway response of mild asthmatic patients to allergen inhalation. Lancet 1994;344:1668–71.

28. Horstman DH, Roger LJ, Kehrl H, et al. Airway sensitivity of asthmatic patients to sulfur dioxide. Toxicol Ind Health 1986;2:289–98.

29. Koenig JQ, Pierson WE, Korike M. The effects of inhaled sulfuric acid on pulmonary function in adolescent asthmatic patients. Am Rev Respir Dis 1983;128:221–5.

30. Utell MJ, Morrow PE, Speers DM, et al. Airway responses to sulfate and sulfuric acid aerosols in asthmatic patients. Am Rev Respir Dis 1983;128:444–50.

31. Petrovic S, Urch B, Liu L, et al. Cardiorespiratory effects following inhalation of concentrated $PM_{2.5}$ with and without ozone in mild asthmatic patients. Am J Respir Crit Care Med 2000;161:A239.

32. Fujieda S, Diaz-Sanchez D, Saxon A. Combined nasal challenge with diesel exhaust particles and allergen induces in vivo IgE isotype switching. Am J Respir Cell Mol Biol 1998;19:507–12.

33. Cockcroft DW, Ruffin RE, Dolovich J, Hargreave FE. Allergen-induced increase in nonallergic bronchial reac-tivity. Clin Allergy 1977;7:503–13.

34. Boulet LP, Cartier A, Thomson NC, et al. Asthma and increases in nonallergic bronchial responsiveness from seasonal pollen exposure. J Allergy Clin Immunol 1983;71:399–406.

35. Deal EC, McFadden ER, Ingram RH, Jaeger JJ. Role of respiratory heat exchange in asthma. J Appl Physiol 1984;57:608–9.

36. Thurston GD, Ito K, Kinney PL, Lippmann M. A multi-year study of air pollution and respiratory hospital admissions in three New York state metropolitan areas: results for 1988 and 1989 summers. J Expos Anal Environ Epidemiol 1992;2:429–50.

37. Thurston GD, Ito K, Hayes CG, et al. Respiratory hospital admissions and summertime haze air pollution in Toronto, Ontario: consideration of the role of acid aerosols. Environ Res 1994;65:271–90.

38. Sheppard L, Levy D, Norris G, et al. Effects of ambient air pollution on nonelderly asthma hospital admissions in Seattle, Washington, 1987–1994. Epidemiol 1999;10:1–4.

39. Ponka A, Virtonen M. Asthma and ambient air pollution in Helsinki. J Epidemiol Community Health 1996;50 Suppl 1:S59–62.

40. Dab W, Medina S, Quenel P, et al. Short term respiratory health effects of ambient air pollution: results of the APHEA project in Paris. J Epidemiol Community Health 1996;40:S42–6.

41. Schouten JP, Vonk JM, deGraaf A. Short term effects of air pollution on emergency hospital admissions for respiratory disease: results of the APHEA project in two major cities in the Netherlands, 1977–89. J Epidemiol Community Health 1996;50 Suppl 1:S22–9.

42. Atkinson RW, Anderson HR, Strachan DP, et al. Short-term associations between outdoor air pollution and visits to accident and emergency departments in London for respiratory complaints. Eur Respir J 1999;13:257–65.

43. Morgan G, Corvett S, Wlodarczyk J. Air pollution and hospital admissions in Sydney, Australia, 1990 to 1994. Am J Public Health 1998;88:1761–6.

44. Cody RP, Weisel CP, Birnbaum G, Lioy PJ. The effect of ozone associated with summertime photochemical smog on the frequency of asthma visits to hospital emergency departments. Environ Res 1992;58:184–94.

45. Stieb DM, Burnett RT, Beveridge RC, Brook JR. Association between ozone and asthma emergency department visits in Saint John, New Brunswick, Canada. Environ Health Perspect 1996;104:1354–60.

46. Romieu I, Meneses F, Sienra-Monge JJL, et al. Effects of urban air pollutants on emergency visits for childhood asthma in Mexico City. Am J Epidemiol 1995;141:546–53.

47. Schwartz J, Slater D, Larson TV, et al. Particulate air pollution and hospital emergency department visits for asthma in Seattle. Am Rev Respir Dis 1993;147:826–31.

48. Lipsett M, Hurley S, Ostro B. Air pollution and emergency department visits for asthma in Santa Clara County, California. Environ Health Perspect 1997;105:216–22.

49. Garty BZ, Kosman E, Ganor I, et al. Emergency department visits of asthmatic children: relation to air pollution, weather and airborne allergens. Ann Allergy Asthma Immunol 1998;81:563–70.

50. Bates DV, Baker-Anderson M, Sizto R. Asthma attack periodicity: a study of hospital emergency visits in Vancouver. Environ Res 1990;51:51–70.

51. Hajat S, Haines A, Goubet SA, et al. Association of air pollution with daily GP consultations for asthma and other lower respiratory conditions in London. Thorax 1999;54:597–605.

52. Castellsague J, Sunyer J, Saez M, Anto JM. Short-term association between air pollution and emergency department visits for asthma in Barcelona. Thorax 1995;50:1051–6.

53. Rossi OVJ, Kinnula VL, Tienari J, Huhti E. Association of severe asthma attacks with weather, pollen, and air pollutants. Thorax 1993;48:244–8.

54. de Diego Damia A, Leon Fabregas M, Perpina Tordera M, Mompte Torrero L. Effects of air pollution and weather conditions on asthma exacerbation. Respiration 1999;66:52–8.

55. Wordley J, Walters S, Aytes JG. Short term variations in hospital admissions and mortality and particulate air pollution. Occup Environ Med 1997;54:108–16.

56. Norris G, Young-Pong SN, Koenig JQ, et al. An association between fine particles and asthma emergency department visits for children in Seattle. Environ Health Perspect 1999;107:489–93.

57. Rosas I, McCartney HA, Payne RW, et al. Analysis of the relationships between environmental factors (aeroallergens, air pollution, and weather) and asthma emergency admissions to a hospital in Mexico City. Allergy 1998;53:394–401.

58. Vedal S, Petkau J, White R, Blair J. Acute effects of ambient inhalable particles in asthmatic and non-asthmatic children. Am J Respir Crit Care Med 1998;157:1034–43.

59. Ostro BD, Lipsett MJ, Wiener MB, Selner JC. Asthmatic responses to airborne acid aerosols. Am J Public Health 1991;81:694–702.

60. Delfino RJ, Zeiger RS, Seltzer JM, et al. The effect of outdoor fungal spore concentrations on daily asthma severity. Environ Health Perspect 1997;105:622–35.

61. Hiltermann TJN, Stolk J, van der Zee SC, et al. Asthma severity and susceptibility to air pollution. Eur Respir J 1998;11:686–93.

62. Boezen HM, van der Zee SC, Postma DS, et al. Effects of ambient air pollution on upper and lower respiratory symptoms and peak expiratory flow in children. Lancet 1999;353:874–8.

63. Peters A, Goldstein IF, Beyer U, et al. Acute health effects of exposure to high levels of air pollution in Eastern Europe. Am J Epidemiol 1996;144:570–81.

64. Forsberg B, Stjernberg N, Linne R, et al. Daily air pollution levels and acute asthma in southern Sweden. Eur Respir J 1998;12:900–5.

65. Pope CA, Dockery DW, Spengler JD, et al. Respiratory health and PM_{10}: a daily time-series analysis. Am Rev Respir Dis 1991;149:668–74.

66. Moseholm L, Taudorf E, Frosig A. Pulmonary function changes in asthmatic patients associated with low-level SO_2 and NO_2 air pollution, weather, and medicine intake. Allergy 1993;48:334–44.

67. Peters A, Dockery DW, Heinrich H, Wichmann HE. Medication use modifies the health effects of particulate sulfate air pollution in children with asthma. Environ Health Perspect 1997;105:430–5.

68. O'Hollaren MT, Yunginger JW, Offord KP, et al. Exposure to an aeroallergen as a possible precipitating factor in respiratory arrest in young patients with asthma. N Engl J Med 1991;324:359–63.

69. Targonski PB, Persky VW, Ramekrishnan V. Effect of environmental molds on risk of death from asthma during the pollen season. J Allergy Clin Immunol 1995;95:955–61.

70. Paulus HJ, Smith TJ. Association of allergic bronchial asthma with certain air pollutants and weather parameters. Int J Biometeorol 1967;11:119–27.

71. Pollart SM, Reid MJ, Fling FA, et al. Epidemiology of emergency department asthma in northern California: association with IgE antibody to ryegrass pollen. J Allergy Clin Immunol 1988;82:224–30.

72. Celenza A, Fothergill J, Kupek I, Shaw RJ. Thunderstorm associated asthma: a detailed analysis of environmental factors. BMJ 1996;312:604–7.

73. Bellomo R, Gigliotti P, Treloar A, et al. Two consecutive thunderstorm associated epidemics of asthma in Melbourne. Med J Aust 1992;156:834–7.

74. Suphioglu C, Singh M, Taylor P, et al. Mechanism of grasspollen-induced asthma. Lancet 1992;339:569–72.

75. Newson R, Strachan D, Archibald E, et al. Effect of thunderstorms and airborne grass pollen on the incidence of acute asthma in England, 1990–94. Thorax 1997;52:680–5.

76. English P, Neutra R, Scalf R, et al. Examining associations between childhood asthma and traffic flow using a geographic information system. Environ Health Perspect 1999;107:761–7.

77. van Vliet P, Knape M, de Hartog J, et al. Motor vehicle exhaust and chronic respiratory symptoms in children living near freeways. Environ Res 1997;74:122–32.

78. Waldron G, Pottle B, Dod J. Asthma and the motorways—one district's experience. J Public Health Med 1995;17:85–9.

CHAPTER 7

Role of Indoor Aeroallergens

Moira Chan-Yeung, MB, FRCPC

It has been shown by Sears et al[1] in a longitudinal study of a birth cohort of New Zealand children to the age of 13 years that sensitivity to indoor allergens, such as house dust mite and cat dander, is a more significant risk for asthma than sensitivity to outdoor allergens. With the construction of homes that are tightly sealed to conserve heat, the use of wall-to-wall carpeting, use of cold water detergents for washing, and the change of lifestyle to sedentary living, exposure to indoor allergens has increased. During the past decade, significant advances have been made in immunochemical and epidemiologic research on indoor allergens. This is a review of the role of indoor allergens in asthma.

HOUSE DUST MITE

There are four major species of house dust mite: *Dermatophagoides* spp, *Euroglyphus maynei, Bloomia tropicalis, Lepidoglyphus destructor*.[2] They thrive best in places with high humidity, moderate temperatures, and an adequate supply of food, which are provided amply by human skin scales. There are two major groups of mite allergens. Group I allergens (*Der p* I and *Der f* I) are proteolytic enzymes secreted from the digestive tract of mites and are found in high concentrations in their fecal pellets. Group II allergens (*Der p* II and *Der f* II) are found both in the fecal pellets and mite bodies.[3] Panels of monoclonal antibodies have been produced against most of the allergens.[4] These monoclonal antibodies have been used extensively for measuring environmental exposure to these allergens using an enzyme-linked immunosorbent assay (ELISA).

Exposure to Allergen, Sensitization, and Development of Asthma

There are many studies providing evidence that house dust mites are an important cause of asthma in many parts of the world.[5] There is an ecologic relationship between the level of house dust mite and the prevalence of sensitization. In cold climates and in places where humidity is low, mite allergen levels are low; the prevalence of sensitization is also low.[2,5] In these areas, sensitization to other indoor or outdoor aeroallergen predominates.[6,7] In places with a hot and humid climate, mite allergen levels are high, and the prevalence of house dust mite sensitization and asthma are high.[8–10]

There is a dose-response relationship between the level of exposure to house dust mite allergen and the risk of sensitization.[9–11] The threshold allergen level for sensitization in atopic children was found to be 2 μg allergen/1 g dust, while the comparable level for nonatopic children was approximately 50 to 80 μg allergen/1 g dust.[11] In Australia, the risk for sensitized children having current asthma doubled with every doubling of levels of *Der p* I between 0.7 and 50 μg allergen/1 g dust.[9] The odds ratios for developing asthma in those sensitized compared to those not sensitized have been found to vary between 2 to 21.[11] In a prospective study, Sporik and colleagues have shown that exposure to high levels of mite allergens during the first year of life is associated with subsequent increased risk for sensitization and for asthma.[12]

The dose-response relationship between exposure to house dust mite allergens and the severity of asthma symptoms is less clear. This is partly due to the fact that measurement of allergens in settled dust samples may not be an accurate index of exposure. In addition, most asthmatic patients are allergic to more than one indoor allergen. Asthma can be worsened by other triggers such as irritants and infection. There have been recent reports of a positive relationship between levels of exposure to mite allergens and heightened airway hyper-responsiveness,[7,13] increase in asthma symptoms, and reduction in peak expiratory flow[14] in sensitized asthmatic patients.

Reduction of exposure to house dust mite allergens has resulted in improvement of symptoms, peak flow FEV_1 (forced expiratory volume in 1 second), and airway hyper-responsiveness,[15,16] and reductions in total and specific IgE.[17] Prolonged allergen avoidance does not decrease allergen sensitivity.[15]

Thus, there is good evidence that exposure to house dust mites is causally related to asthma (Level II). However, it is not clear whether the increase in prevalence of asthma during the last three decades in many parts of the world is due to an increase in exposure to house dust mite allergen.

Assessment of Exposure

The most widely used method of assessing exposure is measuring group I allergens using ELISA methods with specific mAbs to bind the allergen and labeled group-specific antibodies for detection.[4] Measurements of both *Der p* I and *Der f* I are necessary for assessment of total *Dermatophagoides* spp exposure.[2] At present, almost all standards are allergen extracts with a given concentration of specific allergen in absolute values (ng or mg of protein). It is important to express the allergen measurements against a common standard for the results to be comparable.

In assessing exposure, dust samples are collected from reservoirs within a house, such as mattresses, carpets, and sofas, using a vacuum cleaner.[2] The samples are then extracted and assayed for mite allergen level. The results are expressed as units of $\mu g/1$ g dust. However, for studies relating to avoidance measures, the results may best be expressed as ng/unit area (m^3).[18,19] Mite allergens cannot be detected by air sampling in the absence of household disturbance.[2] Because of the size of the particles, allergen concentration in the air falls rapidly after disturbance. So far, it has not been possible to demonstrate a relationship between airborne levels and sensitization or the severity of asthma.[2]

PETS

Pets are found in over 50% of families in Western society.[20,21] In Canada, 34% of homes have pets, consisting mostly of cats and dogs.[22] Allergy to pet allergen is very common. Surveys have shown that 5 to 15% of the general population and 40 to 70% of patients with asthma have positive skin-test reactions to cat and/or dog dander.[23–26] Close human contact accounts for the high prevalence of pet allergy.

Of all pets, cats are the most prevalent cause of pet allergy. Cat allergen has been well characterized. The most important allergen is *Fel d* I, as most of the IgE antibodies in cat-sensitive subjects are directed against this allergen.[27] *Fel d* I is found in salivary glands, hair follicles, saliva, and lacrimal fluid.[28] The existence of B and T cell epitopes in the *Fel d* I molecule has been demonstrated.[29] Recently, dog allergens, *Can f* I and *Can f* II, have been purified.[30] There have been few studies of sensitivity to dog allergen and its relationship with asthma.

Exposure to Allergen, Sensitization, and Development of Asthma

While house dust mite is the most important allergen responsible for sensitization and asthma in humid tropical and subtropical climates, in dry and cold temperate climate, pet allergens are important (Level II). In Scandinavian countries,[31] prairie provinces of Canada,[32] and mountains of New Mexico,[6] where mite levels are low, sensitization to pet allergens and/or to local pollens is important. In Winnipeg and Vancouver, as many as 70% of both adults and children with asthma reacted to cat allergen, while only 45% reacted to house dust mite extract.[32] In Winnipeg, levels of cat allergen reached high levels during winter months in homes with cats.[32] In a population study in Vancouver,[22] those who were sensitized to cats and owned cats had the highest risk for having current asthma compared to those without cats and were not sensitized to cats (OR 14.1, 95%CI 2.9 to 67.8); those who were sensitized to cats but did not have a cat were also at high risk for having current asthma (OR 19, 95%CI 6.8 to 53) (Level II).

Sensitization to cats appears to be more common than sensitization to dogs. Murray et al,[24] in a study of 1,238 children, found significantly more frequent skin-test reactions to cats than to dogs. The higher frequency of sensitization to cats was not caused by exposure to cats in more homes, since dogs outnumbered cats as household pets in their study. It suggested that the greater intimacy of exposure to cats than dogs might be a factor since cats are more often inside the house (Level II).

Assessment of Exposure

Measurement of *Fel d* I is carried out in an mAb-based ELISA assay that has been developed recently.[33] *Fel d* I has been found in dust from floor, mattresses, soft furnishings, and walls and in the air.[34] The wide distribution of the allergen is due to a significant proportion of *Fel d* I present on particles smaller than 2.5 µm in diameter, which readily become airborne and remain in the air for prolonged periods of time, even in undisturbed conditions.[35] Thus, it is possible to measure airborne cat allergen level readily.[2]

Measurable amounts of *Fel d* I have been found in almost every home,[32] including those without cats, and in public buildings.[31,36,37] Studies in Scandinavian schools have shown that while mite allergen levels were low in classrooms, high levels of both cat and dog allergens were found on both smooth and carpeted floors, with approximately 11 times more on carpeted floors.[31] Levels of cat and dog allergens were much higher on chairs than on floors, suggesting that allergens were brought in by students and teachers on their clothing. The investigators estimated that as much as 30 ng *Fel d* I/m³ was brought into the classroom every day. This level can cause asthma in sensitized children with asthma.[31]

Since *Can f* I and *Can f* II have been identified only recently, few exposure studies have been done using these two allergens. It has been found that *Can f* I has aerodynamic characteristics similar to *Fel d* I.[38] Thus, measurement of airborne *Can f* I should be possible. In Scandinavian schools, *Can f* I has been found in as high concentrations as *Fel d* I.[31]

Levels of 8 µg *Fel d* I/1 g dust and 10 µg *Can f* I/1 g dust have been proposed as significant exposure, leading to attacks of asthma.[2]

COCKROACHES

Cockroaches are ubiquitous and are highly allergenic. Two major groups of cockroach allergens have been identified: *Blatella germanica* and *Periplaneta americana*. The allergen *Bla g* II is an aspartic protease, which is a digestive enzyme secreted by cockroach in the feces.[39,40]

Exposure to Allergen, Sensitization, and Development of Asthma

Cockroach populations are highest in crowded urban areas. In a study of dust samples collected from homes of 87 children with moderate to severe asthma, 26% of bedroom dust samples had detectable levels of cockroach allergens.[41] Over 80% of the children whose bedroom *Bla g* I or *Bla g* II levels were greater than 1 U/g dust demonstrated skin sensitivity to the cockroach allergen. The prevalence of sensitization was directly related to the level of bedroom exposure. Exposure to cockroach allergen has been found to be an important cause of hospitalization for acute asthma in inner city areas in Chicago.[42] Similarly, Rosenstreich et al[43] have shown that immediate hypersensitivity to cockroach allergens is common among children with asthma in a large cohort of children living in seven cities in the Northeast and Midwest United States. They also found that the degree of exposure, in children with positive skin tests to cockroach allergen, is correlated with their risk of hospitalization. Thus, there is considerable evidence to support that cockroach is another important indoor allergen contributing to asthma (Level II).

Assessment of Exposure

Assays for cockroach allergens *Bla g* I and *Bla g* II are now available to assess the degree of exposure. During normal domestic activities, cockroach allergens behave similarly to mite allergens; they are present predominantly on particles greater than 10 fm in size that remain in the air for only 20 to 30 minutes.[44] The level found in the air after artificial disturbance is around 40 to 50 ng/m,[3] similar to those reported for mite allergens.[44] Under undisturbed conditions, airborne cockroach allergens are not detectable in air samples.[44] Exposure to *Bla g* II level of ≥ 2 U/1 g dust has been proposed as a significant risk for asthma exacerbation in sensitized subjects.[44]

SUMMARY

The prevalence and morbidity of asthma in developed countries progressively increased over the past three decades.[45] Although there is no clear evidence that the increase in prevalence of asthma is due to increased exposure to indoor allergens, the evidence is overwhelming that exposure to these allergens is associated with sensitization and asthma. Ongoing daily exposure to these allergens leads to perpetuation of the inflammatory process in the airway, which is likely the cause for the persistence of symptoms and airway hyper-responsiveness in sensitized patients. Clinicians should recognize the importance of these allergens in the management of asthma, as avoidance and/or reduction of exposure is an important part of asthma management.

REFERENCES

1.   Sears MR, Herbison GP, Holdaway MD, et al. The relative risks of sensitization to grass pollen, house dust mite and cat dander in the development of childhood asthma. Clin Exp Allergy 1989;19:419–24.

2.   Platts-Mills TAE, Vervlet D, Thomas WR, et al. Indoor allergens and asthma: report of the third international workshop. J Allergy Clin Immunol 1997;100:S1–24.

3.   Platts-Mills TAE, de Weck AL. Dust mite allergens and asthma—a world wide problem. J Allergy Clin Immunol 1989;83:416–27.

4.   Chapman MD, Smith AM, Slint JB, et al. Immunochemical and molecular methods for defining and measuring indoor allergens: in dust and air. Pediatr Allergy Immunol 1995;6:8–12.

5.   Platts-Mills TAE, Thomas WR, Aalberse RC, et al. Dust mite allergens and asthma: report of a second international workshop. J Allergy Clin Immunol 1992;89:1046–60.

6.   Ingram JM, Sporik R, Rose G, et al. Quantitative assessment of exposure to dog (Can f 1) and cat (Fel d 1) allergens: relation to sensitization and asthma among children living in Los Alamos, New Mexico. J Allergy Clin Immunol 1995;96:449–56.

7.   Chan-Yeung M, Manfreda J, Dimich-Ward J, et al. Mite and cat allergen levels in homes and severity of asthma. Am J Respir Crit Care Med 1995;152:1805–11.

8.   Squillace SP, Sporik RB, Rakes G, et al. Sensitization to dust mites as a dominant risk factor for asthma among adolescents living in central Virginia. Am J Respir Crit Care Med 1997;156:1760–4.

9.   Peat JK, Tovey E, Toelle BG, et al. House dust mite allergens. A major risk factor for childhood asthma in Australia. Am J Respir Crit Care Med 1996;153:141–6.

10.   Kuehr J, Frischer T, Meinert R, et al. Mite allergen exposure is a risk for the incidence of specific sensitization. J Allergy Clin Immunol 1994;94:44–52.

11.   Lau S, Falkenhorst G, Weber A, et al. High mite-allergen exposure inceases the risk of sensitization in atopic children and young adults. J Allergy Clin Immunol 1989;84:718–25.

12. Sporik R, Holgate S, Platts-Mills T, Coswell J. Exposure to house-dust mite allergen (Der p 1) and the development of asthma in childhood. N Engl J Med 1992;323:502–7.

13. Kivity S, Solomon A, Soferman R, et al. Mite asthma in childhood: a study of the relationship between exposure to house dust mites and disease activity. J Allergy Clin Immunol 1993;91:844–9.

14. Vervloet D, Charpin D, Haddi E, et al. Medication requirements and house dust mite exposure in mite-sensitive asthmatic patients. Allergy 1991;46:554–8.

15. Peroni DG, Boner AL, Vallone G, et al. Effective allergen avoidance at high altitude reduced allergen-induced bronchial hyperresponsiveness. Am J Respir Crit Care Med 1994;149:1442–6.

16. Simon H, Grotzer M, Nikolaizik W, et al. High altitude climate therapy reduces peripheral blood T lymphocyte activation, eosinophils, and bronchial obstruction in children with house dust mite allergic asthma. Pediatr Pulmonol 1994;17:304–11.

17. Sensi L, Piacentini G, Nobile E, et al. Changes in nasal specific IgE to mites after periods of allergen exposure avoidance: a comparison with serum levels. Clin Exp Allergy 1994;24:377–82.

18. Tan BB, Weald D, Strickland I, Friedmann PS. Double blind controlled trial of effect of house dust mite allergen avoidance on atopic dermatitis. Lancet 1996;347:15–28.

19. Siebers RW, Fitzharris P, Crane J. Beds, bedrooms, bedding and bugs: anything new between the sheets. Clin Exp Allergy 1996;26:1225–7.

20. Kjellman B, Pettersson R. The problem of furred pets in childhood atopic disease. Failure of an information program. Allergy 1983;38:65–73.

21. Warner JA, Little SA, Pollock I. The influence of exposure to house dust mite on sensitization in asthma. Pediatr Allergy Immunol 1991;1:79–86.

22. Noertjojo K, Dimich-Ward H, Obata H, et al. Exposure and sensitization to cat, asthma, asthma-like symptoms among adults. J Allergy Clin Immunol 1999;103:60–5.

23. Wilkie AT, Ford PPK, Pattemore P, et al. Prevalence of childhood asthma symptoms in an industrial suburb of Christchurch. N Z Med J 1995;108:188–90.

24. Murray A, Ferguson A, Morrison B. The frequency and severity of cat allergy vs dog allergy in atopic children. J Allergy Clin Immunol 1983;72:145–9.

25. Vanto T, Koivikko A. Dog hypersensitivity in asthmatic children. Acta Paediatr Scand 1983;72:571–5.

26. Cuijpers CEJ, Swaen GMH, Wesseling G, et al. Adverse effects of the indoor environment on respiratory health in primary school children. Environ Res 1996;68:11–23.

27. Ohman JL, Kendall S, Lowell FC. IgE antibody to cat allergens in an allergic population. J Allergy Clin Immunol 1977;60:317–23.

28. Brown PR, Leitermann KM, Ohman JL. Distribution of cat allergen in tissues and fluids. Int Arch Allergy Appl Immunol 1984;74:67–70.

29. Rogers BL, Mogenstern JP, Garman RD, et al. Recombinant Fel d1: expression, purification, IgE binding and reaction with cat-allergic human T cells. Mol Immunol 1993;30:559–68.

30. Schou C, Svendsen UG, Lowenstein H. Purification and characterization of the major dog allergen, Can f1. Clin Exp Allergy 1991;21:321–8.

31. Munir AKM, Einarsson R, Schou C, Dreberg SKG. Allergens in school dust. I. The amount of the major cat (Fel d1) and dog (Can f1) allergens in dust from Swedish schools is high enough to probably cause perennial symptoms in most children with asthma who are sensitized to cat and dog. J Allergy Clin Immunol 1993;91:1067–74.

32. Quirce S, Dimich-Ward H, Ferguson A, et al. Major cat allergen (Fel d 1) in the homes of patients with asthma and their relationship to sensitization to cat dander. Ann Allergy Asthma Immunol 1995;75:325–30.

33. de Blay F, Chapman MD, Platts-Mills TAE. Airborne cat allergen (Fel d I): environmental control with the cat in situ. Am Rev Respir Dis 1991;143:1334–9.

34. Warner JA. Environmental allergen exposure in homes and schools. Clin Exp Allergy 1992;22:1044–5.

35. Luczynska M, Li Y, Chapman MD, Platts-Mills TAE. Airborne concentrations and particle size distribution of allergen derived from domestic cats (Felis domesticus). Am Rev Respir Dis 1990;141:361–7.

36. Wood RA, Eggleston PA, Lind P, et al. Antigenic analysis of household dust samples. Am Rev Respir Dis 1988;137:358–63.

37. Enberg RN, Shamie SM, McCullough J, Ownby DR. Ubiquitous presence of cat allergen in cat-free buldings: probable dispersal from human clothing. Ann Allergy 1993;70:471–4.

38. Custovic A, Green R, Fletcher A, et al. Aerodynamic properties of the major dog allergen, Can f 1: distribution in homes, concentration and particle size of allergen in the air. Am J Respir Crit Care Med 1997;155:94–8.

39. Arruda LK, Vailes LD, Mann BJ, et al. Molecular cloning of a major cockroach (Blatella germanica) allergen, Bla g2. J Biol Chem 1995;270:19563–8.

40. Bernton HS, Brown H. Insect allergy: the allergenicity of the excrement of the cockroach. Ann Allergy 1970;28:543–7.

41. Sarpong SB, Hamilton RG, Eggleston PA, Adkinson NF. Socioeconomic status and race as risk factors for cockroach allergen exposure and sensitization in children with asthma. J Allergy Clin Immunol 1996;97:1393–401.

42. Kang BC, Johnson J, Veres-Thorner C. Atopic profile of inner-city asthma with a comparative analysis on the cockroach-sensitive and ragweed-sensitive subgroups. J Allergy Clin Immunol 1993;92:802–11.

43. Rosenstreich DL, Eggleston P, Kattan M, et al. The role of cockroach allergy and exposure to cockcroach allergen in causing morbidity among inner city children with asthma. N Engl J Med 1997;336:1356–63.

44. de Blay F, Sanchez J, Hedelin G, et al. Dust and airborne exposure to allergens derived from cockroach (Blatelli germanica) in low cost public housing in Strasbourg (France). J Allergy Clin Immunol 1997;99:107–12.

45. Burney PGJ. Epidemiology trends. In: Barnes PJ, Grunstein MM, Leff AR, Woolcock A, editors. Asthma. Philadelphia: Lippincott-Raven Publishers; 1997. p. 35–47.

CHAPTER 8

Role of Childhood Infection

Joanne B. Clough, DM, FRCA, MRCP, FRCPCH

For decades now, an association between respiratory infections and asthma has been acknowledged. Initially, infection was thought to be implicated in both the inception of asthma and the provocation of established asthma. Recently it has become clear that infections in early life may play an important role in protecting an individual from developing allergy and asthma, although viral infections remain one of the most important triggers to exacerbations of asthma. Thus, a paradox exists, and along with it the potential for confusion. In this chapter, the author will explore the evidence for the role played by infections in both the inception and the provocation of asthma, using data from the multitude of studies in this area performed over the past five decades.

ASSOCIATION BETWEEN RESPIRATORY INFECTIONS AND EXACERBATIONS OF ASTHMA

The existence of an association between respiratory infections and exacerbations of asthma has been acknowledged for many centuries. Sufferers themselves know that an attack of asthma often follows an upper respiratory tract infection, and this is especially true in children. In 1698, Sir John Floyer wrote, "I cannot remember the first occasion of my asthma, but have been told that it was a cold when I first went to school."[1] Until the 1950s it was assumed that these exacerbations were due to bacterial allergy.[2] However, since then, it has become clear that infection with respiratory viruses plays a more important role.

There are several ways in which epidemiologic evidence can be used to substantiate the role of upper respiratory tract virus infections in producing exacerbations of pre-existing asthma. These are as follows:

- Case reports demonstrating a temporal relationship between viral infections and asthma exacerbations
- Time-series studies
- Identification of viruses during exacerbations of asthma
- Prospective longitudinal studies of individuals with asthma

Case Reports

The first reports of asthma exacerbations being caused by viral infection occurred in the late 1950s during epidemics of influenza affecting two large populations.[3,4] This coincided with the description of an infectious agent found both in chimpanzees with coryza and infants with bronchiolitis.[5] This agent was called respiratory syncytial virus (RSV). By the mid 1960s, it was clear that the infectious agents most commonly implicated in causing attacks of asthma were the influenza and parainfluenza viruses and RSV.[6] In the 1970s, a clear association between lower respiratory tract wheezing illness and annual outbreaks of RSV was demonstrated in a large pediatric practice over a period of 11 years.[7] This realization opened the way for detailed study of this phenomenon.

Time-Series Studies

Exacerbations of asthma were first noted to have a marked seasonal variation—the peak occurring during autumn—by Adams in 1939.[8] A number of explanations for this observation have been proposed, including increases in aeroallergen load, weather effects, changes in indoor air quality due to the use of domestic heating, and seasonal exposure to upper respiratory tract infections. The role of upper respiratory tract viral infections in causing asthma exacerbations was originally proposed in a study of hospital asthma admissions in children, in which a relationship between the peak of admissions and the peak of respiratory tract viral infections was observed.[9] To explore this further, Storr and Lenney examined the asthma admission rates at a children's hospital in Brighton, England, over an 11-year period.[10] Low admission rates during the school holidays contrasted with two peaks of hospital admissions during each school term: the first coinciding with the return to school at the beginning of term; the second coinciding with return after the half-term break. This study suggested a link between exacerbations of asthma and upper respiratory tract viral infections.

Ayres et al[11] strengthened the evidence for this relationship by examining general practitioner weekly returns for England and Wales over an 11-year period to determine the temporal association of asthma episodes with viral isolation rates obtained from the Communicable Disease Surveillance Centre of the UK Public Health Laboratory Service. The most striking finding was the demonstration of a temporal association between wheezing illness in children aged 0 to 4 years and identifications of RSV.

In a study of 400,000 preschool children in Toronto, Canada, Dales et al examined seasonal patterns of emergency department visits and hospital admissions for asthma over a 9-year period.[12] These were compared to presentations for non-respiratory illnesses to allow for confounding factors such as hospital bed closures and holiday periods. Large peaks in asthma admissions during the autumn were demonstrated, and no significant correlations were shown between these peaks and aeroallergen levels or levels of outdoor air pollutants measured during this period. In contrast, there was a significant correlation with respiratory infection rates (Level II).

The most detailed analysis of seasonal changes in asthma exacerbations was performed by Johnston et al who examined the pattern of pediatric hospital admissions for asthma over a 12-month period[13] and compared these to viral infection rates assessed using polymerase chain reaction (PCR) technology in a cohort of children investigated as part of another study.[14] This study confirmed the findings of Storr and Lenney[10] that peaks of hospital admissions occurred within 2 to 4 weeks of the start of each school term and, in addition, that a strong correlation existed between half-monthly rates of pediatric asthma admission and viral detection rates from the cohort study ($r = .67$, $p = .001$) (Level II).

Few time-series studies have been performed in adults to examine the link between upper respiratory tract viral infections and asthma exacerbations. However, Johnston et al have demonstrated a correlation between adult asthma admission rates and virus detection rates in their cohort of children ($r = .5$, $p = .013$).[13] Although this correlation is less strong than that for children, it gives an indication that upper respiratory tract viral infection may be an important cause of asthma exacerbations in adults, too.

Virus Identification

The identification of respiratory tract viruses during exacerbations of asthma can provide evidence of association, if not causation, between respiratory infections and asthma or wheezing episodes. However, such studies may be confounded by difficulties in obtaining adequate and early specimens, and by deficiencies in the viral diagnostic methods available.[15] The asymptomatic viral identification rate in both asthmatic patients and nonasthmatic patients appears to be approximately 3%.[16–19] This is in marked contrast to the virus identification rate during exacerbations of asthma which, prior to the development of PCR technology, was shown to be between 10[20] and 49%.[21] However, caution is needed when interpreting these findings, as there is no standard for the definition of an episode of asthma, and virus detection methods vary widely.

Studies of the pathogen identification rate in the same populations, when symptomatic and asymptomatic, provide further evidence of the importance of virus infections in provoking asthma symptoms. However, similar studies of the effects of bacterial infections suggest that bacterial respiratory tract infections are not significantly implicated in causing worsening of asthma symptoms. Bacteria are found in the respiratory tracts of asthmatic subjects as frequently during asymptomatic periods as during exacerbations[18,22] (Table 8–1).

Table 8–1 *Viral and Bacterial Identification Rates during Wheezing and Asymptomatic Periods**

	Year	Identification (ID) Rate (%)		ID Ratio WheezyAsymp
		Wheezy	*Asymptomatic*	
Viruses				
Mitchell et al[17]	1978	14.3	0.8	17.9
Horn et al[16]	1979	26.4	3.2	8.3
Hudgel et al[18]	1979	11.0	3.3	3.3
Jennings et al[19]	1987	18.6	3.3	5.6
Bacteria				
McIntosh et al[22]	1973			
Pneumococcus		26	24	1.1
Haemophilus influenzae		32	37	0.9
β-Hemolytic streptococcus		6	7	0.9
Staphylococcus aureus		18	19	0.9
Enteric bacillus		26	21	1.2
Hudgel et al[18]	1979	9	9	1.0

*Level II.
Reproduced with permission from Pattemore PK, Johnston SL, Bardin PG. Viruses as precipitants of asthma symptoms. 1. Epidemiology. Clin Exp Allergy 1992;22:325–36.

In 1979, Horn et al published two studies which further investigated the role of viral infection in wheezing episodes, this time in children with a diagnosis of wheezy bronchitis. In the first of these, 163 children presenting with 554 episodes of wheezy bronchitis were studied.[16] Nasopharyngeal swabs were taken within 5 days of the development of symptoms, and virus identification was performed using tissue culture methods. Viruses were identified in 26.4% of reported episodes (Rhinovirus 46.1%, parainfluenza virus 14.5%, Enterovirus 14.5%). In the second study, the authors examined sputum, nasal swabs, and throat swabs from 22 children experiencing a total of 72 attacks of wheezy bronchitis.[21] Viruses were identified in 49% of episodes (63% of severe episodes).

Prospective Longitudinal Studies

The most compelling evidence for a link between virus infections and exacerbations of asthma come from prospective studies of individuals with asthma. Until the 1990s, studies in this area were hampered by the relatively poor methodologies available for virus identification. Despite this, the following findings provided strong evidence to support a causal relationship between respiratory virus infections and asthma exacerbations:

- Virus identification rate falls after the acute stage of illness is over.[16]
- Virus identification rate correlates with asthma medication score.[22]

- Virus identification rate correlates with asthma symptom score.[23]
- Virus identification rate correlates with decreases in FEV_1.[24]
- An association exists between virus identification rate and wheezing illness severity (Level II).[21]

The question of whether asthma exacerbations could be due to allergen exposure rather than virus infection was addressed by the observation of Mertsola et al that wheezing in children commenced an average of 43 hours after the first symptoms of respiratory infection and, in patients in whom virus is identified, lasted for an average of 3.8 days.[25] This time course is not consistent with that of acute allergen challenge and the late asthmatic response.

The advent of PCR technology provided techniques with both high specificity and high sensitivity for the identification of respiratory viruses. The most informative study to date is that by Johnston et al.[14] The aim of this study was to evaluate the association between viral infections and acute exacerbations of wheeze in school children. The study included 108 children aged 9 to 11 years who were followed up longitudinally for 13 months. Both upper and lower respiratory symptoms were recorded using daily diary cards, and peak expiratory flow was measured and recorded twice daily. Specimens of blood and nasal mucus were obtained within 48 hours of the occurrence of a symptomatic episode, defined as a predetermined rise in upper or lower respiratory symptoms score or a fall in peak flow of greater than 50 L/min. Viral identification was performed on these specimens using PCR technology. From the longitudinal symptom and peak flow data, episodes of respiratory illness were identified. Viruses were detected in 80% of episodes of reduced peak expiratory flow, 80% of reported episodes of wheeze, and 85% of episodes in which both upper respiratory tract symptoms and fall in peak flow were reported. Rhinoviruses were responsible for 60% of the wheezing episodes. This study supports the hypothesis that the majority of asthma exacerbations in school-aged children are associated with upper respiratory tract viral infections.

In adults, prospective studies of asthmatic individuals have similarly indicated an association between upper respiratory tract viral infection and episodes of asthma, although virus infection seems to be less important as a trigger of exacerbations. Clarke[26] and Hudgel et al[18] demonstrated a viral infection rate of approximately 11% of asthma exacerbations in cohorts of adult asthmatic subjects. Beasley et al demonstrated a similar virus identification rate during episodes of asthma but also demonstrated that virus was found more frequently during severe exacerbations (35.7%) than in mild or moderate exacerbations (5.3%).[20] Using PCR, technology, Nicholson et al demonstrated that viruses appear to be implicated in 44% of symptomatic episodes in a cohort of adult asthmatic volunteers (Level II).[27]

INFECTION AND PROMOTION OF INCEPTION OF ASTHMA

In the past, it has been thought that infection with respiratory viruses in early life might promote the development of asthma. In an uncontrolled prospective study of 48 children with bronchiolitis, 92% were diagnosed as having asthma over the following 5 years.[28] In a later controlled study, in which 73 children admitted to hospital with bronchiolitis were followed for 5.5 years, 42.5% reported wheezing in the final year of study compared to 15.1% of controls.[29] In a prospective study of 140 children, a history of RSV bronchiolitis proved to be the most important risk factor for the development of asthma and raised IgE antibody titers; a family history of asthma or atopy further increased this risk.[30] However, other studies have not supported RSV bronchiolitis being a risk factor for the development of asthma.[31,32] Although it is possible that RSV infection prevents the switching from Th2 to Th1 phenotype in the infant, thus promoting a Th2 response to other viruses in older childhood,[33] a great deal of further investigation is needed in this area. Another possibility is that RSV infection is more likely to trigger a severe wheezing illness in children already predisposed to wheezing and asthma than in children at low risk for the development of wheezing illness. The relationship between infection in early life and subsequent atopy and allergic disease will not be established until thorough prospective studies on childhood infections are undertaken. Such studies would have to take into account age at infection, the type of organism, and the infective dose.

INFECTION AND PROTECTION FROM THE INCEPTION OF ASTHMA

A consistent finding in epidemiologic studies of the prevalence of asthma is the inverse relationship between asthma and the incidence of respiratory tract infections. Anderson noted in the 1970s that asthma was more prevalent in children living in the coastal regions of Papua New Guinea as compared to children living in highland areas, whereas respiratory infections were more common in the highlands and less common in the coastal areas.[34]

Also of interest is the finding that the prevalence of asthma in Tristan da Cunha is extremely high at 46%. For many years this was explained by genetic factors, as the population is highly inbred and some of the original settlers were thought to have asthma. However, when these islanders were evacuated to the United Kingdom because of a volcanic eruption, investigations showed that the islanders had a very low prevalence of serum antibodies against common respiratory viruses. During the 2 years in which they lived in the United Kingdom, the islanders suffered a very high rate of respiratory infection. Further evidence comes from the western Carolina Islands, which are both remote and isolated. Asthma is common, affecting at least one-third of the population, whereas viral infections are uncommon.[35]

The observation that the prevalence of asthma and other allergic diseases in children has risen dramatically in westernized countries in recent years has given rise to the hypothesis that infection in early childhood might be protective against disease. The process of westernization has reduced the incidence of common childhood infections and increased the mean age at which infection occurs, such that successive birth cohorts of children would be expected to progressively lose the protective effects of early life infections.

A number of recent studies have further supported the hypothesis that viral infection in early life may prevent the development of allergic disease. Strachan et al have shown that children from large families are at a reduced risk of developing hayfever.[36,37] Decreased risk was associated with the number of older, but not younger, siblings (Level II).

Unique information arose from studies performed on the unification of Germany in 1990. The impact of West and East European living conditions on the prevalence of respiratory and allergic disorders in two ethnically similar populations was studied.[38] Atopic sensitization was considerably more frequent in West German children than in those from East Germany (36.7% vs 18.2%). The prevalence of current asthma and hayfever was also significantly higher in West German children (5.9% vs 3.9%, 8.6% vs 2.7%, respectively)(Level II). The authors concluded that the difference in lifestyles and the subsequent protection from early life infections in West Germany when compared to East Germany might explain the differences in prevalence of asthma and hayfever between the two parts of the country. They speculated that Western lifestyle is a risk factor for the development of atopy. Von Mutius et al also demonstrated that the prevalence of atopy was inversely related to the number of siblings in the household among both East and West German children.[39]

The evidence from these and other studies proposes an etiologic hypothesis that attributes the sharp rise in prevalence of allergic disease in the past 50 years to the decline in early life viral infection—the "hygiene" hypothesis. This hypothesis has been supported by recent advances in our understanding of T lymphocyte differentiation and by the development of a putative biologic mechanism for such a protective effect. T helper cells can be broadly subdivided into two phenotypes, Th1 and Th2, based on their patterns of cytokine production. Th1-type cells produce predominantly interferon-γ and IL-2, and Th2-type cells produce IL-4, IL-5, and IL-13. Virtually all neonates display Th2-skewed allergen-specific responses at birth,[40] and these responses are quickly restricted in the early postnatal period by maturing

Th1 immunity. This process appears to fail in individuals destined to become atopic. Repeated viral infections, particularly in early life, may selectively enhance the development of Th1-type cells, perhaps due to interferon-γ production by these organisms during infection. Such a response has been shown in vitro to the influenza virus.[41] Further supportive evidence is given by the finding of a strong inverse association between delayed hypersensitivity to *Mycobacterium tuberculosis* and atopy—positive tuberculin responses predicting a lower incidence of asthma.[42]

SUMMARY

Cohort studies are effective for studying the association between upper respiratory tract virus and exacerbations of asthma, since investigators can closely follow up participants and take samples for virus identification early in the illness. Studies in adults and children, both with and without the use of PCR technology, indicate that upper respiratory tract viruses are implicated in a greater proportion of episodes of asthma in children as compared with adults. The use of PCR technology gives much higher rates of virus identification, largely due to the greater detection of Rhinovirus, and would appear to give a better reflection of the importance of upper respiratory tract viruses as causes of exacerbations of asthma than conventional virologic techniques.

The role of viral infections in the inception of asthma has given rise to considerable debate. In the past, viral infections occurring during early life were thought to deleteriously affect the lungs and the immune system, leading to allergic sensitization and persistent bronchial responsiveness. More recent studies suggest that early life viral infections can protect against the development of asthma. Further prospective studies are required to confirm the validity of the "hygiene" hypothesis.

REFERENCES

1.   Floyer J. A treatise of the asthma. London; 1698.
2.   Stevens FA. Acute asthmatic episodes in children caused by upper respiratory bacteria during colds, with and without bacterial sensitization. J Allergy 1953;24:221–6.
3.   Podosin RL, Felton WL. The clinical picture of Far-East influenza occurring at the 4th National Boy Scout Jamboree. N Engl J Med 1958;258:778–82.
4.   Rebhan AW. An outbreak of Asian influenza in a girls' camp. Can Med Assoc J 1957;77:797–9.
5.   Chanock R, Finberg L. Recovery from infants with respiratory illness of a virus related to chimpanzee coryza agent. II. Epidemiologic aspects of infection in infants and young children. Am J Hyg 1957;66:291–300.
6.   Freeman GL. Wheezing associated with respiratory tract infections in children: the role of specific infectious agents in allergic respiratory manifestations. Clin Pediatr 1966;5:586–92.
7.   Henderson FW, Clyde WA, Collier AM, et al. The etiologic and epidemiologic spectrum of bronchiolitis in pediatric practice. J Pediatr 1979;95:183–90.
8.   Adams F. The genuine works of Hippocrates. Baltimore: The Williams and Wilkins Co; 1939.
9.   Disney ME, Matthews R, Williams JD. The role of infection in the morbidity of asthmatic children admitted to hospital. Clin Allergy 1971;1:399–406.
10.   Storr J, Lenney W. School holidays and admissions with asthma. Arch Dis Child 1989;64:103–7.
11.   Ayres JG, Noah ND, Fleming DM. Incidence of episodes of acute asthma and acute bronchitis in general practice 1976–87. Br J Gen Pract 1993;43:361–4.
12.   Dales RE, Schweitzer I, Toogood JH, et al. Respiratory infections and the autumn increase in asthma morbidity. Eur Respir J 1996;9:72–7.
13.   Johnston SL, Pattemore PK, Sanderson G, et al. The relationship between upper and respiratory infections and hospital admissions for asthma: a time trend analysis. Am J Respir Crit Care Med 1996;154:654–60.
14.   Johnston SL, Pattemore PK, Sanderson G, et al. Community study of the role of viral infections in exacerbations of asthma in 9–11 year old children. BMJ 1995;310:1225–8.
15.   Pattemore PK, Johnston SL, Bardin PG. Viruses as precipitants of asthma symptoms. 1. Epidemiology. Clin Exp Allergy 1992;22:325–36.

16. Horn MEC, Brain EA, Gregg I, et al. Respiratory viral infection and wheezy bronchitis in childhood. Thorax 1979;34:23–8.

17. Mitchell I, Inglis JM, Simpson H. Viral infection as a precipitant of wheeze in children: combined home and hospital study. Arch Dis Child 1978;53:106–11.

18. Hudgel DW, Langston L, Selner JC, McIntosh K. Viral and bacterial infections in adults with chronic asthma. Am Rev Respir Dis 1979;120:393–7.

19. Jennings LC, Barns G, Dawson KP. The association of viruses with acute asthma. N Z Med J 1987;100:488–90.

20. Beasley R, Coleman ED, Hermon Y, et al. Viral respiratory tract infection and exacerbations of asthma in adult patients. Thorax 1988;43:679–83.

21. Horn MEC, Reed SA, Taylor P. Role of viruses and bacteria in acute wheezy bronchitis in childhood: a study of sputum. Arch Dis Child 1979;54:587–92.

22. McIntosh K, Ellis EF, Hoffman LS, et al. The association of viral and bacterial respiratory infections with exacerbations of wheezing in young asthmatic children. J Pediatr 1973;82:578–90.

23. Minor TE, Dick EC, DeMeo AN, et al. Viruses as precipitants of asthmatic attacks in children. JAMA 1974;227:292–8.

24. Roldaan AC, Masural N. Viral respiratory infections in asthmatic children staying in a mountain resort. Eur J Respir Dis 1982;63:140–50.

25. Mertsola J, Ziegler T, Ruuskanen O, et al. Recurrent wheezy bronchitis and viral respiratory infections. Arch Dis Child 1991;66:124–9.

26. Clarke CE. Relationship of bacterial and viral infections to exacerbations of asthma. Thorax 1979;34:344–7.

27. Nicholson KG, Kent J, Ireland DC. Respiratory viruses and exacerbations of asthma in adults. BMJ 1993;307:982–6.

28. Sly PD, Hibbert ME. Childhood asthma following hospitalization with acute viral bronchiolitis in infancy. Pediatr Pulmonol 1989;7:153–8.

29. Murray M, Webb MSC, O'Callaghan C, et al. Respiratory status and allergy after bronchiolitis. Arch Dis Child 1992;67:482–7.

30. Sigurs N, Bjarnason R, Sigurbergsson F, et al. Asthma and immunoglobulin E antibodies after respiratory syncytial virus bronchiolitis: a prospective cohort study with matched controls. Pediatrics 1995;95:500–5.

31. Martinez FD, Wright AL, Taussig LM, et al. Asthma and wheezing in the first six years of life. N Engl J Med 1995;323:133–8.

32. Wennergren G, Amark M, Amark K, et al. Wheezing bronchitis reinvestigated at the age of 10 years. Acta Paediatr 1997;86:351–5.

33. Holt PG, Sly PD. Allergic respiratory disease: strategic targets for primary prevention during childhood. Thorax 1997;52:1–4.

34. Anderson HR. Respiratory abnormalities in Papua New Guinea children: the effects of locality and domestic wood smoke pollution. Int J Epidemiol 1978;7:63–72.

35. Brown P, Gajdusek DC. Acute and chronic pulmonary airway disease in Pacific Island Micronesians. Am J Epidemiol 1978;108:266–73.

36. Strachan DP. Hay fever, hygiene and household size. Br Med J 1989;299:1259–60.

37. Strachan DP, Taylor EM, Carpenter RG. Family size, neonatal infection and hay fever in adolescence. Arch Dis Child 1996;74:422–6.

38. Von Mutius E, Martinez FD, Fritzsch C, et al. Prevalence of asthma and atopy in two areas of west and east Germany. Am J Respir Crit Care Med 1994;149:358–64.

39. Von Mutius E, Martinez FD, Fritzsch C, et al. Skin test reactivity and number of siblings. BMJ 1994;308:692–5.

40. Prescott S, Macaubas C, Smallacombe T, et al. Reciprocal age-related patterns of allergen specific T-cell immunity in normal versus atopic infants. Clin Exp Allergy 1998;28:39–44.

41. Romagnani S. Introduction of Th1 and Th2 responses: a key role for the 'natural' immune response? Immunol Today 1992;13:379–81.

42. Shirakawa T, Enomoto T, Shimazu S, Hopkin J. The inverse association between tuberculin responses and atopic disorder. Science 1997;275:77–9.

CHAPTER 9

Diagnosis and Management of Occupational Asthma

André Cartier, MD, FRCP
Catherine Lemière, MD, MSc

Asthma is the most common chronic respiratory disease, affecting about 5 to 10% of the population,[1] and is thus frequently encountered in the workplace. Consequently, physicians may be confronted with patients with either new-onset asthma or with uncontrolled disease for whom it is important to determine if work is responsible.

When asthma is caused by a specific agent, such as airborne dusts, gases, vapors, or fumes, found in the workplace and not stimuli encountered outside the workplace, it is called occupational asthma.[2,3] Two types of occupational asthma have been distinguished by whether they appear after a latency period.[2] The immunologic type, classically referred as occupational asthma (OA), is characterized by work-related asthma appearing after a latency period and includes (1) work-related asthma associated with mostly high- and some low-molecular-weight agents for which an immunologic mechanism (usually immunoglobulin E [IgE] mediated) has been identified and (2) asthma induced by specific occupational agents (eg, isocyanates, red cedar) for which an immunologic mechanism has not been clearly identified. The nonimmunologic type refers to irritant-induced asthma or reactive airways dysfunction syndrome (RADS), which may occur after single or multiple exposures to irritants, such as chlorine, in high concentrations. A previous history of asthma does not exclude the diagnosis of OA.

Occupational asthma thus excludes asthma that is triggered by irritant mechanisms such as cold air, exercise, or exposure to irritants in a poorly controlled or severe asthmatic subject. This exacerbation of asthma needs to be distinguished from OA as its management differs entirely: whereas subjects with OA need to be taken off work to prevent deterioration, most subjects with aggravation of underlying asthma can continue to work with proper asthma management and often with few workplace modifications. Other forms of variable airflow obstruction such as byssinosis (related to exposure to cotton dust) have also been described.[4]

IMMUNOLOGIC OCCUPATIONAL ASTHMA

Prevalence, Etiologies, and Risk Factors

Occupational asthma is the most frequent occupational lung disease.[5,6] The prevalence of occupational asthma among subjects with asthma has been estimated between 3 and 9%.[7–10] Several lists of known occupational agents have been published[11,12] and will need to be upgraded on a regular basis.

Several individual and industrial risk factors have been identified.[13] Among individual factors, atopy is the most important for high-molecular-weight agents (eg, bakers, laboratory animals handlers[14]); atopic individuals develop sensitization earlier and at lower exposures than nonatopic individuals.[15] However, the presence of atopy or skin-test sensitivity to a specific allergen is not sufficiently predictive of disease to justify exclusion of these individuals in high-risk industries.[16] Smoking is a risk factor in certain industries such a crab processing[17] and platinum refineries.[18] The role of nonallergic bronchial responsiveness (NABR) as a predisposing factor is unknown, although it is usually considered as an acquired phenomenon rather than a predisposing factor. Similarly, pre-existing asthma is not considered a risk factor for most low-molecular-weight agents but is associated with a higher risk of developing occupational asthma in atopic asthmatic patients exposed to high-molecular-weight agents. Genetic predispositions to develop occupational asthma are likely important as modulating factors.[19]

Among industrial factors, the type of agent comes first; isocyanates are among the most frequent agents responsible for occupational asthma in most industrial countries,[7,9,20,21] followed by flours and animals (see Table 9–1 for a short list of the most frequent causes). Obviously, the responsible agents will vary among countries in relation to the major industries. Finally, spills and high exposure to sensitizing agents are associated with higher risk of developing sensitization and disease.[15,22–24]

Table 9–1 *Frequent Causes of Occupational Asthma*

Type of Agent	*Occupations/Work Implements*
High molecular weight	
Flours, cereals	Bakers, millers
Animal danders and urine	Animal handlers
Latex	Dental hygienists, nurses
Enzymes—particularly α-amylase	Bakers
Enzymes and antibiotics	Pharmaceutical staff
Psyllium	Nurses, personnel of nursing homes
Crab	Crab processors
Low molecular weight	
Isocyanates (HDI, MDI, TDI, IPDI)	Spray paint, insulation, foam, glues
Wood dusts (red cedar, exotic woods)	Forest workers, carpenters (windows and doors)
Methacrylate, cyanoacrylates	Glues, dental prostheses
Dyes	Plastics, textiles
Phtalic anhydrides, phtalates	Paint, plastics
Colophony (flux)	Electronic solder

HDI = hexamethylene diisocyanate; MDI = methylene diphenyl isocyanate; TDI = toluene diisocyanate; IPDI = isophorone diisocyanate.

Investigation

As opposed to the traditional pneumoconiosis of which the diagnosis is based only on exposure history and chest radiograph abnormalities, occupational asthma can and should be confirmed by objective means (Level IIIA). Indeed, the social consequences of making or refuting such a diagnosis are important for both the worker and the employer. On one hand, to prevent further deterioration of asthma, it is essential to withdraw the worker from exposure to the offending agent;[25–27] this imposes a serious stress to the worker and his family and may mean loss of job or benefits or even moving to another town. On the other hand, removing from exposure a worker who does not have occupational asthma is not necessary adequate as environmental control (eg, reduction of exposure to irritants), and better control of asthma may be sufficient to allow the worker to continue his job without loss of income.

To avoid loss of income and frustration, a worker suspected of having occupational asthma should not automatically be withdrawn from work before the investigation is completed. If the asthma is too severe, it may be necessary to withdraw temporarily the worker from his job, but monitoring of the asthma, including spirometry, peak expiratory flows (PEF), and assessment of NABR should be started without any delay.

As reviewed elsewhere,[3,28,29] the steps to perform in the investigation of occupational asthma are history, pulmonary function tests, details on the workplace, immunologic tests, combined monitoring of PEF and NABR, and specific bronchial challenges.

History

The questionnaire is the essential tool used in most epidemiologic surveys and all individual assessments. The classic history of occupational asthma is one of a worker whose asthma is worse at work and improves over weekends or holidays. However, this pattern is often absent as symptoms also are usually present outside the workplace, triggered by exposure to irritants such as cold air or fumes, or upon exercise. In many cases, symptoms are more severe at home, awaking the subject at night, and weekends may not be long enough to allow recovery. A previous history of asthma may also postpone the diagnosis.

The concomitant occurrence of rhinoconjunctivitis at work and occasionally of skin rash (urticaria), especially in a worker exposed to high-molecular-weight chemicals who develops asthma, is suggestive of occupational asthma. Chan-Yeung and Desjardins recently showed that rhinitis occurring in workers exposed to red cedar may be a predisposing factor for developing occupational asthma.[23] Furthermore, rhinitis often precedes or coincides with the development of occupational asthma, especially for those working with high-molecular-weight chemicals.[30] Symptoms may develop after only a few weeks or after several years; duration of exposure tends to be shorter for low-molecular-weight chemicals.[31]

However, a history suggestive of occupational asthma, even in a worker exposed to a known sensitizer, is not sufficient to make the diagnosis (Level IIA). Indeed, even in the hands of expert physicians, we showed in a prospective study of 162 workers referred for occupational asthma that the predictive value of a positive questionnaire was only 63%, whereas the predictive value of a negative questionnaire was 83%.[32] Therefore, in more than one-third of cases, objective testing showed that the subjects did not have occupational asthma even though the initial questionnaire had been highly suggestive.

Pulmonary Function Tests

Although the diagnosis of asthma can be confirmed by the presence of reversible airflow obstruction, for example, increase of forced expiratory volume in 1 second (FEV_1) greater than 12 to 15% after β_2-agonist inhalation, most workers investigated for occupational asthma have normal spirometry when seen in the clinic. Pre- and post-shift monitoring of FEV_1 has not proven sensitive or specific enough to be a useful tool in the investigation of occupational asthma.[33–35]

Increased NABR is the hallmark of asthma, but it is also present in other conditions such as rhinitis and chronic obstructive pulmonary disease (COPD). Therefore, the presence of increased NABR does not make the diagnosis of occupational asthma (Level IIA). It may suggest that the subject has occupational asthma, common asthma, or other conditions with increased NABR. There is a need for further confirmation of work-related asthma.

The absence of increased NABR as assessed shortly (minutes or hours) after a work shift in a worker who complains of symptoms virtually excludes occupational asthma (Level IIIB; although, in rare instances, specific inhalation challenges have been positive in workers without increased NABR[36–38]). However, even in the presence of occupational asthma, NABR may be normal in a worker who has left work for several days (a weekend may be enough[39]), weeks, or months. Return to work or specific inhalation tests can then increase the bronchial responsiveness in the asthmatic range.[36,40,41]

Details on the Workplace

It is essential to obtain a list of the different agents used at work by the subject and colleagues to try to identify the product or process that is likely the cause. Material safety data sheets (MSDS) of the different products used in the plant may help to identify potential sensitizers, ,but, unfortunately, some of these MSDS do not give information on products that are found in concentrations lower than 1%, even though these may be potent sensitizers. Enquiring about other workers with respiratory complaints may also increase the suspicion of occupational asthma.

Immunologic Testing

The presence of immediate skin reactivity or increased specific IgE or IgG antibodies may reflect exposure and/or sensitization to a suspected agent, but it does not imply that the target organs (the bronchi in this instance) are involved (Level IIA). This has been shown for common allergens and occupational sensitizers such as snow crab,[42] psyllium,[34] and isocyanates.[43] With high-molecular-weight agents for which good extracts are available, such as cereals, latex, or psyllium, negative skin tests to these allergens cannot entirely exclude the diagnosis of occupational asthma, but they make it unlikely; however, the worker may be sensitized to another agent found in the workplace or the extract may not be available or adequate. Indeed, in snow crab processors, the odds for the presence of occupational asthma in a subject with positive skin tests to snow crab extract or radioallergosorbent test [RAST] ratio > 4.5 were respectively 69% and 79%, whereas the odds for the absence of occupational asthma in a subject with negative skin test or RAST ratio < 4.5 were 76% and 73%, respectively.[42] With low-molecular-weight agents such as isocyanates and red cedar, negative skin tests or specific IgE or IgG do not refute or make the diagnosis of occupational asthma;[43,44] furthermore, skin tests are most often unavailable.

Monitoring of PEF and NABR

The availability of portable, inexpensive devices has allowed physicians to monitor PEF at and away from work. This approach was first used in the investigation of work-related asthma by Burge et al.[45,46] The usefulness of PEF monitoring in diagnosing occupational asthma has been recently reviewed.[47,48]

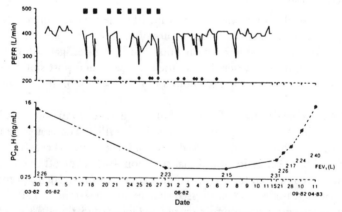

Figure 9–1 Combined monitoring of PEF rate (PEFR) (*upper panel*) and PC$_{20}$ (*lower panel*) in the same subject before and after return to work. *Squares* represent the time spent at work, whereas *diamonds* illustrate the use of inhaled salbutamol (albuterol). Baseline FEV$_1$ values before each histamine inhalation test are illustrated. They vary by no more than 6% from one test to another. (Reproduced with permission from Cartier A, Malo JL, Forest F, et al. Occupational asthma in snow crab–processing workers. J Allergy Clin Immunol 1984;74:261–9.)

The patient should be carefully instructed in the correct use of the PEF meter and asked to perform readings at least four times a day (preferably every 2 hours[49]) during several weeks at and away from work. On each occasion, three readings should be done and recorded in a diary. Records are interpreted by either plotting the individual PEF recordings against time, with working hours identified (Figure 9–1), or by plotting the recordings as maximum, mean, and minimum against time, as proposed by Gannon and Burge.[50] The sensitivity and specificity of PEF monitoring in confirming occupational asthma were assessed prospectively in two studies using specific inhalation challenges as the gold standard for diagnosing occupational asthma.[51,52] Sensitivity and specificity were 81 to 89% and 74 to 89%, respectively. Similar findings have been shown by others,[53] although Burge et al[45,46] showed a greater sensitivity of 100% and a specificity of 77%. "Eyeballing" the deterioration of asthma while at work is still the best way to evaluate changes in PEF.[52,54] Worsening of PEF at work versus PEF away from work suggests occupational asthma; no objective criterion has been universally accepted, but diurnal variation of PEF greater than 20% is suggestive of asthma, and if it occurs more frequently on working days, it may suggest occupational asthma. A computer-assisted diagnostic aid (OASYS-2) has been developed by Gannon et al[55] and is based on a scoring system developed from visual analysis; this system may help the clinician to interpret these results.

The poor sensitivity or specificity of PEF monitoring in certain subjects as compared to specific bronchial challenges can be explained by several means. Even if performed under close supervision of a technician, PEF monitoring may greatly underestimate or overestimate changes in airway caliber as assessed by FEV_1.[56–58] Furthermore, PEFs are effort dependent, and thus require collaboration of the worker, which is not always obtained due to fear of losing the job or malingering to get some compensation benefit. Two recent studies, in which subjects were unaware that PEF data was being stored on a computer chip, have shown that many workers will falsify their records: approximately 50% of values are inaccurately reported on diaries either in terms of the recorded value or the timing of the measurement.[59,60]

The minimum period of monitoring should be at least 2 weeks at work and 2 weeks away from work to be able to draw some conclusions. In certain situations, particularly when asthma is severe or when the nature of the offending agent is unknown and intermittent, the interpretation of the monitoring may be difficult.[52] Subjects should be asked to take their β_2-agonists on demand only and should continue their regular inhaled corticosteroids and, if taken, their theophylline at the same dosage throughout the entire monitoring period; the use of long-acting β_2-agonists or leukotriene receptor antagonists may mask significant changes due to work and usually is not recommended unless the asthma is not controlled. Reduction of corticosteroids upon return to work may be associated with deterioration of asthma and mistaken as being diagnostic of occupational asthma. In severe asthmatic patients, it may be necessary to withdraw the subject from work until the asthma is under control with minimum treatment; deterioration of asthma upon return to work may then suggest that asthma is caused by work.

Coupling PEF monitoring and changes in NABR for periods at and away from work has also been proposed.[51,52,61] Nonallergic bronchial responsiveness can be assessed by several means, but methacholine and histamine inhalation challenges with determination of the provocative concentration inducing a 20% fall in FEV_1 (PC_{20}) are the most reliable, and they are well standardized. Indeed, whereas exposure to irritants does not induce marked and prolonged changes in NABR, except in cases of RADS, occupational asthma may be associated with significant and often long-lasting changes in NABR.[62] Even if PC_{20} monitoring at and away from work does not improve the sensitivity or specificity of PEF monitoring in diagnosing occupational asthma,[51,52] many investigators recommend that monitoring of PEF is coupled to monitoring of NABR: when changes in PEF are associated with parallel changes in NABR, the diagnosis of occupational asthma is highly probable, and there is no need for further investigation if the suspected agent is known (Level IA). When monitoring of PEF and NABR shows no evidence of asthma in a symptomatic subject while at work, the diagnosis of occupational asthma usually can be excluded (Level IIA). If the monitoring of PEF and NABR are discordant, further investigations should be completed such as specific bronchial challenges in the workplace or in the laboratory (Level IIB). Worsening of PEF at work with no changes in PC_{20} may support a diagnosis of asthma aggravated at work by an irritant exposure (Level IIIB).

Although monitoring of PEF and NABR are useful tools, they are time consuming, require subjects' collaboration, and may be hazardous in workers with a history of severe asthma at work, as exposure may not be titrated as easily as when the challenge is done in the laboratory. Monitoring of PEF and NABR is particularly useful as a screening procedure, when the worker is exposed to several sensitizers or when the offending agent is unknown, but they do not identify the sensitizing agent.

Specific Inhalation Challenges

Specific inhalation challenges are considered the gold standard to confirm the diagnosis of occupational asthma.[28,63–66] Originally done in the laboratory and aimed at mimicking work exposure,[67] they are now often done in the workplace.[17,68]

These tests are safe when performed under the close supervision of an expert physician and by trained personnel and are thus limited to specialized centers. Resuscitative measures should be available. When performed in the laboratory, the exposure chambers should be well ventilated and enclosed to minimize exposure to the personnel. In most subjects, the tests can be carried out on an outpatient basis.

Although there is no standardized protocol, the methodology is well developed.[64–66] Drugs should be withheld before specific bronchial challenges according to standard recommendations.[65] In all cases, spirometry (FEV_1 and forced vital capacity [FVC]) should be monitored for at least 8 hours on a control day to ensure stability of airway caliber. If the subject shows too much variability of his FEV_1 (> 10%) or if the FEV_1 is too low, the tests should be postponed, and asthma should be controlled by adjusting the medication. At the end of the control day, a methacholine challenge test is done to determine the PC_{20}. This value may help to determine the starting concentration to the offending agent on the next day—the lower the PC_{20}, the lower the exposure. Whereas FEV_1 is the standard parameter used to assess airway caliber, PEF is not reliable enough, as it may underestimate or overestimate changes;[56] measures of airway resistance (Raw) are also not reliable enough.

When performed in the laboratory, specific bronchial challenges can be done in several ways, depending on the nature of the agent (ie, powder, aerosol, liquid, or gas). With powders, such as flour, psyllium, or red cedar, the subject may be exposed to a fine dust, mimicking work exposure,[67] either by pouring the dust from one tray to another or by using dust generators[69–71] that allow proper monitoring, regulation of exposure, and establishment of dose-response curves, and reduce the risk of severe or irritant reactions. Alternatively, the worker may be exposed to an aerosol of a crude extract. Exposure to nonpowder agents is usually done by reproducing work environment, for example, by nebulizing an aerosol of the isocyanate hardener or by having the worker breathe over a bottle of methacrylate glue. Isocyanates and other gases can also be generated in their gaseous or aerosolized form in a small chamber to improve safety of exposure.[69–71] Whenever possible, the level of exposure should be monitored to avoid high exposure and, therefore, irritant reactions. In most cases, exposure is done in an open fashion, with the subject knowing the nature of the exposure. Baseline spirometry on each exposure day should be reproducible (ie, ± 10% of the control day). Exposure should always be progressive, the total duration of exposure being a function of the type of agent and the history given by the subject; rarely, total exposure is more than 2 hours and this may be achieved over 1 or several days. If there is no significant change in FEV_1

on the last exposure day, a significant change in PC_{20}, as assessed at the end of that day, may suggest that an additional exposure may then trigger an asthmatic reaction.[72]

Tests in the workplace are particularly useful when the relevant agent at work is unknown, when there are several potential sensitizing agents, or when there is discordance between PEF and NABR monitoring. They are also done stepwise, although usually total exposure equals the length of a work shift. Spirometry is followed in the same way throughout the day.[17,68] Exposure to the offending agent is, however, less well controlled than in the laboratory, and it may be difficult to ensure that the subject really is exposed to the relevant agent at work. However, this may be the only way to confirm the diagnosis of occupational asthma, especially in cases in which the nature of the offending agent is unknown.

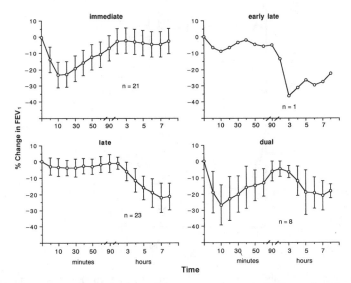

Figure 9–2 Mean ± SD or individual values of the percent change in FEV_1 as a function of time since exposure for the four typical patterns of reactions. The numbers of individuals for each pattern are presented. (Reproduced with permission from Perrin B, Cartier A, Ghezzo H, et al. Reassessment of the temporal patterns of bronchial obstruction after exposure to occupational sensitizing agents. J Allergy Clin Immunol 1991;87:630–9.)

A significant reaction is defined as a 20% fall in FEV_1. Typical patterns of bronchial reactions have been described (Figure 9–2).[67,73] Immediate reactions are maximal between 10 and 30 minutes after exposure with complete recovery within 1 to 2 hours; although usually readily reversible by inhaled β_2-agonists, they actually are the most dangerous as they can be severe and unpredictable, particularly in subjects for whom skin tests with the suspecting agent are not possible, stressing the importance of progressive exposure. Late reactions develop slowly and progressively either 1 to 2 hours ("early late") or 4 to 8 hours (late) after exposure; they may occasionally be accompanied by fever and general malaise, but extrinsic alveolitis should be then considered. Contrary to popular belief, they generally respond well to inhaled β_2-agonist, although the response may be of shorter duration in some subjects.[74] Dual reactions are a combination of early and late. A recurrent nocturnal asthma pattern has also been described and is likely related to an increase in NABR following exposure.[75]

Atypical patterns (Figure 9–3) have also been described (particularly with isocyanates):[73] they include the progressive type (starting within minutes after end of exposure and progressing over the next 7 to 8 hours), the square-waved reaction (with no recovery between the immediate and late components of the reaction), and, finally, the prolonged immediate type with slow recovery. Irritant reactions have not been well defined yet, but falls in FEV_1 that

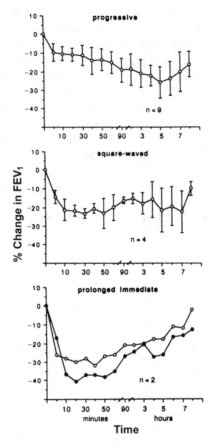

Figure 9–3 Mean ± SD or individual values of the percent change in FEV$_1$ as a function of time since exposure for the three atypical patterns of reactions. The numbers of individuals for each pattern are presented. (Reproduced with permission from Perrin B, Cartier A, Ghezzo H, et al. Reassessment of the temporal patterns of bronchial obstruction after exposure to occupational sensitizing agents. J Allergy Clin Immunol 1991;87:630–9.)

recover rapidly within 10 or 20 minutes are suggestive of an irritant pattern. It may be impossible to interpret results of specific bronchial challenges in a subject with too much variability of FEV$_1$, stressing the importance of an adequate control day.

A positive test confirms the diagnosis of occupational asthma (Level IA), whereas a negative test in the workplace, or in the laboratory, does not absolutely rule out the diagnosis of occupational asthma in a worker who has not been exposed to work for several months (Level IIB), as he may have become "desensitized";[17,41,72] this is particularly true if there is a change in PC$_{20}$ following the specific challenges.[41,72] The worker should be returned to work with monitoring of PEF and bronchial responsiveness for at least a few weeks before excluding the diagnosis. False-negative challenges in the laboratory may also be due to exposure to the wrong agent or administration of a preventive drug (such as an inhaled β$_2$-agonist) before the test. However, if the subject had symptoms during the challenge procedure without any change in spirometry, these tests are conclusive and exclude the diagnosis of occupational asthma (Level IIIA).

Prognosis

Occupational asthma is not a self-limited disease; it can induce long-lasting sequelae, with more than 50% of workers still being symptomatic after leaving work and the majority still showing abnormal PC$_{20}$.[26,76–78] A plateau of improvement in pulmonary function tests may be seen after 2 years,[79,80] although some workers still show a greater improvement at 5 years.[81] Severity of asthma at the time of diagnosis (as assessed by FEV_1 and PC_{20}) as well as duration of exposure after onset of symptoms are the major determinants of clinical outcome.[81,82] The majority of workers who continue their exposure, even if reduced, will show a deterioration of their spirometry and NABR.[83] Long-term protective equipment such as a mask has yet to be proven effective.[83,84] Early and complete withdrawal from exposure to the sensitizing agent is thus essential to prevent permanent sequelae. There is some evidence that early administration of inhaled corticosteroids may improve the outcome of affected workers.[85,86]

Management

Although affected individuals should be removed completely from exposure to the sensitizing agent as early as possible to obtain the best outcome of their asthma, this should not be done until the diagnosis is confirmed objectively, unless the worker is too sick (Level IIIA). When the investigation is done, the treatment of asthma should be appropriately adjusted. Referral to specialized centers may facilitate the investigation. Proper rehabilitation programs should be offered to these workers. Appropriate referral to Workers' Compensation Boards should be done when indicated. In determining whether compensation should be given to the affected worker, level of airways obstruction, PC_{20}, and need of medication to control symptoms should be considered.[5,87–89]

Screening and Surveillance

Pre-employment screening including skin tests to common or specific allergens and assessment of PC_{20} should not be used to exclude subjects from employment;[90] however, they may serve as a reference if a worker develops symptoms. In high-risk industries, surveillance programs should be implemented, although the value of this approach has only been proven in the case of isocyanate asthma.[91] These programs should include information for the worker and employers. A simple questionnaire is probably the most sensitive index for surveillance, the prospective use of spirometry and PC_{20} still being research tools; in certain industries, prospective skin testing (eg, with detergent enzymes) have proven useful to detect early sensitization and progression of disease. Identification of a worker with occupational asthma should be viewed as an alerting event[92] and prompt collaborative efforts between occupational physicians and company management to identify other cases of occupational asthma and to improve work hygiene to avoid or limit workers' exposure. Primary prevention of occupational asthma can be achieved only by reducing exposure to sensitizing agents, for example, by improving ventilation or by reducing direct exposure through modification of processes.

Conclusion

Asthma is one of the most frequent occupational lung diseases. Its diagnosis should be based on objective means and cannot rely only on history or even on confirmation of the presence of asthma and exposure to a known sensitizing agent. Monitoring of PEF and PC_{20} is a useful tool, but it may not be sufficiently sensitive or specific in certain cases. Specific inhalation challenges in the laboratory or workplace are the gold standard for confirming the diagnosis of occupational asthma, but they should be done under the supervision of expert physicians. Early withdrawal from exposure is essential to improve the outcome of occupational asthma, but this should not be done before the diagnosis is confirmed to avoid unnecessary loss of income and frustration.

IRRITANT-INDUCED ASTHMA

Reactive airway dysfunction syndrome (RADS; nonimmunologic) was first described in 1985 as the occurrence of asthmatic symptoms within 24 hours after a single high-level exposure to an irritant gas, vapor, or fume with persistence of reversible airflow obstruction and/or air-way responsiveness for several months.[93] The original diagnosis criteria have been modified and extended to the occurrence of asthmatic symptoms following repetitive exposure to moderate to high levels of an irritant agent.[94–96] This condition has been labeled "irritant-induced asthma."

Prevalence

The prevalence of RADS or irritant-induced asthma is difficult to assess. Some cohort stud-ies tried to determine the prevalence of irritant-induced asthma in workers exposed repeti-tively to chlorine. They found little impact of gassing events on the respiratory function in nonsmokers and were not able to determine a prevalence of irritant-induced asthma because of minimal physiologic alterations found in the subjects.[97,98] However, there was a tendency to increased airway responsiveness with increasing levels of exposure (Level IIA).[98] In the cohort assessed by Gautrin et al,[98] 13 subjects were assessed after gassing events that led to treatment in first aid unit. Two subjects had a significant increase in airway responsiveness, and 1 had a 9.5% fall in his FEV_1.[99] Therefore, 2 subjects of 13 (15.4%) met the criteria for diagnosis of irritant-induced asthma. Review of files of workers referred to the Ontario Workers' Compensation Board suggested that 6% of cases were caused by high-level irritant exposure at work.[78]

Diagnosis

The diagnosis of irritant-induced asthma or RADS is based mostly on retrospective history and two findings: (1) the onset of asthma-like symptoms within 24 hours after exposure to a high concentration of irritant agent in a subject without previous history of respiratory symptoms and (2) the persistence of airway obstruction or hyper-responsiveness. Specific inhalation challenges or monitoring of PEF and PC_{20} at and away from work are not useful, nor are they indicated unless there is a suspicion of immunologic occupational asthma.

Outcome

The time course of irritant-induced asthma is variable. Some subjects report improvement of symptoms and become completely asymptomatic within a few months.[100–103] Others complain of persistent asthma for several years after the offending exposure.[93,104–106] A case-control study of 15 subjects with RADS assessed 12 months after the initial exposure to an irritant compared with 30 subjects with occupational asthma showed that subjects with RADS had a lower reversibility of their FEV_1 after short acting β_2-agonists than subjects with occupational asthma (Level IIB).[106]

Predisposing Factors

Pre-existing airway hyper-responsiveness has been thought to be a predisposing factor to development RADS.[107] However, it has been shown in firefighters[108] that airway hyper-respon-siveness does not predispose to the development of RADS (Level IID). Recently, Brooks et al differentiated two groups of subjects with irritant-induced asthma: subjects with sudden onset of asthma with development of asthmatic symptoms within 24 hours after exposure (initially called RADS) and subjects with not-so-sudden onset of asthma whose the symp-toms occurred over longer periods of lesser exposure.[109] There was a higher rate of atopic asthma among subjects with not-so-sudden onset of asthma (88%) compared with those with sudden onset of asthma (52%). Forty percent of subjects reporting not-so-sudden onset of asthma had pre-existing asthma versus 21% of those reporting a sudden onset. It seems that atopic status and pre-existing asthma are important risks factors for developing irritant-induced asthma (Level IIB). Smoking and gassing might also interact to induce airflow limi-tation (Level IIB).[97]

Treatment

Subjects with RADS should be treated as are any other asthmatic patients. Although some reports suggest that early use of oral or inhaled corticosteroids after the accidental exposure could improve outcome,[110,111] prospective randomized control trials are lacking.

Management

In contrast to patients with immunologic occupational asthma, those with RADS or irritant-induced asthma can generally continue the same work, if provisions are made to reduce the risk of a similar accident, if environmental control ensures proper reduced levels of irritants in the air, and if asthma is properly managed. Follow-up of these workers is required to ensure that exposure did not also result in sensitization, particularly with potent sensitizers such as isocyanates.[104,112]

REFERENCES

1. Lebowitz MD. The trends in airway obstructive disease morbidity in the Tucson Epidemiological Study. Am Rev Respir Dis 1989;140:S35–41.

2. Bernstein IL, Chan-Yeung M, Malo JL, et al. Definition and classification of asthma. In: Bernstein IL, Chan-Yeung M, Malo JL, Bernstein DI, editors. Asthma in the work place. New York: Marcel Dekker Inc; 1993. p. 1–4.

3. Tarlo SM, Boulet LP, Cartier A, et al. Canadian Thoracic Society. Guidelines for occupational asthma. Can Respir J 1998;5:289–300.

4. Merchant JA, Bernstein IL. Cotton and other textile dusts. In: Bernstein IL, Chan-Yeung M, Malo JL, Bernstein DI, editors. Asthma in the workplace. New York: Marcel Dekker Inc; 1993. p. 551–76.

5. Malo JL. Compensation for occupational asthma in Quebec. Chest 1990;98:236–9S.

6. Meyer JD, Holt DL, Cherry NM, McDonald JC. SWORD '98: surveillance of work-related and occupational respiratory disease in the UK. Occup Med 1999;49:485–9.

7. Meredith S, Nordman H. Occupational asthma: measures of frequency from four countries. Thorax 1996;51:435–40.

8. Reijula K, Haahtela T, Klaukka T, Rantanen J. Incidence of occupational asthma and persistent asthma in young adults has increased in Finland. Chest 1996;110:58–61.

9. Kogevinas M, Anto JM, Soriano JB, et al. The risk of asthma attributable to occupational exposures. A population-based study in Spain. Spanish Group of the European Asthma Study. Am J Respir Crit Care Med 1996;154:137–43.

10. Blanc PD, Toren K. How much adult asthma can be attributed to occupational factors? Am J Med 1999;107:580–7.

11. Chan-Yeung M, Malo JL. Aetiological agents in occupational asthma. Eur Respir J 1994;7:346–71.

12. Chan-Yeung M, Malo JL. Tables of major inducers of occupational asthma. In: Bernstein IL, Chan-Yeung M, Malo JL, Bernstein DI, editors. Asthma in the workplace. New York: Marcel Dekker Inc; 1999. p. 683–720.

13. Malo JL, Chan-Yeung M. Population surveys of occupational asthma. In: Bernstein IL, Chan-Yeung M, Malo JL, Bernstein DI, editors. Asthma in the workplace. New York: Marcel Dekker Inc; 1993. p. 145–70.

14. Aoyama K, Ueda A, Manda F, et al. Allergy to laboratory animals: an epidemiological study. Br J Indust Med 1992;49:41–7.

15. Houba R, Heederik DJ, Doekes G, van Run PE. Exposure-sensitization relationship for alpha-amylase allergens in the baking industry. Am J Respir Crit Care Med 1996;154:130–6.

16. What are the health risks of employees with a history of asthma when placed as handlers in an animal research facility? J Occup Med 1994;36:296–7.

17. Cartier A, Malo JL, Forest F, et al. Occupational asthma in snow crab–processing workers. J Allergy Clin Immunol 1984;74:261–9.

18. Calverley AE, Rees D, Dowdeswell RJ, et al. Platinum salt sensitivity in refinery workers—incidence and effects of smoking and exposure. Occup Environ Med 1995;52:661–6.

19. Newman Taylor AJ. Genetics and occupational asthma. In: Bernstein IL, Chan-Yeung M, Malo JL, Bernstein DI, editors. Asthma in the workplace. New York: Marcel Dekker Inc; 1999. p. 67–80.

20. Keynes HL, Ross DJ, McDonald JC. SWORD '95—surveillance of work-related and occupational respiratory disease in the UK. Occup Med (Oxf) 1996;46:379–81.

21. Ross DJ, Sallie BA, McDonald JC. SWORD '94—surveillance of work-related and occupational respiratory disease in the UK. Occup Med (Oxf) 1995;45:175–8.

22. Butcher B, Jones R, O'Neil C, et al. Longitudinal study of workers employed in the manufacture of toluene diisocyanate. Am Rev Respir Dis 1977;116:411–21.

23. Chan-Yeung M, Desjardins A. Bronchial hyperresponsiveness and level of exposure in occupational asthma due to western red cedar (Thuja plicata). Serial observations before and after development of symptoms. Am Rev Respir Dis 1992;146:1606–9.

24. Cullinan P, Cook A, Gordon S, et al. Allergen exposure, atopy and smoking as determinants of allergy to rats in a cohort of laboratory employees. Eur Respir J 1999;13:1139–43.

25. Pisati G, Baruffini A, Zedda S. Toluene diisocyanate induced asthma: outcome according to persistence or cessation of exposure. Br J Ind Med 1993;50:60–4.

26. Paggiaro PL, Vagaggini B, Bacci E, et al. Prognosis of occupational asthma. Eur Respir J 1994;7:761–7.

27. Chan-Yeung M, Malo JL. Natural history of occupational asthma. In: Bernstein IL, Chan-Yeung M, Malo JL, Bernstein DI, editors. Asthma in the workplace. New York: Marcel Dekker Inc; 1999. p. 129–43.

28. Chan-Yeung M, Malo JL. Occupational asthma. Chest 1987;91:130–6S.

29. Cartier A. Definition and diagnosis of occupational asthma. Eur Respir J 1994;7:153–60.

30. Lemière C, Malo JL, Desjardins A, et al. Symptoms of rhinoconjunctivitis are often associated with occupational asthma, are generally milder and do not precede its onset in the case low-molecular-weight agents [abstract]. J Allergy Clin Immunol 1997;99 (Pt 2):S80.

31. Malo JL, Ghezzo H, D'Aquino C, et al. Natural history of occupational asthma: relevance of type of agent and other factors in the rate of development of symptoms in affected subjects. J Allergy Clin Immunol 1992;90:937–44.

32. Malo JL, Ghezzo H, L'Archevêque J, et al. Is the clinical history a satisfactory means of diagnosing occupational asthma? Am Rev Respir Dis 1991;143:528–32.

33. Malo JL, Cartier A. Occupational asthma in workers of a pharmaceutical company processing spiramycin. Thorax 1988;43:371–7.

34. Bardy JD, Malo JL, Séguin P, et al. Occupational asthma and IgE sensitization in a pharmaceutical company processing psyllium. Am Rev Respir Dis 1987;135:1033–8.

35. Burge PS. Single and serial measurements of lung function in the diagnosis of occupational asthma. Eur J Respir Dis 1982;63 Suppl 123:47–59.

36. Smith AB, Brooks SM, Blanchard J, et al. Absence of airway hyperreactivity to methacholine in a worker sensitized to toluene diisocyanate. J Occup Med 1980;22:327–31.

37. Banks DE, Barkman WHJ, Butcher BT, et al. Absence of hyperresponsiveness to methacholine in a worker with methylene diphenyl diisocyanate (MDI)-induced asthma. Chest 1986;89:389–93.

38. Weytjens K, Cartier A, Lemière C, Malo JL. Occupational asthma to diacrylate. Allergy 1999;54:289–90.

39. Cockcroft DW, Mink JT. Isocyanate-induced asthma in an automobile spray painter. Can Med Assoc J 1979;121:602–4.

40. Hargreave FE, Ramsdale EH, Pugsley SO. Occupational asthma without bronchial hyperresponsiveness. Am Rev Respir Dis 1984;130:513–5.

41. Lemière C, Cartier A, Dolovich J, et al. Outcome of specific bronchial responsiveness to occupational agents after removal from exposure. Am J Respir Crit Care Med 1996;154:329–33.

42. Cartier A, Malo JL, Ghezzo H, et al. IgE sensitization in snow crab–processing workers. J Allergy Clin Immunol 1986;78:344–8.

43. Cartier A, Grammer L, Malo JL, et al. Specific serum antibodies against isocyanates: association with occupational asthma. J Allergy Clin Immunol 1989;84:507–14.

44. Tse KS, Chan H, Chan-Yeung M. Specific IgE antibodies in workers with occupational asthma due to western red cedar. Clin Allergy 1982;12:249–58.

45. Burge PS, O'Brien I, Harries M. Peak flow rate records in the diagnosis of occupational asthma due to isocyanates. Thorax 1979;34:317–23.

46. Burge PS, O'Brien I, Harries M. Peak flow rate records in the diagnosis of occupational asthma due to colophony. Thorax 1979;34:308–16.

47. Moscato G, Godnic-Cvar J, Maestrelli P. Statement on self-monitoring of peak expiratory flows in the investigation of occupational asthma. Subcommittee on Occupational Allergy of European Academy of Allergy and Clinical Immunology. J Allergy Clin Immunol 1995;96:295–301.

48. Bright P, Burge PS. Occupational lung disease. The diagnosis of occupational asthma from serial measurements of lung function at and away from work. Thorax 1996;51:857–63.

49. Malo JL, Côté J, Cartier A, et al. How many times per day should peak expiratory flows be assessed when investigating occupational asthma? Thorax 1993;48:1211–7.

50. Gannon PFG, Burge PS. Serial peak expiratory flow measurement in the diagnosis of occupational asthma [abstract]. Eur Respir J 1997;10 Suppl 24:57–63s.

51. Côté J, Kennedy S, Chan-Yeung M. Sensitivity and specificity of PC20 and peak expiratory flow in cedar asthma. J Allergy Clin Immunol 1990;85:592–8.

52. Perrin B, Lagier F, L'Archevêque J, et al. Occupational asthma: validity of monitoring of peak expiratory flows and non-allergic bronchial responsiveness as compared to specific inhalation challenge. Eur Respir J 1992;5:40–8.

53. Liss GM, Tarlo SM. peak expiratory flows in possible occupational asthma. Chest 1991;100:63–9.

54. Côté J, Kennedy S, Chan-Yeung M. Quantitative versus qualitative analysis of peak expiratory flow in occupational asthma. Thorax 1993;48:48–51.

55. Gannon PFG, Newton DT, Belcher J, et al. Development of OASYS-2—a system for the analysis of serial measurement of peak expiratory flow in workers with suspected occupational asthma. Thorax 1996; 51:484–9.

56. Bérubé D, Cartier A, L'Archevêque J, Ghezzo H, Malo JL. Comparison of peak expiratory flow and FEV_1 in assessing bronchomotor tone after challenges with occupational sensitizers. Chest 1991;99:831–6.

57. Gautrin D, D'Aquino LC, Gagnon G, et al. Comparison between peak expiratory flow rates (PEFR) and FEV_1 in the monitoring of asthmatic subjects at the outpatient clinic. Chest 1994;106:1419–26.

58. Moscato G, Dellabianca A, Paggiaro P, et al. Peak expiratory flow monitoring and airway response to specific bronchial provocation tests in asthmatic patients. Monaldi Arch Chest Dis 1993;48:23–8.

59. Malo JL, Trudeau C, Ghezzo H, et al. Do subjects investigated for occupational asthma through serial peak expiratory flow measurements falsify their results? J Allergy Clin Immunol 1995;96:601–7.

60. Quirce S, Contreras G, Dybuncio A, Chan-Yeung M. Peak expiratory flow monitoring is not a reliable method for establishing the diagnosis of occupational asthma. Am J Respir Crit Care Med 1995;152:1100–2.

61. Cartier A, Pineau L, Malo JL. Monitoring of maximum expiratory peak flow rates and histamine inhalation tests in the investigation of occupational asthma. Clin Allergy 1984;14:193–6.

62. Chan-Yeung M. Nonspecific bronchial hyperresponsiveness. In: Bernstein IL, Chan-Yeung M, Malo JL, Bernstein DI, editors. Asthma in the workplace. New York: Marcel Dekker Inc; 1993. p.189–214.

63. Canadian Thoracic Society. Occupational asthma: recommendations for diagnosis, management and assessment of impairment. Can Med Assoc J 1989;140:1029–32.

64. Cartier A, Malo JL. Occupational challenge tests. In: Bernstein IL, Chan-Yeung M, Malo JL, Bernstein DI, editors. Asthma in the workplace. New York: Marcel Dekker Inc; 1993. p. 215–48.

65. Cartier A, Bernstein IL, Burge PS, et al. Guidelines for bronchoprovocation on the investigation of occupational asthma. Report of the Subcommittee on Bronchoprovocation for Occupational Asthma. J Allergy Clin Immunol 1989;84:823–9.

66. EAACI. Guidelines for the diagnosis of occupational asthma. Subcommittee on "Occupational Allergy" of the European Academy of Allergology and Clinical Immunology. Clin Exp Allergy 1992;22:103–8.

67. Pepys J, Hutchcroft BJ. Bronchial provocation tests in etiologic diagnosis and analysis of asthma. Am Rev Respir Dis 1975;112:829–59.

68. Chan-Yeung M, McMurren T, Catonio-Begley F, Lam S. Occupational asthma in a technologist exposed to glutaraldehyde. J Allergy Clin Immunol 1993;91:974–8.

69. Cloutier Y, Malo JL. Update on an exposure system for particles in the diagnosis of occupational asthma. Eur Respir J 1992;5:887–90.

70. Cloutier Y, Lagier F, Cartier A, Malo JL. Validation of an exposure system to particles for the diagnosis of occupational asthma. Chest 1992;102:402–7.

71. Cloutier Y, Lagier F, Lemieux R, et al. New methodology for specific inhalation challenges with occupational agents in powder form. Eur Respir J 1989;2:769–77.

72. Vandenplas O, Delwiche JP, Jamart J, Vandeweyer R. Increase in non-specific bronchial hyperresponsiveness as an early marker of bronchial response to occupational agents during specific inhalation challenges. Thorax 1996;51:472–8.

73. Perrin B, Cartier A, Ghezzo H, et al. Reassessment of the temporal patterns of bronchial obstruction after exposure to occupational sensitizing agents. J Allergy Clin Immunol 1991;87:630–9.

74. Malo JL, Ghezzo H, L'Archevêque J, Cartier A. Late asthmatic reactions to occupational sensitizing agents: frequency of changes in nonspecific bronchial responsiveness and of response to inhaled beta 2-adrenergic agent. J Allergy Clin Immunol 1990;85:834–42.

75. Cockcroft DW, Hoeppner VH, Werner GD. Recurrent nocturnal asthma after bronchoprovocation with western red cedar sawdust: association with acute increase in nonallergic bronchial responsiveness. Clin Allergy 1984;14:61–8.

76. Chan-Yeung M, Malo JL. Natural history of occupational asthma. In: Bernstein IL, Chan-Yeung M, Malo JL, Bernstein DI, editors. Asthma in the workplace. New York: Marcel Dekker Inc; 1993. p. 299–322.

77. Pauli G, Kopferschmitt-Kubler MC, Gassman V, et al. Asthme professionnel: pronostic médical et social. Rev Pneumol Clin 1996;52:104–9.

78. Tarlo SM, Liss G, Corey P, Broder I. A workers compensation claim population for occupational asthma—comparison of subgroups. Chest 1995;107:634–41.

79. Malo JL, Cartier A, Ghezzo H, et al. Patterns of improvement in spirometry, bronchial hyperresponsiveness, and specific IgE antibody levels after cessation of exposure in occupational asthma caused by snow-crab processing. Am Rev Respir Dis 1988;138:807–12.

80. Allard C, Cartier A, Ghezzo H, Malo JL. Occupational asthma due to various agents. Absence of clinical and functional improvement at an interval of four or more years after cessation of exposure. Chest 1989;96:1046–9.

81. Perfetti L, Cartier A, Ghezzo H, et al. Follow-up of occupational asthma after removal from or diminution of exposure to the responsible agent—relevance of the length of the interval from cessation of exposure. Chest 1998;114:398–403.

82. Chan-Yeung M, Maclean L, Paggiaro PL. Follow-up study of 232 patients with occupational asthma caused by western red cedar (Thuja plicata). J Allergy Clin Immunol 1987;79:792–6.

83. Côté J, Kennedy S, Chan-Yeung M. Outcome of patients with cedar asthma with continuous exposure. Am Rev Respir Dis 1990;141:373–6.

84. Obase Y, Shimoda T, Mitsuta K, et al. Two patients with occupational asthma who returned to work with dust respirators. Occup Environ Med 2000;57:62–4.

85. Maestrelli P, De Marzo N, Saetta M, et al. Effects of inhaled beclomethasone on airway responsiveness in occupational asthma. Placebo-controlled study of subjects sensitized to toluene diisocyanate. Am Rev Respir Dis 1993;148:407–12.

86. Malo JL, Cartier A, Côté J, et al. Influence of inhaled corticosteroids on recovery from occupational asthma after cessation of exposure: an 18-month double-blind crossover study. Am J Respir Crit Care Med 1996;153:953–60.

87. Malo JL. Législation québécoise en matière de maladies professionnelles pulmonaires: application spécifique à l'asthme professionnel. Rev Mal Respir 1990;7 Suppl 2:R121–5.

88. American Thoracic Society Guidelines for the evaluation of impairment/disability in patients with asthma. ATS. Medical Section of the American Lung Association. Am Rev Respir Dis 1993;147:1056–61.

89. Chan-Yeung M, Malo JL. Evaluation of impairment/disability in subjects with occupational asthma. In: Bernstein IL, Chan-Yeung M, Malo JL, Bernstein DI, editors. Asthma in the workplace. New York: Marcel Dekker Inc; 1993. p. 341–58.

90. Slovak AJM, Hill RN. Does atopy have any predictive value for laboratory animal allergy? A comparison of different concepts of atopy. Br J Ind Med 1987;44:129–32.

91. Tarlo SM, Banks D, Liss G, Broder I. Outcome determinants for isocyanate induced occupational asthma among compensation claimants. Occup Environ Med 1997;54:756–61.

92. Mullan RJ, Murthy LI. Occupational sentinel health events: an up-dated list for physician recognition and public health surveillance. Am J Ind Med 1991;19:775–99.

93. Brooks S, Weiss M, Bernstein I. Reactive airways dysfunction syndrome (RADS): persistent asthma syndrome after high level irritant exposures. Chest 1985;88:376–84.

94. Tarlo SM, Broder I. Irritant-induced occupational asthma. Chest 1989;96:297–300.

95. Bherer L, Cushman R, Courteau JP, et al. Survey of construction workers repeatedly exposed to chlorine over a three to six month period in a pulpmill: ii. Follow up of affected workers by questionnaire, spirometry, and assessment of bronchial responsiveness 18 to 24 months after exposure ended. Occup Environ Med 1994;51:225–8.

96. Chan-Yeung M, Lam S, Kennedy SM, Frew AJ. Persistent asthma after repeated exposure to high concentrations of gases in pulpmills. Am J Respir Crit Care Med 1994;149:1676–80.

97. Henneberger PK, Lax MB, Ferris BG Jr. Decrements in spirometry values associated with chlorine gassing events and pulp mill work. Am J Respir Crit Care Med 1996;153:225–31.

98. Gautrin D, Leroyer C, L'Archevêque J, et al. Cross-sectional assessment of workers with repeated exposure to chlorine over a three year period. Eur Respir J 1995;8:2046–54.

99. Leroyer C, Malo JL, Infanterivard C, et al. Changes in airway function and bronchial responsiveness after acute occupational exposure to chlorine leading to treatment in a first aid unit. Occup Environ Med 1998;55:356–9.

100. Weill H, George R, Schwarz M, Ziskind M. Late evaluation of pulmonary function after acute exposure to chlorine gas. Am Rev Respir Dis 1969;99:374–9.

101. Hasan F, Gehshan A, Fuleihan F. Resolution of pulmonary dysfunction following acute chlorine exposure. Arch Environ Health 1983;38:76–80.

102. Courteau JP, Cushman R, Bouchard F, et al. Survey of construction workers repeatedly exposed to chlorine over a three to six month period in a pulpmill: i. exposure and symptomatology. Occup Environ Med 1994;51:219–24.

103. Das R, Blanc PD. Chlorine gas exposure and the lung: a review. Toxicol Ind Health 1993;9:439–55.

104. Boulet LP. Increases in airway responsiveness following acute exposure to respiratory irritants. Reactive airway dysfunction syndrome or occupational asthma? Chest 1988;94:476–81.

105. Moisan TC. Prolonged asthma after smoke inhalation: a report of three cases and a review of previous reports. J Occup Med 1991;33:458–61.

106. Gautrin D, Boulet LP, Boutet M, et al. Is reactive airways dysfunction syndrome a variant of occupational asthma? J Allergy Clin Immunol 1994;93:12–22.

107. Kennedy SM. Acquired airway hyperresponsiveness from nonimmunogenic irritant exposure. Occup Med 1992;7:287–300.

109. Brooks SM, Hammad Y, Richards I, et al. The spectrum of irritant-induced asthma: sudden and not-so-sudden onset and the role of allergy. Chest 1998;113:42–9.

110. Chester E, Schwartz H, Payne C, Greenstein S. Phthalic anhydride asthma. Clin Allergy 1977;7:15–20.

111. Lemière C, Malo JL, Boutet M. Reactive airways dysfunction syndrome due to chlorine—sequential bronchial biopsies and functional assessment. Eur Respir J 1997;10:241–4.

112. Leroyer C, Perfetti L, Cartier A, Malo JL. Can reactive airways dysfunction syndrome (RADS) transform into occupational asthma due to sensitisation to isocyanates? Thorax 1998;53:152–3.

CHAPTER 10

Principles of Asthma Management in Adults

Donald W. Cockcroft, MD, FRCPC

Over the past decade, numerous guidelines on asthma management have emerged.[1–3] These guidelines are based on scientific studies (Level I or Level II) of individual aspects of asthma treatment which will be covered in greater detail in subsequent chapters. The integration of these data into an overall approach to asthma management, however, is a *consensus* of experts and must be considered Level IIIA/B.

Current consensus regarding asthma treatment in various countries is remarkably similar. The approach outlined in the current chapter is based on the Canadian Asthma Guidelines,[3] updated in 1999. The only major difference between the Canadian Guidelines and other guidelines is that they regard asthma severity and its treatment as a *continuum* from mild to severe (Figure 10–1), rather than as a series of *steps*, as suggested by several other

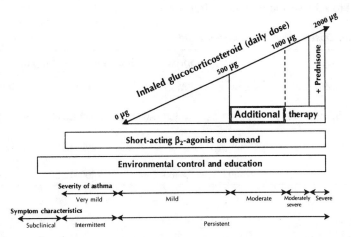

Figure 10–1 Asthma continuum. The severity of asthma in an individual patient is judged by the frequency and chronicity of symptoms, the presence of persistent airflow limitation, and the medication required to maintain control. Indications of severe asthma included previous near-fatal episode (loss of consciousness, intubation), recent hospitalization or emergency room visit, night-time symptoms, limitation of daily activities, need for β_2-agonist several times per day or at night, forced expiratory volume in 1 second (FEV_1) or peak expiratory flow (PEF) less than 60% predicted. β_2-Agonist should not be required daily; if used more than twice per week, institute anti-inflammatory or preventive therapy. The usual initial dose of inhaled corticosteroid is 400 to 800 μg/day of budesonide or the equivalent. The initial dose in children may be lower, that is, budesonide 200 to 400 μg or equivalent. If asthma is mild, or if control is achieved with beclomethasone less than 400 μg or equivalent, a trial of sodium cromoglycate (children) or nedocromil may be warranted. Additional therapy is indicated for patients with unsatisfactory symptom control, despite a moderate (fluticasone 500 μg/d, budesonide 800 μg/d) to high (fluticasone 1,000 μg/d, budesonide 1,600 μg/d) dose of inhaled corticosteroid. Additional therapies include trials of long-acting inhaled β_2-agonists, ingested sustained-release theophylline, or ingested leukotriene receptor antagonist. (Reprinted with permission from Boulet LP, Becker A, Berube D, et al. Summary of recommendations from the Canadian Asthma Consensus Report 1999. Can Med Assoc J 1999;161:S1–12.)

guidelines.[1,2] An integrated approach to asthma management must focus on three main components, patient education, environmental control, and drug therapy. It is important to assess both the correctness and the completeness of the diagnosis and to reassess this from time to time, particularly if the asthma fails to come under control easily.

DIAGNOSIS AND ASSESSMENT OF SEVERITY

The diagnosis of asthma is based on the three cardinal features contained within the definition of asthma, namely, symptoms, airway dysfunction (variable airflow obstruction and airway hyper-responsiveness), and eosinophilic airway inflammation. Individuals with asthma should have all three features (Level III); there is uncertainty as to how best to label and treat individuals who have only two (or perhaps only one) of these three cardinal features of asthma. Since asthma symptoms (chest tightness, dyspnea, cough, shortness of breath) are not specific for asthma,[4] it is recommended that whenever possible, asthma should be documented objectively by demonstration of variable airflow obstruction and/or airway hyper-responsiveness (Level IIIA). This becomes mandatory when asthma symptoms fail to respond to usual therapy (see below).

Asthma severity is assessed in different ways before and after treatment has been introduced. Prior to treatment, asthma severity is based on frequency and severity of symptoms both by day and by night, amount of rescue inhaled β_2-agonist required, severity of airflow obstruction, and asthma morbidity (eg, days away from work or school, emergency department visits, hospitalizations, previous intubations).[1–3] Following treatment, asthma severity is best assessed by the *minimum* amount of therapy, chiefly inhaled corticosteroids (Table 10–1), required to achieve and maintain ideal control.[1,5]

Table 10–1 *Daily Doses of Inhaled Corticosteroid*

Inhaled Corticosteroid	Approximate Equivalent Doses (µg/d)			
	Low	*Moderate*	*High*	*Very High*
Beclomethasone dipropionate	≤500	>500–1,000	>1,000–2,000	N/A
Fluticasone propionate	≤250	>250–500	>500–1,000	>1,000–2,000
Budesonide	≤400	>400–800	>800–1,600	>1,600–3,200

N/A = not applicable.

ASTHMA CONTROL

It is considered important to define, achieve, and maintain ideal asthma control. Ideal asthma control has been defined as follows (Level IIIA):[1–3]

- Daytime symptoms—nil to ≤ thrice a week
- Night-time symptoms—nil
- Lifestyle including physical activity—normal (except where proscribed by environmental control)
- Exacerbations—nil to mild
- Absenteeism—nil
- β_2-Agonist requirement (as needed)—nil to ≤ thrice a week
- Forced expiratory volume in 1 second (FEV$_1$), peak expiratory flow (PEF)—normal to > 90% of personal best

The criteria used to define well-controlled asthma are the opposite of those used to define pretreatment asthma severity. This has led to some confusion and, we believe, inappropriate misuse of the term "severe asthma" when a more appropriate term would be "poorly controlled asthma" (Level IIIB):[5] the two are not synonymous. A suggested schema for defining asthma severity based on minimum medication requirements to achieve good control is outlined in Table 10–2.

Table 10–2 *Asthma Severity Based on Minimum Treatment Requirements*

Asthma Severity	Asthma Control	Minimum Chronic Medication Requirements		
		Inhaled β_2-Agonist	Corticosteroid	Additional Medication
Very mild	Well controlled	Nil to rare	Nil	Nil
Mild	Well controlled	Nil to ≤ 3/wk	Nil to low dose inhaled	Nil
Moderate	Well controlled	Nil to ≤ 3/wk	Moderate–high dose inhaled	Occasional
Severe	Well controlled	Nil to ≤ 3/wk	High–very high inhaled + oral	Usual
Very severe	Not well controlled	≥ 3/wk	Very high dose inhaled + oral	Always

PATIENT EDUCATION

It is widely accepted that patient education and patient involvement in asthma management is a critical first step in overall asthma management.[6] There is no universal agreement as to how this should be achieved. This concept is relevant to any chronic disease; however, since asthma is both controllable and highly variable from time to time, it is particularly amenable to patient education.

We believe patients should have an understanding of the basic concepts of the disease (airway inflammation, bronchospasm), the various triggers (those which cause inflammation vs those which cause only bronchoconstriction), the medications and how they work (anti-inflammatory or controller vs bronchodilator or reliever), and medication side effects. Of special relevance to asthmatic patients is the issue of correct use of inhalation devices. These devices are frequently misused. It is important to have subjects repeatedly demonstrate their inhaler technique and to educate and often re-educate them regarding appropriate technique. This includes issues such as the use of large volume spacer devices and the need to rinse out the mouth following the use of inhaled corticosteroids.

The three most important aspects of asthma education center around defining, achieving, and maintaining ideal control (Level IIIA). These three are inter-related and include the following:

1. *Understanding and achieving ideal control.* The patient with asthma must understand the definition of ideal asthma control if there is to be any hope of achieving such control. In our experience, we often have to correct many patient (and physician) misconceptions, occasionally misconceptions that have been present for years.
2. *Recognition of worsened control.* The recognition by the patient of worsened asthma control, that is, the recognition that asthma is exacerbating, is the critical first step toward initiating treatment changes. This involves recognition that asthma symptoms are occurring with increasing frequency and that the as-needed inhaled β_2-agonist requirements are increasing likewise. This may be accompanied by objective documentation of changes in self-measured PEF. In well-controlled asthmatic patients, symptoms are probably more sensitive as indicators of exacerbation than changes in PEF or airway hyper-responsiveness.

3. *Exacerbation treatment.* Early treatment of worsened asthma control follows logically upon early identification of worsened asthma control. This is generally accomplished by increasing anti-inflammatory therapy based on the severity of the exacerbation; this should be based on an individualized *action plan* (see below).

ENVIRONMENTAL CONTROL

Attention to the patient's environment is important both diagnostically and therapeutically. Allergens and low-molecular-weight chemical sensitizers are now recognized as *causes* of asthma by their role as *inducers* of airway inflammation and secondary airway hyper-responsiveness.[7,8] The majority of asthmatic patients are atopic, including adult asthmatic patients— particularly those whose asthma started in childhood. The prevalence of occupational asthma in patients whose asthma starts in adulthood is significant. These facts should be considered in the historic work-up and investigation of all asthmatic patients. Skin testing or serologic testing for allergen-specific IgE against inhaled allergens relevant to the subject is indicated in most, if not all, asthmatic patients (Level IIIA).[3] More detailed and specialized investigations may be required to confirm or exclude occupational causes for asthma.[9]

Early environmental control in both allergen-induced asthma and occupational asthma can markedly improve symptoms, airway inflammation,[10] and airway hyper-responsiveness.[11,12] In cases of isolated single sensitization, environmental control can be curative. This requires, of course, accurate diagnostic procedures as well as patient education regarding the importance of these so-called inducers and subsequent avoidance. When faced with unexplained deterioration in asthma control, re-evaluation of the patient's environment can occasionally be very informative.

BASIC DRUG THERAPY

The overall approach to asthma management including basic drug therapy is a continuum and is outlined in Figure 10–2.[3] Symptoms should be treated as they arise with a bronchodilator, generally an inhaled β_2-agonist. In occasional subjects, inhaled anticholinergic may be used because of adverse effects of even low doses of inhaled β_2-agonists. Bronchodilators may be used prophylactically to prevent exercise-induced bronchospasm.

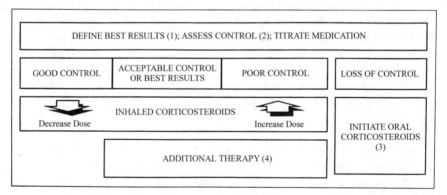

Figure 10–2 Assessment of control. *(1)* Best results are defined as a minimum of symptoms, ability to carry out all normal activities, absence of need for bronchodilators, maximal attainable forced expiratory volume in 1 second (FEV_1) or peak expiratory flow (PEF), and no or minimal side effects from medication. *(2)* Criteria for control are listed in Table 10–2. *(3)* In some cases, when loss of control is neither severe or of long duration, a doubling of the dose of inhaled corticosteroid may be attempted in lieu of oral corticosteroids. *(4)* Strong consideration should be given to removing additional therapy before decreasing the dose of inhaled corticosteroid. (Reproduced with permission from Ernst P, FitzGerald JM, Spier S, editors. Canadian Asthma Consensus Conference: summary of recommendations. Can Respir J 1996;3(2):89–100.

When symptoms and β_2-agonist requirements exceed a minimum (thrice a week has been recommended; Level III), anti-inflammatory therapy is indicated. Inhaled corticosteroids are the anti-inflammatory therapy of choice. Approximate comparative doses of the most commonly used inhaled corticosteroids are outlined in Table 10–1. The usual starting dose in adults would be in the moderate (800 µg/d budesonide, 500 µg/d fluticasone propionate) to high (1,600 µg/d budesonide, 1,000 µg/d fluticasone propionate) dose range. Following achievement of control, inhaled corticosteroid dose should be tapered to identify the lowest maintenance dose that will maintain control (Figure 10–2). The approach of gaining control with moderate- to high-dose inhaled corticosteroids and then tapering to a maintenance dose is generally accepted (Level IIIA). The majority of asthmatic patients should be controllable with inhaled β_2-agonist and a variable dose of inhaled corticosteroids, with occasional ingested corticosteroids for more severe exacerbations. When this is not possible, reassessment regarding additional or alternative therapies and/or additional or alternative diagnoses is recommended.

REASSESSMENT

When to Reassess

It is recommended that asthma treatment and possibly asthma diagnosis be reassessed when control is not easily achieved. The threshold for reassessment will vary from patient to patient and clinician to clinician. Reassessment is reasonable when asthma fails to be controlled with moderate-dose inhaled corticosteroid and strongly recommended if asthma cannot be controlled with high-dose inhaled corticosteroid or greater (see Table 10–1).

Reasons for Reassessment

There are at least three reasons why the diagnosis and treatment of asthma should be reassessed at these levels. These include the following:

- *Inhaled corticosteroid safety.* There continue to be concerns regarding safety of long-term use of inhaled corticosteroids. The major theoretic medical concern regarding systemic side effects is the potential effect on bone metabolism (growth in children, osteoporosis in adults).[13] The risk has neither been clarified nor quantitated. The risk likely relates both to dose and duration of therapy as well as (and perhaps more importantly) the need for intercurrent ingested corticosteroid. Doses of inhaled corticosteroids defined as moderate (see Table 10–1) are considered safe for chronic use in adults.[14] Until the risk of osteoporosis with inhaled corticosteroids can be clarified, it seems prudent to maintain dosing at the lowest possible levels.[13,14]
- *Efficacy of inhaled corticosteroids.* Group mean data show that inhaled corticosteroid dose response is steep and plateaus at a low dose.[14] It is probably not appropriate to carry over such data to individual subjects or to subjects during an exacerbation; however, it has become generally accepted that increasing doses of inhaled corticosteroids above the low to moderate level achieves diminishing returns regarding asthma control. This may have several, not mutually exclusive, explanations including corticosteroid refractoriness of asthma, coexistence of nonasthmatic confounders, and failure to increase the dose of inhaled corticosteroids geometrically (ie, by a factor of two- to fourfold).
- *Noncorticosteroid responsive conditions.* Asthma is a common condition that may coexist with one or more noncorticosteroid responsive conditions that can mimic asthma and simulate suboptimal control (Table 10–3). These are outlined below.

Table 10–3 *Causes of Poor Response of Asthma to Inhaled Corticosteroid*

Noncompliance
Noneosinophilic airway inflammation
Habitual β_2-agonist overuse
β_2-Agonist-induced poor control
Gastroesophageal reflux
Sinusitis
Paradoxical vocal cord function
Hyperventilation
Other concomitant diseases, such as:
Diffuse airway disease (bronchitis, bronchiectasis, CAL)
Focal airway disease (larynx, subglottic, trachea)
Pulmonary thromboembolic disease
Obstructive sleep apnea
Cardiac (angina, heart failure)
Severe asthma

CAL = chronic airflow limitation.

Procedures

A standardized approach to reassessment of the asthmatic who fails to come under control (or who requires an unacceptable dose of inhaled corticosteroids) is indicated. The circumstances outlined in Table 10–3 should be given careful consideration and excluded or treated, insofar as is possible, prior to increasing asthma therapy.

- *Noncompliance.* Noncompliance is the most common reason for suboptimal asthma control. Aspects of compliance that need to be assessed include environmental control, technical aspects of medication use, and frequency of medication use.
- *Noneosinophilic airway inflammation.* Asthma inflammation is usually eosinophilic. Occasionally, the airway inflammation is primarily neutrophilic. The prevalence of this is uncertain; however, it appears to be particularly common in steroid-resistant asthmatic patients[15] and may be more common during exacerbations.[16,17]
- *Habitual β_2-agonist abuse.* The habitual, unnecessary use of inhaled β_2-agonist in mild asthmatic patients will simulate poor control. This may be difficult to identify, and the prevalence of habitual β_2-agonist use is not known. Two reasons for suspecting this condition are expiratory flow rates that are better than expected and lack of nocturnal symptoms (Level III).
- *Inhaled β_2-agonist-induced worsened asthma control.* Regular use of conventional inhaled β_2-agonists four times daily can cause slight[18] to modest[19] worsening of asthma control. Larger doses may have a greater effect. This must always be a consideration in subjects who use a very large dose of inhaled β_2-agonist (Level I).
- *Gastroesophageal reflux.* Gastroesophageal reflux is common in asthmatic subjects and may be worsened by frequent coughing, corticosteroid-associated weight gain, and, possibly, ingested theophylline. Gastroesophageal reflux may worsen asthma control.[20] It is possible that gastroesophageal reflux could be otherwise silent (Level II).
- *Sinusitis.* Rhinitis is almost universal among asthma subjects, and sinusitis is a common complication of chronic rhinitis. It is widely accepted that uncontrolled sinusitis may worsen asthma control.[21]
- *Paradoxical vocal cord function.* Paradoxical vocal cord function may mimic or compli-

cate asthma.[22] Paradoxical vocal cord dysfunction may be more common in subjects with gastroesophageal reflux (Level IIIC).

- *Hyperventilation.* Inappropriate ventilation may occur alone in psychogenic dyspnea, anxiety hyperventilation, and frank panic attacks. Hyperventilation is a common complicating factor in asthma and can contribute both to worsened bronchospasm and nonresponse to asthma therapy (Level IIB).[23]
- *Other concomitant diseases.* Other diseases causing continuous or episodic dyspnea or chest tightness should always be considered when asthma fails to respond to appropriate therapy. These are listed in Table 10–3 and include both diffuse and focal airway disease, pulmonary thromboembolic disease, obstructive sleep apnea, cardiac conditions.

It is therefore important to objectively confirm and, in some cases, objectively reconfirm the presence of variable airflow obstruction and/or airway hyper-responsiveness. If there are suspicions that symptoms might not be due to airflow obstruction (eg, habitual β_2-agonist use, anxiety hyperventilation), home measurement of PEF during symptoms can prove helpful.

ADDITIONAL THERAPY

When asthma fails to come under control with moderate to high doses of inhaled corticosteroids or requires an unacceptable dose of inhaled corticosteroids (high to very high, with or without ingested corticosteroid), and confounding problems as outlined in Table 10–3 have been excluded as best as possible, additional therapy is indicated. The goals of additional therapy are improved asthma control and, in many cases, reduced corticosteroid requirement. The specifics of additional therapies are outlined in subsequent chapters and include the following:

- *Ultra-long-acting inhaled β_2-agonists.* Addition of either salmeterol or formoterol twice daily has been shown to be at least as effective in symptom control as doubling the dose of inhaled corticosteroids in suboptimally controlled asthmatic patients (Level IA).[24–26] The use of long-acting β_2-agonists in conjunction with low to moderate doses of inhaled corticosteroids does not result in increased exacerbation rates (Level IA).[26] At this point, inhaled long-acting β_2-agonists appear to be the most popular additional therapy considered.
- *Sustained-release theophylline.* Ingested theophylline has fallen out of favor in recent years. However, low-dose (or doses producing low therapeutic levels) ingested theophylline provides similar benefits to long-acting inhaled β_2-agonists when combined with inhaled corticosteroids (Level IA).[27] Advantages include both ease and cost of administration.
- *Leukotriene receptor antagonists (LTRAs).* Leukotriene receptor antagonists have recently become available.[28] These are ingested agents with bronchodilator and possibly some anti-inflammatory activity. The current consensus recommendations suggest they should be used as add-on therapy as an alternate agent to long-acting β_2-agonists. They may be particularly helpful in subjects with aspirin-sensitive asthma. Leukotriene receptor antagonists may have an advantage over long-acting β_2-agonists in exercise-induced bronchospasm, since significant tolerance does not occur (Level IA);[29] this contrasts with the marked tolerance to the bronchoprotective effect of the long-acting β_2-agonists (Level IA).[30] A further advantage is the fact that this is an ingested agent, rather than a third inhaler; it is speculated that this might improve compliance.
- *Cromones.* Sodium cromoglycate and nedocromil inhibit exercise-[31] and allergen-induced bronchospasm (both Level IA),[32] and have a prophylactic anti-inflammatory effect in allergen-exposed individuals;[33] nedocromil may also be anti-inflammatory in

nonatopic asthmatic patients.[34] The anti-inflammatory effect is hypothesized by the effect on airway hyper-responsiveness. The major use of these drugs is as an adjunct to the management of exercise-induced bronchospasm in subjects requiring overly frequent inhaled β_2-agonists. Sodium cromoglycate is occasionally preferred as an anti-inflammatory in young, mild, atopic asthmatic patients and nedocromil occasionally in adults. These drugs are not frequently helpful as add-on therapy in poorly controlled asthma.

- *Anticholinergics.* Anticholinergic bronchodilators are used infrequently in maintenance therapy of asthma. Their most frequent use appears to be as an alternative reliever in subjects who, for one reason or another, cannot or will not use inhaled β_2-agonists. Anticholinergic drugs are commonly used in combination with inhaled β_2-agonists in the management of acute exacerbations. By contrast, anticholinergic bronchodilators have become front-line therapy for the management of airflow obstruction in subjects with chronic airflow limitation.

- *Immunosuppressants.* Nonsteroid immunosuppressant drugs (including methotrexate,[35] gold,[36] cyclosporine,[37] hydroxychloroquine,[38] and others) have a prednisone-sparing effect in severe refractory asthma. These agents are required rarely. They require close monitoring for side effects. It is recommended that subjects requiring these agents be followed up in specialized centers and ideally should be part of a clinical investigation.

TREATMENT OF EXACERBATIONS

A structured approach to treatment of exacerbations based on early identification of worsened asthma control and the severity thereof should be outlined in an individual action plan. Treatment of exacerbations is most often accomplished by geometrically increasing the dose of inhaled corticosteroids by a factor of two- to fourfold and, if the exacerbation is more severe or nonresponsive to the increased inhaled corticosteroid, adding ingested corticosteroids (Level I). Exacerbations that are more severe as assessed by frequency and severity of symptoms, frequency and effectiveness (or lack thereof) of inhaled β_2-agonists, and, if available, severity of PEF drop, may require a phone call to the physician or an immediate visit to a hospital emergency department.

When asthma is well controlled, asthma therapy can be cautiously withdrawn to identify the lowest effective level. Consideration should be given to reducing additional therapy (if present) prior to reducing or further reducing inhaled corticosteroids (see Figure 10–2).

Identification of the cause of exacerbation rarely alters the immediate medical treatment. Exceptions are the use of epinephrine and H_1 blockers where asthma exacerbation is a component of a systemic allergic (anaphylactic) reaction, and inhaled or parenteral anticholinergics where asthma exacerbation is caused by β-blocker use. Identification of the cause of the exacerbation is, however, important, both for understanding the nature of the asthma and for preventing future episodes.

SUMMARY

A standardized approach to asthma therapy focusing on patient self-involvement in management can reduce asthma morbidity and, hopefully, mortality to a great extent. The cornerstones of management are patient education, environmental control, and drug therapy, usually limited to as-needed inhaled β_2-agonists and inhaled corticosteroid in variable doses. When asthma control cannot be easily achieved, it is important to objectively confirm both the accuracy and completeness of the diagnosis, and treat any additional diagnoses before considering additional or alternate asthma therapy. These difficult cases are in the minority, and should probably be managed with the aid of a consultant who specializes in the condition.

The author wishes to thank Jacquie Bramley for her assistance in the preparation of this manuscript.

REFERENCES

1. National Heart, Lung, and Blood Institute. International consensus report on diagnosis and management of asthma. Bethesda (MD): NHLBI; 1992 Publication No.:92-3091.

2. Barnes PJ, Barnett AH, Brewis RAL, et al. Chronic asthma in adults and children. Thorax 1993;48:S1–24.

3. Boulet LP, Becker A, Berube D, et al. Summary of recommendations from the Canadian Asthma Consensus Report 1999. Can Med Assoc J 1999;161:S1–12.

4. Adelroth E, Hargreave FE, Ramsdale EH. Do physicians need objective measurements to diagnose asthma? Am Rev Respir Dis 1986;134:704–7.

5. Cockcroft DW, Swystun VA. Asthma control versus asthma severity. J Allergy Clin Immunol 1996;98:1016–8.

6. Boulet L-P, Chapman KR (chairpersons). Proceedings of the 2nd National Conference on Asthma and Education. Can Respir J 1996;3:1–47A.

7. Dolovich J, Hargreave FE. The asthma syndrome: inciters, inducers, and host characteristics. Thorax 1981;36:641–4.

8. Platts-Mills TAE, Vervloet D, Thomas WR, et al. Indoor allergens and asthma: report of the third international workshop. J Allergy Clin Immunol 1997;100:S1–24.

9. Tarlo SM, Boulet L-P, Cartier A, et al. Canadian Thoracic Society: guidelines for occupational asthma. Can Respir J 1998;5:289–300.

10. Piacentini GL, Martinati L, Mingoni S, Boner AL. Influence of allergen avoidance on the eosinophil phase of airway inflammation in children with allergic asthma. J Allergy Clin Immunol 1996;97:1079–84.

11. Chan-Yeung M. Fate of occupational asthma. A follow-up study of patients with occupational asthma due to Western Red Cedar (Thuja plicata). Am Rev Respir Dis 1977;116:1023–9.

12. Platts-Mills TAE, Mitchell EB, Nock P, et al. Reduction of bronchial hyperreactivity during prolonged allergen avoidance. Lancet 1982;2:675–8.

13. Ledford D, Apter A, Brenner AM, et al. Osteoporosis in the corticosteroid-treated patient with asthma. J Allergy Clin Immunol 1998;102:353–62.

14. Barnes PJ, Pedersen S, Busse WW. Efficacy and safety of inhaled corticosteroids: new developments. Am J Respir Crit Care Med 1998;157:S1–53.

15. Jayaram L, Pizzichini MMM, Pizzichini E, et al. Sputum in steroid resistant asthma: a comparison with prednisone dependent asthma [abstract]. Am J Respir Crit Care Med 1999;159:A703.

16. Fahy JV, Kim KW, Liu J, Boushey HA. Prominent neutrophilic inflammation in sputum from subjects with asthma exacerbation. J Allergy Clin Immunol 1995;95:843–52.

17. Turner MO, Hussack P, Sears MR, et al. Exacerbations of asthma without sputum eosinophilia. Thorax 1995;50:1057–61.

18. Drazen JM, Israel E, Boushey HA, et al. Comparison of regularly scheduled with as-needed use of albuterol in mild asthma. N Engl J Med 1996;335:841–7.

19. Sears MR, Taylor DR, Print CG, et al. Regular inhaled beta-agonist treatment in bronchial asthma. Lancet 1990;336:1391–6.

20. Simpson WG. Gastroesophageal reflux disease and asthma: diagnosis and management. Arch Intern Med 1995:155:798–804.

21. Zimmerman B, Gold M. Role of sinusitis in asthma. The Pediatrician 1991;18:312–6.

22. O'Connell MA, Sklarew PR, Goodman DL. Spectrum of presentation of paradoxical vocal cord motion in ambulatory patients. Ann Allergy 1995;74:341–4.

23. Demeter SL, Cordasco EM. Hyperventilation syndrome and asthma. Am J Med 1986;81:989–94.

24. Greening AP, Ing PW, Northfield M, Shaw G. Treatment of adult asthmatic patients symptomatic on low dose inhaled salmeterol to existing inhaled corticosteroid therapy with increasing dose of inhaled corticosteroids. Lancet 1994;344:219–24.

25. Woolcock A, Lundback B, Ringdal N, Jacques LA. Comparison of addition of salmeterol to inhaled corticosteroids with doubling of the dose of inhaled corticosteroids. Am J Respir Crit Care Med 1996;153:1481–8.

26. Pauwels RA, Lofdahl C-G, Postma DS, et al. Effect of inhaled formoterol and budesonide on exacerbations of asthma. N Engl J Med 1997;337:1405–11.

27. Evans DJ, Taylor DA, Zetterstrom O, et al. A comparison of low-dose inhaled budesonide plus theophylline and

high-dose inhaled budesonide for moderate asthma. N Engl J Med 1997;337:1412–8.

28. Holgate ST, Bradding P, Sampson AP. Leukotriene antagonists and synthesis inhibitors: new directions in asthma therapy. J Allergy Clin Immunol 1996;98:1–13.

29. Leff JA, Busse WW, Pearlman D, et al. Montelukast, a leukotriene-receptor antagonist for the treatment of mild asthma and exercise-induced bronchoconstriction. N Engl J Med 1998;339:147–52.

30. Simons FER, Gerstner TV, Cheang MS, Math M. Tolerance to the bronchoprotective effect of salmeterol in adolescents with exercise-induced asthma using concurrent inhaled glucocorticoid treatment. Pediatrics 1997;99:655–9.

31. Anderson SD. Issues in exercise-induced asthma. J Allergy Clin Immunol 1985;76:763–72.

32. Cockcroft DW, Murdock KY. Comparative effects of inhaled salbutamol, sodium cromoglycate and beclomethasone dipropionate on allergen-induced early asthmatic responses, late asthmatic responses and increased bronchial responsiveness to histamine. J Allergy Clin Immunol 1987;79:734–40.

33. Lowhagen O, Rak S. Modification of bronchial hyperreactivity after treatment with sodium cromoglycate during pollen season. J Allergy Clin Immunol 1985;75:460–7.

34. Bel EH, Timmers MC, Hermans J, et al. The long-term effects of nedocromil sodium and beclomethasone dipropionate on bronchial responsiveness to methacholine in nonatopic asthmatic subjects. Am Rev Respir Dis 1990;141:21–8.

35. Marin MG. Low dose methotrexate spares steroid usage in steroid-dependent asthmatic patients: a meta-analysis. Chest 1997;112(1):29–33.

36. Nierop G, Gijzel WP, Bell EH, et al. Auranofin in the treatment of steroid dependent asthma: a double-blind study. Thorax 1992;47:349–54.

37. Lock SH, Kay AB, Barnes NC. Double-blind, placebo-controlled study of cyclosporin A as a corticosteroid-sparing agent in corticosteroid-dependent asthma. Am J Respir Crit Care Med 1996;153:509–14.

38. Charous BL, Halpern EF, Steven GC. Hydroxychloroquine improves airflow and lowers circulating IgE levels in subjects with moderate symptomatic asthma. J Allergy Clin Immunol 1998;102:198–203.

CHAPTER 11

Management of Persistent Asthma in Childhood

F. Estelle R. Simons, MD, FRCPC

In children, as in adults, the primary goal of asthma treatment is to prevent the symptoms of coughing, wheezing, and breathlessness at all times and, by so doing, to minimize the need for urgent care visits, emergency department visits, or hospitalizations. Additional goals are to improve pulmonary function as much as possible, avoid adverse effects from treatment, and meet patients' and families' expectations.[1–3]

In childhood asthma, there are unique considerations. Identification of high-risk allergic infants who have not yet developed wheezing and coughing may offer an opportunity for prevention or delay of asthma, either by avoidance of environmental allergens and irritants[4] or by pharmacologic intervention.[5] Diagnosis of asthma, especially differentiation from bronchiolitis in children under age 3 years, may present a challenge and may have implications for management and for prognosis.[6]

In children, increased duration of asthma correlates directly with reduced lung function.[7] Some physicians report that prompt control of persistent allergic inflammation in the lower airways improves the eventual outcome;[8] however, others who have monitored children with asthma of varying severity over several decades find that mild asthma remains mild regardless of the treatment administered.[9–11]

Two issues about which there is complete agreement are that evaluation of the benefit-to-risk ratio of all forms of asthma treatment in children must include consideration of potential adverse effects on growth and development;[1–3] and that as most young people with asthma also have allergies, control of allergic rhinitis and other upper airway allergic disorders facilitates control of asthma.[12]

The management of persistent asthma in children includes medications, avoidance of environmental allergens and respiratory irritants, patient and family education, and, in selected patients, allergen vaccinations (formerly known as immunotherapy). Most current guidelines for asthma management in children are not evidence based. In this chapter, we evaluate relevant publications and, where available, systematic reviews or meta-analyses, using published definitions of levels of evidence.[13] We adopt a broad view of evidence-based medicine, as "the conscientious, explicit, and judicious use of current best evidence in making decisions about the care of individual patients...integration of clinical expertise, external evidence, and the patient's values and expectations."[14]

The evidence base for asthma treatment in children younger than age 12 years, and especially in those younger than age 6 years, differs in some respects from the evidence base for asthma treatment in adults. Fewer large randomized clinical trials have been performed in children. Pulmonary function tests and other objective measurements are difficult to obtain in very young children, and are consequently less often included as outcome measures in clinical trials. In some respects, the quality of the evidence available regarding asthma treatment is inversely proportional to the age of the child being studied. Use of an evidence-based approach to decision-making is of critical importance in childhood asthma, as it facilitates identification of inadequately studied therapies.

A summary of key recommendations for asthma management in children is presented in Table 11–1.

Table 11–1 *Summary of Key Recommendations*

Management Component	Evidence-Based Recommendation
Medications	
Inhaled glucocorticoids	The most effective medications for prevention of asthma symptoms (Level IA); their use must be individualized in each child with regard to benefit-to-risk ratio
Inhaled anti-allergics (cromolyn or nedocromil)	Less effective than glucocorticoids but are the safest medications available for long-term use (Level IC)
Short-acting β_2-adrenergic agonists	Used to prevent exercise-induced asthma and to relieve acute asthma symptoms (Level IA)
Long-acting β_2-adrenergic agonists	Potentially useful as steroid-sparing agents; further studies are needed in children (Level IB)
Cysteinyl leukotriene antagonists	Emerging role in mild asthma, exercise-induced asthma and as steroid-sparing agents; further studies are needed in children (Level IA)
Theophylline	A relatively inexpensive steroid-sparing agent; is seldom used now in many countries but remains on the World Health Organization list of essential medications for asthma due to its low cost (Level IC)
H_1 receptor antagonists	Not first choice medications for asthma treatment; however, they are not harmful when used for concurrent allergic rhinitis treatment; their role in asthma prevention in infants requires further investigation (Level IB)
Avoidance of airborne allergens and respiratory irritants	The foundation of all asthma treatment in children; understudied and underused (Level IB)
Asthma education	The evidence base for its importance is increasing (Level IB)
Allergen vaccinations (immunotherapy)	Invasive treatment that remains controversial in asthma a century after it was introduced (Level IC)

PHARMACOLOGIC TREATMENT

General Considerations

The keys to successful pharmacotherapy of asthma in children are to use it in the context of a comprehensive approach involving allergen avoidance and education, to avoid polypharmacy, and to recommend medication(s) in the lowest doses that prevent and control symptoms.[1–3]

In children, as in adults, a stepwise approach to pharmacotherapy is recommended (Level III).[1-3] Children with mild intermittent asthma who have symptoms only two or three times weekly require only one medication: a short-acting β_2-adrenergic agonist to prevent exercise-induced symptoms and to use for occasional breakthrough wheezing. Children with mild or moderate persistent asthma generally require an anti-inflammatory medication such as a low-dose inhaled glucocorticoid for prevention of symptoms, and a short-acting inhaled β_2-adrenergic agonist for breakthrough symptoms. Children with severe persistent asthma may require two medications for prevention of symptoms—an inhaled glucocorticoid and a steroid-sparing medication such as a long-acting inhaled β_2-adrenergic agonist, a cysteinyl leukotriene$_1$ antagonist, or theophylline—along with a short-acting β_2-agonist for breakthrough symptoms. In any child with asthma, an oral glucocorticoid may be required intermittently for relief of acute exacerbations.[1-3]

Inhaled Glucocorticoids

Efficacy

Glucocorticoids inhaled once or twice daily regularly, although not a cure for asthma, are more effective than any other anti-inflammatory medications available for treatment of persistent asthma (Figure 11–1) (Level IA).[15-30] In children, there are few comprehensive studies in which the efficacy of currently available inhaled glucocorticoids has been compared directly on a μg/μg basis, and equipotent doses are not optimally defined.[15,16] Although all medications in this class are effective, they have distinctive pharmacologic and pharmacokinetic profiles. Recent meta-analyses suggest that they may not be equally effective,[17,18] and their benefit-to-risk ratios may differ considerably (Level I).[15,16]

The most common reasons for apparent failure of response to inhaled glucocorticoid treatment are continued massive exposure to allergens or respiratory irritants such as ciga-

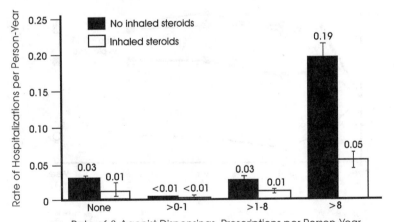

Figure 11–1 A retrospective cohort study in a health maintenance organization was performed to determine if anti-inflammatory treatment for asthma reduced the risk of hospitalization for asthma (the main outcome). Of the 16,941 eligible persons, 742 (4.4%) were hospitalized during a 3-year period. The overall relative risk of hospitalization among those who received inhaled steroids was 0.5 (95% CI 0.4 to 0.6, after adjustment for β_2-adrenergic agonist dispensing). The steroid-associated protection was most marked among individuals who received the largest amount of β_2-adrenergic agonist. In the children, but not in the adults in this study, cromolyn was similarly associated with a reduced risk of hospitalization for asthma (OR 0.8, 95% CI 0.7 to 0.9) (not shown). (Reproduced with permission from Donahue JG, Weiss ST, Livingston JM, et al. Inhaled steroids and the risk of hospitalization for asthma. JAMA 1997;277:887–91.)

rette smoke, lack of adherence to a treatment regimen of regular inhalations, or poor inhaler technique. Fortunately, true steroid-resistant asthma is uncommon.[19]

Children using inhaled glucocorticoids for treatment of persistent asthma have fewer hospitalizations, fewer symptoms, reduced need for "rescue" β_2-agonist medication, improved pulmonary function, and decreased bronchial airway hyperresponsiveness, including improved exercise tolerance (Level IA).[8,20–31] In those with mild or moderate persistent asthma, these beneficial effects usually occur with a total daily beclomethasone dipropionate dose of $\leq$400 μg or an equivalent dose of other inhaled glucocorticoid. The dose-response curve for inhaled glucocorticoid efficacy is relatively flat.[21–24] In some studies, statistically significant and clinically important differences among doses have been shown for symptom control, improvement in pulmonary function (Figure 11–2),[23] and prevention of exercise-induced bronchospasm.[24] The dose needed to normalize airway responsiveness to bronchoconstricting agents and to eliminate exercise-induced bronchospasm is generally higher than that needed to reduce symptoms at rest and to improve baseline pulmonary function.

Inhaled glucocorticoid treatment may be more effective if started early during the course of childhood asthma in an attempt to stop the inflammatory process, rather than after symptoms have been present for several years (Level IIB).[8] It is not easy to identify with absolute certainty all young children who will benefit from early introduction of inhaled glucocorticoid treatment and at the same time avoid giving inhaled glucocorticoids unnecessarily to those whose asthma will disappear or remain mild, and who may not benefit.[9–11]

Coughing, wheezing, and breathlessness begin to improve within 1 day of starting an inhaled glucocorticoid, but complete control of symptoms and maximum improvement in pulmonary function takes weeks or months, and airway hyperresponsiveness continues to improve even after years of regular treatment.[25–30] Tachyphylaxis does not occur during long-term inhaled glucocorticoid treatment; however, benefits begin to disappear within weeks of discontinuing the inhaled glucocorticoid (Level I) (Figure 11–3A).[27,31]

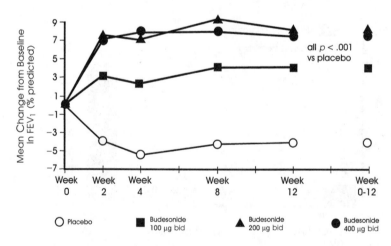

Figure 11–2 In a randomized, multicenter, double-blind, parallel-group, 12-week placebo-controlled study in 404 children, mean age approximately 12 years, budesonide administered via Turbuhaler in total daily doses of 100 μg, 200 μg, or 400 μg was more effective than placebo in improving lung function and asthma symptoms; it did not significantly decrease inhaled short-acting β_2-adrenergic agonist use. The 400-μg dose was significantly more effective than the 100-μg dose in improving FEV$_1$, morning peak expiratory flow, daytime but not evening asthma symptoms, and β_2-adrenergic agonist use. There was a statistically significant difference between the 100- and 200-μg total daily dose. (Reproduced with permission from Shapiro G, Bronsky EA, LaForce CF, et al. Dose-related efficacy of budesonide administered via a dry powder inhaler in the treatment of children with moderate to severe persistent asthma. J Pediatr 1998;132:976–82.)

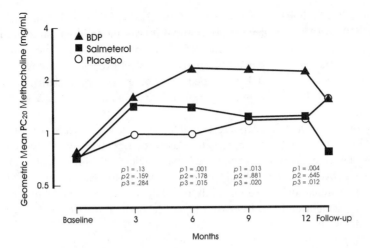

Figure 11–3*A* In a one-year, randomized, double-blind, multicenter, parallel-group, placebo-controlled study in 241 glucocorticoid-naive children aged 9.3 ± 2 years, beclomethasone dipropionate (BDP) 200 μg twice daily was compared with salmeterol 50 μg twice daily. Placebo and study medications were administered using a dry-powder inhaler, followed by rinsing and expectorating. The primary outcome measure, airway hyperresponsiveness to methacholine, was evaluated before and after 3, 6, 9, and 12 months of treatment. Beclomethasone dipropionate had a significantly greater effect than salmeterol or placebo in reducing airway hyperreactivity, but this was lost 2 weeks after treatment was discontinued. Although BDP and salmeterol both improved airway patency significantly, as evidenced by spirometry and twice-daily home monitoring of peak expiratory flows, BDP was significantly more effective than salmeterol for decreasing symptoms, decreasing "rescue" short-acting β_2-adrenergic agonist use, and improving quality of life. *p*1 indicates BDP vs placebo; *p*2 indicates salmeterol vs placebo; *p*3 indicates salmeterol vs BDP.

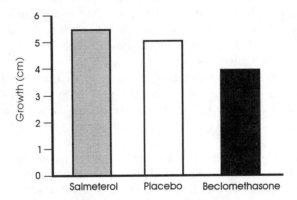

Figure 11–3*B* Mean height increases in children treated with BDP, salmeterol, or placebo for 1 year were 3.96, 5.4, and 5.04 cm, respectively (p = .018 BDP vs placebo; p = .004 BDP vs salmeterol). Inhaled glucocorticoids have a satisfactory benefit-to-risk ratio in children. (Reproduced with permission from Simons FER and the Canadian Beclomethasone Dipropionate–Salmeterol Xinafoate Study Group. A comparison of beclomethasone, salmeterol, and placebo in children with asthma. N Engl J Med 1997;337:1659–65.)

Delivery Systems

Comprehensive comparative studies of inhalation devices in children have not been published. Available evidence suggests that delivery systems differ markedly in their efficiency; for example, there are significant differences in dose output from different combinations of pressurized metered-dose inhalers and spacers.[32] Metered-dose inhalers, in conjunction with small-volume (100 mL) spacer devices are optimal for young children; large-volume (750 mL) spacer devices are more efficient for older children, although rather cumbersome. Metered-dose inhalers containing hydrofluoroalkane (HFA) propellants are replacing those containing chlorofluorocarbon (CFC) propellants. Some HFA propellants may enhance inhaled glucocorticoid deposition in the peripheral airways and necessitate glucocorticoid dose reduction.[33]

A variety of dry-powder inhalers are available, some of which are more child friendly than others. The Turbuhaler, for example, can be used correctly by 55% of children aged 5 to 8 years and by 96% of children older than age 8 years.[33] Nebulized formulations are the least efficient form of delivery available. Physicians should be able to demonstrate the optimal use of age-appropriate inhalation devices to children and their caregivers and be prepared to provide repeated assessment and coaching with regard to optimal use of inhaler devices in all children and adolescents.[1–3]

Adverse Effects

Local adverse effects of inhaled glucocorticoids, including oropharyngeal candidiasis, hoarseness, throat irritation, and coughing are not usually troublesome and seldom, if ever, result in discontinuation of treatment.[15,16,34] Serious systemic adverse effects are also uncommon.[15,16,34–41] The risk of any systemic adverse effect is significantly less during inhaled glucocorticoid treatment than during oral glucocorticoid treatment.

The potential adverse effects on growth are of greatest importance. Height measurements must be interpreted carefully, as persistent asthma itself may result in delayed onset of puberty and preadolescent deceleration of height velocity. Randomized, double-blind, placebo-controlled studies of at least 6 months' duration have shown that growth delay may occur with beclomethasone or budesonide dipropionate doses as low as 400 µg/day,[26–28,36] and that this effect can be measured within the first 6 to 12 weeks of treatment (Level IC) (Figure 11–3B).[27,36] Delayed intermediate-term growth (growth over at least 6 months) is not associated with decreased growth hormone secretion or impaired hypothalamic-pituitary-adrenal (HPA) axis function; however, osteoblasts are affected and type I and type III collagen turnover is suppressed.[26,35,36] Some new inhaled glucocorticoids are said to be free from significant adverse effects on growth, at least in low doses.[37]

There are no prospective, randomized, rigorously controlled, double-blind studies of the effect of inhaled glucocorticoids on long-term linear growth (to adulthood). A retrospective cohort study suggests that the attained adult height of asthmatic children treated with glucocorticoids is not significantly different from the adult height of those not treated with these medications (Level II).[38]

During treatment with recommended doses of inhaled glucocorticoids, most tests of HPA axis function are within normal limits. Highly sensitive tests, such as serial early morning cortisol measurements, the area under the curve of 24-hour serum cortisol measurements, or 24-hour urine-free cortisol measurements, may show evidence of HPA axis suppression after 400 µg beclomethasone dipropionate or equivalent.[39] Clinical manifestations of adrenal insufficiency are rare.

Other systemic effects from inhaled glucocorticoids are extremely uncommon[15,16,34,40,41] if recommended doses are used and if supplementary courses of oral or intravenous glucocorticoids are required infrequently. Posterior subcapsular cataracts, for example, were not found in any young subjects with a median age of 13.8 years inhaling a median dose of beclomethasone dipropionate or budesonide of 750 µg/d (12.9 µg/kg/d) for a median duration of 5 years, with infrequent supplemental oral glucocorticoids (Level IIB).[40] Rarely, reports of behavioural disturbances and other adverse central nervous system effects, or disseminated infection with varicella[41] or other viruses are published (Level IV). Carbohydrate and lipid metabolism may be altered when high doses of inhaled glucocorticoids are administered. Effects on collagen synthesis in the skin can be documented, but skin thinning or excessive bruising are more of a theoretical concern than a practical problem in children.[15]

Anti-allergics

The inhaled anti-allergic medications cromolyn or nedocromil are still used for the treatment of children with mild or moderate persistent asthma.[42–48] Cromolyn is less effective than an inhaled glucocorticoid (Level IIA)[20,29] and has the disadvantage of needing to be administered three or four times daily during initiation of treatment. A CFC-free metered-dose inhaler formulation is available.[42]

In the open follow-up to the original placebo-controlled efficacy study of cromolyn in children, 2 or 3 of the 46 children remained well over 5 years, as assessed by lack of need for further inhaled glucocorticoid treatment (Level IIA).[43] In another study, data were reviewed from 175 children who had been monitored for up to 16.8 years (mean 8.4 years). Pulmonary function improved to normal values in the children treated with cromolyn sodium as well as in those treated with inhaled glucocorticoids (Level IIB).[44] In a study of very young children, however, cromolyn sodium 10 mg administered by face mask and nebulizer three times daily was found to be no more effective than placebo (Level IA),[45] and in a recent meta-analysis of studies conducted in young subjects, cromolyn was found to be no more effective than placebo (Level I).[46]

Nedocromil sodium 4 mg twice daily prevents exercise-induced bronchoconstriction in children (Level IB),[47] and can be used on a regular twice-daily basis to prevent asthma symptoms, as an alternative to inhaled glucocorticoids.[48] A 5-year, prospective, randomized, placebo-controlled comparative study of nedocromil sodium and budesonide in approximately 1,000 children and adolescents has recently been completed and will provide Level IA evidence of the relative efficacy of these medications.[30]

Cromolyn and nedocromil have excellent safety profiles and are well tolerated. Systemic concentrations are extremely low after inhalation; only 10% of the dose enters the lungs, and 90% enters the gastrointestinal tract, from which minimal absorption takes place. Some children complain that nedocromil has an unpleasant taste.

β_2-Adrenergic Agonists

Short-Acting β_2-Adrenergic Agonists

Short-acting β_2-adrenergic agonists such as salbutamol or terbutaline, potent and rapidly acting bronchodilators, are generally administered by inhalation from a pressurized metered-dose inhaler or a dry-powder inhaler (Level IA).[1–3,49–51] In persistent asthma treatment, they are no longer recommended for regular use three to four times daily. Increasing use of a short-acting β_2-adrenergic agonist, or lack of effect of a short-acting β_2-adrenergic agonist, indicates inadequate asthma control[1–3,51] and the need for a regular anti-inflammatory medication such as an inhaled glucocorticoid or, if the child is already taking such a medication, the need for review and modification of the drug and/or the dose.

Salbutamol and some other β_2-adrenergic agonists are also available in oral formulations that, compared to inhaled formulations, have a slow onset of action and a less favorable benefit-to-risk ratio. They have generally been studied during regular administration three or four times daily rather than during intermittent use for relief of breakthrough asthma symptoms. As they are palatable and easy to administer, they are still prescribed for infants and children who refuse inhaled medications or whose parents are unable to learn how to administer medications by inhalation (Level III).[3] Adverse effects of β_2-adrenergic agonists include tachycardia, tremor, and headache.

Long-Acting β_2-Adrenergic Agonists

The long-acting β_2-adrenergic agonists salmeterol and formoterol have been reasonably well

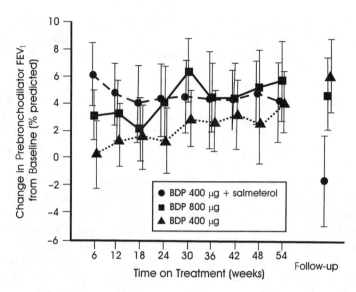

Figure 11–4 In a randomized, multicenter, double-blind, parallel-group, placebo-controlled 1-year study in 177 children, mean age approximately 11 years, salmeterol 50 μg twice daily plus beclomethasone dipropionate (BDP) 200 μg twice daily was no more effective than BDP 200 μg twice daily alone or BDP 400 μg twice daily alone, with regard to FEV$_1$ (shown), bronchial hyperresponsiveness to methacholine, symptom scores, or exacerbation rates. (Reproduced with permission from Verberne AAPH, Frost C, Duiverman EJ, et al. Addition of salmeterol versus doubling the dose of beclomethasone in children with asthma. Am J Respir Crit Care Med 1998;158:213–9.)

studied in adolescents and children over age 6 years but not in very young children or in infants. They provide excellent bronchodilation for 12 to 24 hours; salmeterol, but not formoterol, has a slightly slower onset of action than salbutamol. In studies of up to 1 year of duration, salmeterol 25 μg or 50 μg twice daily regularly, in contrast to salbutamol 200 μg twice daily regularly, has decreased the need for "rescue" bronchodilator treatment and improved nocturnal asthma symptoms and morning peak expiratory flows (Level IA).[52]

Salmeterol or formoterol, used as monotherapy, have a comparable bronchodilator effect to inhaled glucocorticoids, but otherwise are less effective (Level IA).[27,28] In salmeterol studies of 1 year duration, in which bronchial hyperreactivity to methacholine was the main outcome measure, no loss of bronchoprotection, rebound bronchial hyperreactivity (see Figure 11–3A), decrease in bronchodilation, or worsening of symptoms was found (Level IA).[27,28] The role of salbutamol and formoterol as steroid-sparing agents has not been as clearly documented in children as it has been in adults (Figure 11–4) (Level IC);[53] however, studies of salmeterol in a fixed-dose combination in the same inhaler with fluticasone propionate[54] are in progress in children.

A single dose of salmeterol 25 to 50 μg or formoterol 12 μg provides excellent protection against methacholine-induced bronchospasm or exercise-induced bronchospasm for 12 to 24 hours. As with short-acting β$_2$-adrenergic agonists, the long-acting β$_2$-adrenergic agonists shift the stimulus response curve to exercise in a beneficial direction. Unlike the short-acting medications, which do not entirely eliminate airflow obstruction, the long-acting β$_2$-adrenergic agonists may almost completely abolish the post-exercise decrease in peak expiratory flow or FEV$_1$ throughout the dosing interval, thus providing protection against exercise-induced bronchospasm throughout the school day. Slight loss of the bronchoprotective effect of the long-acting β$_2$-adrenergic agonists against exercise-induced bronchospasm may develop during chronic use (Figure 11–5) (Level IA).[55]

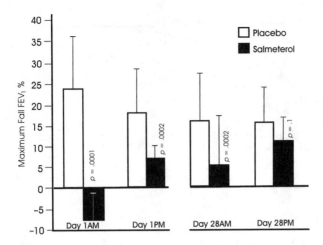

Figure 11–5 In a randomized, double-blind, crossover study in 12 adolescents, mean age 13 years, salmeterol 50 μg was compared with placebo, both treatments being administered once daily by a Nebulizer Chronolog that recorded the date, hour, and minute of dose. On Day 1 of treatment, salmeterol provided excellent protection against exercise-induced bronchospasm 1 and 9 hours after dosing. On Day 28 of treatment, although it remained highly protective 1 hour after treatment (mean maximum fall in FEV_1, 4% ± 12%), protection 9 hours after treatment (mean maximum fall in FEV_1, 10% ± 6%) was no longer statistically significant. (Reproduced with permission from Simons FER, Gerstner TV, Cheang MS. Tolerance to the bronchoprotective effect of salmeterol in adolescents with exercise-induced asthma using concurrent inhaled glucocorticoid treatment. Pediatrics 1997; 99:655–9.)

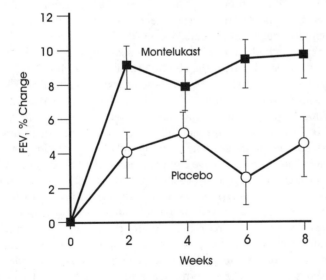

Figure 11–6 In an 8-week, randomized, double-blind, multicenter, parallel-group study in 336 asthmatics aged 6 to 14 years, montelukast 5 mg at bedtime was compared with placebo. In both groups, pretreatment baseline FEV_1 was 72% predicted (1.85 L). The primary outcome, FEV_1 % change from baseline, increased by 8.23% in montelukast-treated children and by 3.58% in placebo-treated children ($p < .001$). (Reproduced with permission from Knorr B, Matz J, Bernstein JA, et al. Montelukast for chronic asthma in 6- to 14-year-old children. A randomized, double-blind trial. JAMA 1998;279:1181–6.)

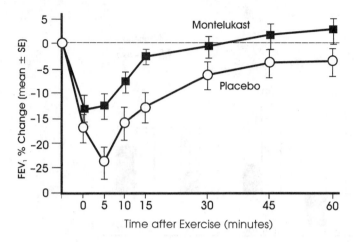

Figure 11–7 In a two-period, double-blind, multicenter, crossover study, 27 children with an FEV_1 ≥ 70% of predicted and a fall in FEV_1 ≥ 20% after exercise received montelukast 5 mg or placebo once daily for 2 days, with at least 4 days between treatment periods. Standardized exercise challenges were performed 20 to 24 hours after the last dose in each period. Montelukast attenuated exercise-induced bronchospasm; that is, it significantly reduced the maximum percent fall (by 18% vs 26% for placebo, $p \leq .05$) and reduced the post-exercise FEV_1 % fall versus time curve (265%/minute vs 590%/minute, $p \leq .05$). (Reproduced with permission from Kemp JP, Dockhorn RJ, Shapiro GG, et al. Montelukast once daily inhibits exercise-induced bronchoconstriction in 6- to 14-year-old children with asthma. J Pediatr 1998;133:424–8.)

Leukotriene Modifiers

Cysteinyl leukotriene$_1$ antagonists offer a new option for treatment of persistent asthma and for prevention of exercise-induced bronchospasm.[56–62] In persistent asthma, montelukast 5 mg has been compared with placebo in a prospective, randomized, double-blind, crossover 8-week study in 336 children aged 6 to 14 years, one-third of whom were using inhaled glucocorticoids regularly. The children receiving montelukast had a significantly greater improvement in FEV_1 from baseline than the children receiving placebo (8.23% vs 3.58%) throughout the study (Figure 11–6) (Level IA).[59] Those receiving montelukast also had significantly decreased short-acting β_2-agonist use, fewer asthma exacerbations, decreased peripheral blood eosinophil counts, and improved asthma-specific quality of life, compared to those receiving placebo. There was no significant difference between the two groups for other outcomes, such as peak flow monitored at home morning and evening, daytime asthma symptoms, and nocturnal awakenings. In school-age children, montelukast 5 mg daily added to the budesonide 200 µg bid has a modest glucocorticoid-sparing effect.[61] Studies of montelukast in children aged 2 to 5 years who have persistent asthma, have recently been completed, and in many countries, montelukast is now approved for use in children aged 2 years and older.

Montelukast 5 mg daily prevents exercise-induced bronchospasm, as confirmed in a randomized, double-blind, placebo-controlled 2-day crossover study in 6- to 14-year-old children. Twenty to twenty-four hours postdose, montelukast decreased the area under the curve for FEV_1 following exercise bronchoprovocation by approximately 50% and also decreased the maximum fall in FEV_1 (18%, 27% during the placebo treatment) (Figure 11–7) (Level IB).[60] The time to recovery was not significantly different between the montelukast- and placebo-treated groups.

Zafirlukast is approved for children aged 12 years or older and also protects against exercise-induced bronchospasm. In doses greater than the 20 mg twice daily dose recommended by the manufacturer for this age group, there may be a slightly increased risk of transaminase elevations and of interactions with other medications.[62]

Theophylline

During the past decade the use of theophylline has diminished considerably, and it is now more likely to be used for its modest immunomodulatory effects as a glucocorticoid-sparing medication in children with severe persistent asthma than for its modest bronchodilator effect.[63–65] When compared directly with beclomethasone dipropionate, it is less effective in reducing symptoms and improving pulmonary function (Level IA).[26]

Theophylline metabolism is relatively rapid, and maintenance of stable serum concentrations requires administration as a reliably absorbed slow-release formulation.[63,64] Rates of elimination vary over a fourfold range among individuals but usually remain stable within the same patient, except when altered by interaction with other medications or by physiologic changes produced by intercurrent illness, for example, viral infection with high fever. Dosage must be individualized, guided by intermittent monitoring of serum concentrations,[63,64] and patients and their parents should be advised of the potential for adverse effects and medication interactions.

The optimal therapeutic range of serum theophylline concentrations is now considered to be 5 to 10 µg/mL, not 10 to 20 µg/mL, as recommended years ago.[63,64] Potential pharmacokinetic interactions involving theophylline and medications such as clarithromycin, erythromycin, ciprofloxacin, or cimetidine may result in a >20% increase in serum theophylline concentrations and lead to toxicity. If concentrations exceed 20 µg/mL, nausea, vomiting, headache, irritability, and insomnia may occur, and at very high concentrations, there is a risk of seizures, toxic encephalopathy, brain damage, cardiac arrhythmias, and death.

Histamine$_1$ Receptor Antagonists

Antihistamines (H$_1$ receptor antagonists) are not generally recommended for asthma treatment.[66] Asthma and allergic rhinitis often coexist as an "allergic rhinobronchitis,"[67] however, and when needed for the management of concurrent allergic rhinitis, H$_1$ antagonists in usual doses may improve mild asthma symptoms and pulmonary function tests (Level IB);[68] further proof of this is needed in children.

In moderate persistent asthma, the H$_1$ antagonist doses required to decrease symptoms, decrease "rescue" bronchodilator use, and increase peak expiratory flows may be 2 to 3 times those ordinarily recommended for allergic rhinitis treatment. The response is similar in magnitude to that produced by inhaled cromolyn (Level IC).[69] Antihistamines have been demonstrated to have a glucocorticoid-sparing effect in asthma in some, but not all, studies (Level IC).[70]

The role of H$_1$ antagonists in prevention or delay of asthma symptoms in atopic children who have not yet developed wheezing is currently of considerable interest. In placebo-controlled studies of 1- and 3-years duration in infants with atopic dermatitis and/or elevated serum IgE and a family history of atopy, who are at high risk for development of asthma, ketotifen appeared to delay the development of asthma (Level IB).[71,72] In a recent study, cetirizine was also found to modify the onset of asthma in at-risk young children with atopic dermatitis and sensitization to house dust mite and/or grass pollen; no adverse effects were reported despite the high doses administered (Level IB).[5,73]

Other Medications

The inhaled anticholinergic/antimuscarinic ipratropium bromide has no role in the management of persistent asthma in children. Also, antibiotics have no role in asthma treatment, as the upper respiratory tract infections that trigger asthma exacerbations are viral, rather than bacterial (Level III).[1–3] In severe, oral steroid–dependent asthma, high-dose intravenous immunoglobulin (Level IIB)[74] or cyclosporin[75] are advocated as steroid-sparing agents. New immunomodulators such as anti-IgE and soluble recombinant human IL-4-receptor are currently being investigated in adults and adolescents with asthma,[76,77] but have not yet been studied in young children.

NONPHARMACOLOGIC TREATMENT

Avoidance of Trigger Factors for Asthma Symptoms

Control of environmental allergens and respiratory irritants is easier said than done and easier done than maintained over many years. Environmental allergens have been identified as potential trigger factors for fatal asthma attacks in young people.[78] Control of airborne allergens in the environment should be based on objective evidence of sensitization to allergens, obtained using skin-prick tests, in every child with asthma (Level III).[79] Specific measures such as washing bed sheets in hot water at least twice monthly to get rid of house dust mites are associated with significantly reduced hospitalization rates for asthma (in house dust mite–sensitive children) (Level IIA).[80] A recent meta-analysis that failed to find evidence to support house dust mite control included studies in which the physical or chemical interventions failed to reduce the environmental mite content and, thus, could not have been expected to decrease symptoms.[81] Lack of avoidance of trigger factors, especially cigarette smoke, is a major barrier to successful asthma treatment in many children.[82] Unfortunately, avoidance of viral upper respiratory tract infections, a common trigger for many acute asthma episodes in childhood, is difficult.

The one trigger factor for asthma that should not be avoided is exercise; indeed, the adequacy of asthma control can often be assessed by a child's ability to keep up with his or her peers in physical education classes or while participating in extracurricular athletic activities.

Education

Asthma education is based on the following principles: anticipation of exacerbations, determination of an appropriate response, and rehearsal of solutions,[83] for example, when, why, and how to take or increase medications; and if age- or disease severity–appropriate, when, why, and how to monitor peak expiratory flows. It is most successful when targeted to children of specific age groups and their families, such as preschoolers, school-aged children, and adolescents.[84]

Asthma educators must be cognizant of self-identified learning needs and preferred learning methods of patients and their families, particularly where adolescents are concerned.[85] The importance of a written Asthma Action Plan (a mutual agreement by the child or adolescent, the family, and the physician[s]) cannot be overemphasized. Having a self-management plan and increasing medications promptly at the onset of "colds" are associated with reduced odds of having an emergency department visit for asthma (Level IIA).[80] Asthma education sessions also offer the opportunity for discussion of general maintenance of good health, including nutritional[86] and lifestyle issues.

Allergen Vaccinations (Immunotherapy)

Immunotherapy for asthma associated with allergy to airborne substances such as house dust mites or tree, grass, and weed pollens that are impossible to avoid in the outdoor environment, remains more controversial in asthma than in other allergic disorders such as rhinoconjunctivitis. A meta-analysis of immunotherapy studies in asthma (Level I)[87] and a review of immunotherapy in childhood asthma[88] suggest efficacy, especially for house dust mite–allergic patients. At this time, immunotherapy is not recommended for young children.[79] Improvement in asthma after immunotherapy is related to the allergen dose that can be administered during a defined time frame and is thus easier to achieve when only one allergen is being injected. Long-term, low-dose, multiple antigen immunotherapy is reported to add little to treatment involving optimal control of environmental allergens and optimal pharmacotherapy including inhaled glucocorticoids (Level ID).[89]

REFERENCES

1. Murphy S, Sheffer AL, Pauwels RA. National Asthma Education and Prevention Program. Expert panel report II: guidelines for the diagnosis and management of asthma. Bethesda (MD): National Heart, Lung, and Blood Institute; 1997. Publication No.: 97-4051.

2. Boulet LP, Becker A, Bérubé D, et al, on behalf of the Canadian Asthma Consensus Group. Summary of recommendations from the Canadian Consensus Guidelines for Asthma Care 1999. Can Med Assoc J 1999;161:S3–12.

3. Warner JO, Naspitz CK, Cropp GJA, et al. Third international pediatric consensus statement on the management of childhood asthma. Pediatr Pulmonol 1998;25:1–17.

4. Arshad SH, Stevens M, Hide DW. The effect of genetic and environmental factors on the prevalence of allergic disorders at the age of two years. Clin Exp Allergy 1993;23:504–11.

5. Wahn U for the ETAC Study Group. Allergic factors associated with the development of asthma and the influence of cetirizine in a double-blind, randomised, placebo-controlled trial: first results of ETAC. Pediatr Allergy Immunol 1998;9:116–24.

6. Martinez FD, Wright AL, Taussig LM, et al. Asthma and wheezing in the first six years of life. N Engl J Med 1995;332:133–8.

7. Zeiger RS, Dawson C, Weiss S for the Childhood Asthma Management Program (CAMP) Research Group. Relationships between duration of asthma and asthma severity among children in the Childhood Asthma Management Program (CAMP). J Allergy Clin Immunol 1999;103:376–87.

8. Agertoft L, Pedersen S. Effects of long-term treatment with an inhaled corticosteroid on growth and pulmonary function in asthmatic children. Respir Med 1994;88:373–81.

9. Godden DJ, Ross S, Abdalla M, et al. Outcome of wheeze in childhood. Symptoms and pulmonary function 25 years later. Am J Respir Crit Care Med 1994;149:106–12.

10. Panhuysen CIM, Vonk JM, Koëter GH, et al. Adult patients may outgrow their asthma. A 25-year follow-up study. Am J Respir Crit Care Med 1997;155:1267–72.

11. Oswald H, Phelan PD, Lanigan A, et al. Childhood asthma and lung function in mid-adult life. Pediatr Pulmonol 1997;23:14–20.

12. Watson WTA, Becker AB, Simons FER. Treatment of allergic rhinitis with intranasal corticosteroids in patients with mild asthma: effect on lower airway responsiveness. J Allergy Clin Immunol 1993;91:97–101.

13. Cook DJ, Guyatt GH, Laupacis A, et al. Clinical recommendations using levels of evidence for antithrombotic agents. Chest 1995;108 Suppl:227–305S.

14. Sackett DL. Apply overviews and meta-analyses at the bedside. J Clin Epidemiol 1995;48:61–6.

15. Pedersen S, O'Byrne P. A comparison of the efficacy and safety of inhaled corticosteroids in asthma. Allergy 1997;52 Suppl 39:1–34.

16. Simons FER. Benefits and risks of inhaled glucocorticoids in children with persistent asthma. J Allergy Clin Immunol 1998;102:S77–84.

17. Adams NP, Bestall JC, Jones PW. Efficacy of inhaled beclomethasone dipropionate and budesonide in the treatment of chronic asthma: a meta-analysis. Eur Respir J 1999;14:1s.

18. Bestall JC, Adams NP, Jones PW. Meta-analysis of the efficacy of fluticasone propionate versus placebo in the treatment of chronic asthma for measures of FEV_1 and PEFR. Eur Respir J 1999;14:1–2s.

19. Szefler SJ, Leung DYM. Glucocorticoid-resistant asthma: pathogenesis and clinical implications for management. Eur Respir J 1997;10:1640–7.

20. Donahue JG, Weiss ST, Livingston JM, et al. Inhaled steroids and the risk of hospitalization for asthma. JAMA 1997;277:887–91.

21. Baker JW, Mellon M, Wald J, et al. A multiple-dosing, placebo-controlled study of budesonide inhalation suspension given once or twice daily for treatment of persistent asthma in young children and infants. Pediatrics 1999;103:414–21.

22. Shapiro G, Mendelson L, Kraemer MJ, et al. Efficacy and safety of budesonide inhalation suspension (Pulmicort Respules) in young children with inhaled steroid-dependent, persistent asthma. J Allergy Clin Immunol 1998;102:789–96.

23. Shapiro G, Bronsky EA, LaForce CF, et al. Dose-related efficacy of budesonide administered via a dry powder inhaler in the treatment of children with moderate to severe persistent asthma. J Pediatr 1998;132:976–82.

24. Pedersen S, Hansen OR. Budesonide treatment of moderate and severe asthma in children: a dose-response study. J Allergy Clin Immunol 1995;95:29–33.

25. Van Essen-Zandvliet EE, Hughes MD, Waalkens HJ, et al, and the Dutch Chronic Non-Specific Lung Disease Study Group. Effects of 22 months of treatment with inhaled corticosteroids and/or beta-2-agonists on lung function, airway responsiveness, and symptoms in children with asthma. Am Rev Respir Dis 1992;146:547–54.

26. Tinkelman DG, Reed CE, Nelson HS, Offord KP. Aerosol beclomethasone dipropionate compared with theophylline as primary treatment of chronic, mild to moderately severe asthma in children. Pediatrics 1993;92:64–77.

27. Simons FER and the Canadian Beclomethasone Dipropionate–Salmeterol Xinafoate Study Group. A comparison of beclomethasone, salmeterol, and placebo in children with asthma. N Engl J Med 1997;337:1659–65.

28. Verberne AAPH, Frost C, Roorda RJ, et al, and the Dutch Paediatric Asthma Study Group. One year treatment with salmeterol compared with beclomethasone in children with asthma. Am J Respir Crit Care Med 1997;156:688–95.

29. Price JF, Russell G, Hindmarsh PC, et al. Growth during one year of treatment with fluticasone propionate or sodium cromoglycate in children with asthma. Pediatr Pulmonol 1997;24:178–86.

30. CAMP corporate paper. The Childhood Asthma Management Program (CAMP): design, rationale, and methods. Control Clin Trials 1999;20:91–120.

31. Waalkens HJ, Van Essen-Zandvliet EE, Hughes MD, et al, and the Dutch CNSLD Study Group. Cessation of long-term treatment with inhaled corticosteroid (budesonide) in children with asthma results in deterioration. Am Rev Respir Dis 1993;148:1252–7.

32. Berg E, Madsen J, Bisgaard H. In vitro performance of three combinations of spacers and pressurized metered dose inhalers for treatment in children. Eur Respir J 1998;12:472–6.

33. De Boeck K, Alifier M, Warnier G. Is the correct use of a dry powder inhaler (Turbuhaler) age dependent? J Allergy Clin Immunol 1999;103:763–7.

34. Agertoft L, Larsen FE, Pedersen S. Posterior subcapsular cataracts, bruises and hoarseness in children with asthma receiving long-term treatment with inhaled budesonide. Eur Respir J 1998;12:130–5.

35. Crowley S, Hindmarsh PC, Matthews DR, Brook CGD. Growth and the growth hormone axis in prepubertal children with asthma. J Pediatr 1995;126:297–303.

36. Doull IJM, Freezer NJ, Holgate ST. Growth of prepubertal children with mild asthma treated with inhaled beclomethasone dipropionate. Am J Respir Crit Care Med 1995;151:1715–9.

37. Allen DB, Bronsky EA, LaForce CF, et al, and the Fluticasone Propionate Asthma Study Group. Growth in asthmatic children treated with fluticasone propionate. J Pediatr 1998;132:472–7.

38. Silverstein MD, Yunginger JW, Reed CE, et al. Attained adult height after childhood asthma: effect of glucocorticoid therapy. J Allergy Clin Immunol 1997;99:466–74.

39. Nicolaizik WH, Marchant JL, Preece MA, Warner JO. Endocrine and lung function in asthmatic children on inhaled corticosteroids. Am J Respir Crit Care Med 1994;150:624–8.

40. Simons FER, Persaud MP, Gillespie CA, et al. Absence of posterior subcapsular cataracts in young patients treated with inhaled glucocorticoids. Lancet 1993;342:776–8.

41. Choong K, Zwaigenbaum L, Onyett H. Severe varicella after low dose inhaled corticosteroids. Pediatr Infect Dis J 1995;14:809–11.

42. Furukawa C, Atkinson D, Forster TJ, et al, for the Intal Study Group. Controlled trial of two formulations of cromolyn sodium in the treatment of asthmatic patients >12 years of age. Chest 1999;116:65–72.

43. Godfrey S, Balfour-Lynn L, König P. The place of cromolyn sodium in the long-term management of childhood asthma based on a 3- to 5-year follow-up. J Pediatr 1975;87:465–73.

44. König P, Shaffer J. The effect of drug therapy on long-term outcome of childhood asthma: a possible preview of the international guidelines. J Allergy Clin Immunol 1996;98:1103–11.

45. Tasche MJA, van der Wouden JC, Uijen JHJM, et al. Randomised placebo-controlled trial of inhaled sodium cromoglycate in 1–4-year-old children with moderate asthma. Lancet 1997;350:1060–4.

46. van der Wouden JC, Tasche MJ, Uijen JH, et al. Systematic review of inhaled sodium cromoglycate in childhood asthma. Eur Respir J 1999;14:12s.

47. de Benedictis FM, Tuteri G, Pazzelli P, et al. Cromolyn versus nedocromil: duration of action in exercise-induced asthma in children. J Allergy Clin Immunol 1995;96:510–4.

48. Armenio L, Baldini G, Bardare M, et al. Double blind, placebo controlled study of nedocromil sodium in asthma. Arch Dis Child 1993;68:193–7.

49. Nelson HS. β-adrenergic bronchodilators. J Allergy Clin Immunol 1995;333:499–506.

50. Drazen JM, Israel E, Boushey HA, et al. Comparison of regularly scheduled with as-needed use of albuterol in mild asthma. N Engl J Med 1996;335:841–7.

51. Spitzer WO, Suissa S, Ernst P, et al. The use of β-agonists and the risk of death and near death from asthma. N Engl J Med 1992;326:501–6.

52. Verberne AAPH, Hop WCJ, Creyghton FBM, et al. Airway responsiveness after a single dose of salmeterol and during four months of treatment in children with asthma. J Allergy Clin Immunol 1996;97:938–46.

53. Verberne AAPH, Frost C, Duiverman EJ, et al, and the Dutch Paediatric Asthma Study Group. Addition of salmeterol versus doubling the dose of beclomethasone in children with asthma. Am J Respir Crit Care Med 1998;158:213–9.

54. Spencer CM, Jarvis B. Salmeterol/fluticasone propionate combination. Drugs 1999;57:933–40.

55. Simons FER, Gerstner TV, Cheang MS. Tolerance to the bronchoprotective effect of salmeterol in adolescents with exercise-induced asthma using concurrent inhaled glucocorticoid treatment. Pediatrics 1997;99:655–9.

56. Lipworth BJ. Leukotriene-receptor antagonists. Lancet 1999;353:57–62.

57. Drazen JM, Israel E, O'Byrne PM. Treatment of asthma with drugs modifying the leukotriene pathway. N Engl J Med 1999;340:197–206.

58. Horwitz RJ, McGill KA, Busse WW. The role of leukotriene modifiers in the treatment of asthma. Am J Respir Crit Care Med 1998;157:1363–71.

59. Knorr B, Matz J, Bernstein JA, et al, for the Pediatric Montelukast Study Group. Montelukast for chronic asthma in 6- to 14-year-old children. A randomized, double-blind trial. JAMA 1998;279:1181–6.

60. Kemp JP, Dockhorn RJ, Shapiro GG, et al. Montelukast once daily inhibits exercise-induced bronchoconstriction in 6- to 14-year-old children with asthma. J Pediatr 1998;133:424–8.

61. Simons FER, Villa JR, Lee BW, et al. Montelukast added to budesonide in children with persistent asthma: results of a multicenter, randomized, double-blind, crossover study. Allergy 55 2000;S63:1–2.

62. Adkins JC, Brodgen RN. Zafirlukast. A review of its pharmacology and therapeutic potential in the management of asthma. Drugs 1998;55:121–44.

63. Weinberger M, Hendeles L. Theophylline in asthma. N Engl J Med 1996;334:1380–94.

64. Hendeles L, Weinberger M, Szefler S, Ellis E. Safety and efficacy of theophylline in children with asthma. J Pediatr 1992;120:177–83.

65. Kidney J, Dominguez M, Taylor PM, et al. Immunomodulation by theophylline in asthma. Am J Respir Crit Care Med 1995;151:1907–14.

66. Simons FER, Simons KJ. The pharmacology and use of H_1-receptor antagonist drugs. N Engl J Med 1994;330:1663–70.

67. Simons FER. Allergic rhinobronchitis. The asthma/allergic rhinitis link. J Allergy Clin Immunol 1999;104:534–7.

68. Corren J, Harris AG, Aaronson D, et al. Efficacy and safety of loratadine plus pseudoephedrine in patients with seasonal allergic rhinitis and mild asthma. J Allergy Clin Immunol 1997;100:781–8.

69. Menardo JL, Wessel F, Cougnard J, Czarlewski W. Prophylactic treatment with loratadine versus cromolyn sodium in children with mild-to-moderate perennial allergic asthma. Curr Ther Res 1998;59:567–78.

70. Canny GJ, Reisman J, Levison H. Does ketotifen have a steroid-sparing effect in childhood asthma? Eur Respir J 1997;10:65–70.

71. Iikura Y, Naspitz CK, Mikawa H, et al. Prevention of asthma by ketotifen in infants with atopic dermatitis. Ann Allergy 1992;68:233–6.

72. Bustos GJ, Bustos D, Bustos GJ, Romero O. Prevention of asthma with ketotifen in preasthmatic children: a three-year follow-up study. Clin Exp Allergy 1995;25:568–73.

73. Simons FER, on behalf of the ETAC Study Group. Prospective, long-term safety evaluation of the H_1-receptor antagonist cetirizine in very young children with atopic dermatitis. J Allergy Clin Immunol 1999;104:433–40.

74. Landwehr LP, Jeppson JD, Katlan MG, et al. Benefits of high-dose intravenous immunoglobulin in patients with severe steroid-dependent asthma. Chest 1998;114:1349–56.

75. Coren ME, Rosenthal M, Bush A. The use of cyclosporin in corticosteroid-dependent asthma. Arch Dis Child 1997;77:522–3.

76. Milgrom H, Fick RB Jr, Su JQ, et al. Treatment of allergic asthma with monoclonal anti-IgE antibody. rhuMAb-E25 Study Group. N Engl J Med 1999;341:1966-73.

77. Borish LC, Nelson HS, Lanz MJ, et al. Interleukin-4 receptor in moderate atopic asthma. A phase I/II randomized, placebo-controlled trial. Am J Respir Crit Care Med 1999;160:1816–23.

78. O'Hollaren MT, Yunginger JW, Offord KP, et al. Exposure to an aeroallergen as a possible precipitating factor in respiratory arrest in young patients with asthma. N Engl J Med 1991;324:359–63.

79. Ownby DR, Adinoff AD. The appropriate use of skin testing and allergen immunotherapy in young children. J Allergy Clin Immunol 1994;94:662–5.

80. Lieu TA, Quesenberry CP Jr, Capra AM, et al. Outpatient management practices associated with reduced risk of pediatric asthma hospitalization and Emergency Department visits. Pediatrics 1997;100:334–41.

81. Gotzsche P, Hammarquist C, Burr M. House dust mite control measures in the management of asthma: meta-analysis. BMJ 1998;317:1105–10.

82. DiFranza JR, Lew RA. Morbidity and mortality in children associated with the use of tobacco products by other people. Pediatrics 1996;97:560–8.

83. Childhood Asthma Management Program Research Group. Design and implementation of a patient education center for the childhood asthma management program. Ann Allergy Asthma Immunol 1998;81:571–81.

84. Bender B, Milgrom H, Rand C. Nonadherence in asthmatic patients: is there a solution to the problem? Ann Allergy Asthma Immunol 1997;79:177–86.

85. Gillespie C, Kudlak M, Ernst F, et al. Self-identified learning needs and preferred learning methods of adolescents with asthma. J Allergy Clin Immunol 1999;103:S6.

86. Cook DG, Carey IM, Whincup PH, et al. Effect of fresh fruit consumption on lung function and wheeze in children. Thorax 1997;52:628–33.

87. Abramson MJ, Puy RM, Weiner JM. Is allergen immunotherapy effective in asthma? A meta-analysis of randomized controlled trials. Am J Respir Crit Care Med 1995;151:969–74.

88. Sigman K, Mazer B. Immunotherapy for childhood asthma: is there a rationale for its use? Ann Allergy Asthma Immunol 1996;76:299–309.

89. Adkinson NF Jr, Eggleston PA, Eney D, et al. A controlled trial of immunotherapy for asthma in allergic children. N Engl J Med 1997;336:324–31.

CHAPTER 12

Mechanisms of Action of β-Agonists and Short-Acting β₂ Therapy

Tony R. Bai, MD, MRCP, FACP, FRACP, FRCPC

Short-acting β-adrenoceptor agonists have been used since 1903 to treat asthma, following the isolation of epinephrine. Evaluation of a large volume of data generated in the study of β-adrenergic pharmacology enabled Lands et al in 1967 to suggest a division of the β-adrenergic receptor (βAR) response into subtypes termed β_1 and β_2.[1] This distinction was based on the relative potency of the naturally occurring catecholamines, epinephrine and norepinephrine. β_1 responses are equally sensitive to these two agonists; β_2 responses are more potently stimulated by epinephrine. Generally, but not invariably, β_1 responses appear to be initiated by the neurotransmitter, norepinephrine, in innervated tissues, whereas β_2 responses are triggered by the circulating hormone epinephrine.[2] Soon after the subdivision into β_1 and β_2 responses, relatively selective β_2-adrenergic agonists were developed; they remain the most widely prescribed class of asthma medication today.

β-ADRENOCEPTOR BIOLOGY

Molecular Biology and Mechanisms of Agonist Action

The β_2AR gene lacks introns, maps to chromosome five, and encodes a protein of 413 amino acids, only 54% of which are shared with β_1ARs.[3–6] The mature messenger ribonucleic acid (mRNA) transcript for the β_2AR is 2.2 kilobases. Studies of the regulation of gene transcription show that glucocorticoids increase mRNA levels by increasing the rate of gene transcription.[7] Isoproterenol decreases mRNA levels by decreasing stability of the mature mRNA.[8,9] Gene transcription increases following cytokines such as interleukin-1 (IL-1)-β.[10] Adrenergic receptors belong to the G protein-linked, rhodopsin-related receptor superfamily, one of at least three cell membrane receptor superfamilies. The current model of this cell membrane–associated receptor indicates seven transmembrane segments connected by alternating intracellular and extracellular loops. Homology among all the members of the seven transmembrane (serpentine) receptor family is greatest in the transmembrane spanning domains. Genetic and biochemical manipulation of the β_2AR has identified that the ligand-binding domain is a pocket buried within the membrane bilayer; agonists interact specifically with amino acids in transmembrane helixes III and V.[3,11] Antagonists do not bind to the same amino acids.

Binding of an agonist to the β_2AR, coupled to the stimulatory guanine-nucleotide binding protein, G_s, catalyzes the release of guanosine diphosphate (GDP) from the β subunit of the G protein (β_s), allowing the binding of guanosine triphosphate (GTP); this leads to the direct activation of adenylyl cyclase by βs-GTP. Adenylyl cyclase catalyzes the formation of the second messenger cyclic adenosine monophosphate (cAMP), so that levels of cAMP up to 400-fold over basal levels can occur within minutes of agonist exposure.[3,11–14] Upon removal of agonist, the activation of adenylyl cyclase persists until the intrinsic GTPase activity of β_s hydrolyzes the bound nucleotide.[11,13] Cell relaxation is primarily determined by generation of cAMP and activation of cAMP-dependent kinases, which have several actions including shifting myosin light-chain kinase to a less active form. However, stimulation of β_2ARs has other effects (Table 12–1). The rise in cAMP leads to calcium reuptake into the sarcoplasmic reticulum and organelles, and calcium extrusion from the cell. Cyclic AMP also causes suppression of inositol triphosphate (IP3) formation. Finally, activation of β_2ARs stimulates a calcium-activated large conductance potassium channel (KCa) in the cell membrane which leads to hyperpolarization of the membrane and cell relaxation.[15,16] This effect is mediated by a cAMP-dependent protein kinase. Antagonism of β_2AR-mediated relaxation by muscarinic agonists may occur in part by opposing effects of stimulatory versus inhibitory G proteins at the level of KCa channels.[16,17] Such an effect could be clinically important in asthma exacerbations under conditions in which acetylcholine release is increased, because the end result could be decreased efficacy of exogenous β_2 agonists.

Table 12–1 *Mechanisms of Smooth Muscle Relaxation by β_2-Agonists*

Stimulation of cAMP and subsequent reduction of MLCK activity

cAMP inhibition of PLC with reduction of IP3 formation

Stimulation of calcium extrusion pumps

Stimulation of a calcium-activated potassium channel

Inhibition of acetylcholine release from cholinergic nerve terminals

cAMP = cyclic adenosine monophosphate; MLCK = myosin light chain kinase; PLC = phospholipase C; IP3 = inositol triphosphate.

Molecular Basis of Agonist Desensitization

β_2-Adrenoceptor desensitization, that is, waning of the stimulated response in the face of continuous agonist exposure, can occur by several mechanisms.[13,18,19] These include uncoupling, which is most rapid, intracellular sequestration [internalization] of the receptor, and finally, after hours of continuous stimulation, downregulation of receptor number by lysozymal degradation.

β_2-Adrenoceptor Localization and Physiologic Effects of Short-Acting β_2-Agonists in Human Lung

Hamid et al have reported the distribution of β_2AR mRNA in human lung by in situ hybridization and correlated this with receptor autoradiographic distribution.[20] They report striking differences between the density of labeling with the two techniques in different cell types. Pulmonary vascular and airway smooth muscle showed a high intensity of mRNA but only a low density of receptors, and the converse was reported for the alveolar epithelium. These investigators speculate the differences may be due to either a rapid rate of β_2AR synthesis or high stability of mRNA in the airways, and this observation may explain the difficulty in demonstrating desensitization in airway smooth muscle.[21,22]

β_1-Adrenoceptors are found in lung parenchyma, heart, and brain, whereas β_2 receptors are found in airways, nose, heart, blood vessels, inflammatory cells, guts, kidney, liver, pancreas, spleen, uterus, brain, and nonadrenergic and cholinergic nerve terminals.

Organ bath and autoradiographic studies have demonstrated that the airway smooth muscle relaxant effect of βAR agonists is largely via β_2ARs directly on the muscle surface.[18,23,24] This is not unexpected, given that β_1 receptors are found at sites of sympathetic innervation responding to norepinephrine release, and there is no direct sympathetic innervation of human airway smooth muscle.[18,25] Similarly, the receptors on mucous and serous glands and inflammatory cells are largely of the β_2 type.[18,26] β_2-Adrenoceptors also predominate on epithelium, type I and II pneumocytes, and vascular smooth muscle; they make up 70% of the βARs in the human lung—the other 30% being β_1ARs on alveolar walls. β_2-Adrenoceptors are, in general, low-abundance receptors (500 to 5,000 sites/cell), but the density of receptors increases from the large to small airways and is much greater on alveolar walls than on other structures in the lung.[24]

Although, in vivo, the most obvious and therapeutic effect of β_2AR stimulation is bronchodilation mediated by airway smooth muscle relaxation; a number of other effects also occur (Table 12–2).[27–35]

Table 12–2 *Physiologic Effects of β_2-Adrenoceptor Stimulation in Human Lung*

Airway smooth muscle relaxation[35]

Prejunctional inhibition of acetylcholine release from parasympathetic neurons in
    airway smooth muscle[35]

Stimulation of mucous and serous cell secretion[28]

Stimulation of chloride ion secretion across the apical membrane of airway
    epithelial cells[30]

Increase in ciliary beat frequency[29]

Stimulation of surfactant secretion from alveolar type II cells[31]

Inhibition of mediator release from lung mast cells and neutrophils[27]

? Reduction in microvascular permeability (animal models)[32]

? Increase in bronchial blood flow (animal models)[33,34]

β_2-Adrenoceptors are present on a variety of inflammatory cells which passage through or reside in the lung.[36–39] Short-acting β_2AR agonists do not prevent mediator release from activated human alveolar macrophages.[40] There is some evidence that β_2AR agonists reduce the release of histamine from mast cells and that this is part of their mechanism of action in abating the early response to allergic bronchial challenge, in addition to being functional antagonists of the airway smooth muscle contraction induced by release of mediators.[18,41] β_2-Adrenoceptor agonists may also inhibit mediator release from basophils.[18] Both alveolar macrophages and eosinophils are thought to be important effector cells in the pathogenesis of asthma, and the lack of influence of short-acting β_2AR agonists on these cell types may explain in part the poor efficacy of these agents as monotherapy in asthma (see below).

β-Adrenoceptors are present in peribronchial parasympathetic ganglia, which receive direct sympathetic innervation,[18] and β_2ARs are also present on cholinergic nerve terminals in airway smooth muscle and act here to inhibit acetylcholine release (prejunctional inhibition), thereby reducing the cholinergic component of bronchoconstriction.[35,42] It is possible that propranolol induces asthma attacks not only by reducing the tonic effect of epinephrine on airway smooth muscle in maintaining airway patency, but also by blocking the effect of epinephrine on cholinergic nerve terminals leading to the exuberant release of acetylcholine. In support of this hypothesis, cholinergic antagonists have been shown to partially reverse propranolol-induced bronchoconstriction.[43]

The role of β_2ARs in the pathogenesis of asthma has been a subject of intense speculation and investigation for more than three decades. β_2-Adrenoceptors are present in normal or increased numbers on asthmatic airway smooth muscle. They are uncoupled in severe asthma, leading to functional hyporesponsiveness, probably due to the effects of inflammatory mediators.[23] There is also evidence for dysfunction of β_2ARs on circulating inflammatory cells following mediator release. There is heterogeneity in the structure of β_2ARs in the human population, and polymorphisms that impart an accelerated agonist-promoted downregulation are over-represented in steroid-dependent and nocturnal asthma and may contribute to the severity of airway responsiveness.

β-Adrenoceptor Agonists

Structure and Metabolism

Commonly used agonists are shown in Table 12–3. The term catecholamine refers to all compounds with a catechol nucleus (benzene plus two adjacent hydroxyl groups) and an amine group. The three principal naturally occurring catecholamines are dopamine (dihydroxyphenylethylamine) and the metabolic products of dopamine, norepinephrine, and epinephrine. Monoamine oxidase, predominantly an intraneuronal enzyme, and catechol O-methyltransferase, predominantly an extraneuronal enzyme, are the two enzymes primarily responsible for degradation of catecholamines. Ligand receptor interactions are stereospecific. All the commonly used β-agonists exist in racemic mixtures of optical isomers referred to as R and S (or [−] and [+]) enantiomers. The agonist activity lies predominantly in the R enantiomers. There has been speculation that the S enantiomers possess adverse effects in clinical usage but this remains unclear.[44] Preparations of R enantiomers alone will soon be available for commercial usage.

Table 12–3 β-Agonists in Clinical Use

Short-Acting (β₂ Selective)	Long-Acting (β₂ Selective)	Catecholamines
Salbutamol	Salmeterol	Epinephrine (adrenaline)
Terbutaline	Formoterol	Isoproterenol (isoprenaline)
Fenoterol		Isoetharine
Metaproterenol (orciprenaline)		
Clenbuterol		
Pirbuterol		
Bitolterol		
Procaterol		

Both salbutamol and terbutaline, the first of the current generation of "short-acting" relatively β₂-adrenoceptor-specific agonists used in the treatment of asthma were synthesized and characterized before the report of Lands et al subtyping β-adrenoceptors.[1] Since the 1960s, a number of other β₂-agonists have been developed as therapeutic agents. The key substitutions to the β-phenylethylamine parent have been to the catechol ring, or related structure, to make the compounds resistant to metabolism by endogenous methyltransferases and monoamine oxidase, and addition of a monoethanolamine side chain of varying length. Such alterations prolong half-life and increase the selectivity of these agents for β₂-adrenoceptors. In clinical research, a short-acting, β₂-selective compound metabolized by endogenous enzymes is sometimes useful and rimiterol is one such compound, although only modestly β₂ selective.

The prototypic short-acting β₂-agonists salbutamol and terbutaline, despite the subsequent development of many other compounds such as fenoterol, clenbuterol, and procaterol (see Table 12–3), remain the most widely prescribed of this class of drug. The major shortcoming of these medications is duration of action. Agents such as pirbuterol and clenbuterol have been reported to possess a significantly longer duration of action but this is marginal at best and, in the case of clenbuterol, exists only after oral administration. A more recently developed compound, bambuterol, does have a more extended duration of action but this drug is a pro-drug of terbutaline and is effective only after oral administration, which is the least preferred route of administration due to systemic side effects.

All the commonly used β_2-agonists are excreted either unchanged in the urine or in a conjugated fashion. For example, salbutamol and terbutaline are susceptible to 4-0'-sulfate conjugation in intestinal wall and liver (when administered by the oral route).[45,46] Following aerosol administration, the significant proportion that impacts in the oropharynx and is swallowed is also conjugated in the intestinal wall. Following intravenous administration, more of the free drug is excreted compared with the oral and aerosolized routes. Fenoterol is also susceptible to 5-0'-sulfation.

Selectivity, Affinity, and Efficacy

The basis of β_1-/β_2-adrenoceptor selectivity may be in differences in the amino acid sequences of the two adrenoceptors.[47] Selectivity is determined by comparing the potency of β-agonists on preparations containing primarily β_1-adrenoceptors (eg, atrial inotropic responses) versus preparations containing primarily β_2-adrenoceptors (eg, bronchial relaxant responses). In this situation, agents are ranked compared to the effect of a completely nonselective β-adrenoceptor agonist, usually isoproterenol (Table 12–4). The ratio of the relative potencies at β_2 versus β_1 sites gives the selectivity ratio.[2,48,49] Using these criteria, the long-acting agent salmeterol is the most β_2-selective agent in common use, and fenoterol is the least selective.

The potency of a given agonist is usually measured as the concentration of the drug required to cause 50% of maximum response to that agonist. Potency is a function of both receptor affinity and efficacy and of tissue-related factors such as receptor density and efficiency of G protein coupling. Affinity describes the degree of attraction of a ligand for a receptor, as determined by binding studies. A radiolabeled version of agonist is used in increasing concentrations until the maximum is reached for bound label compared to labeling in the presence of a high concentration of unlabeled agonist. Efficacy describes the ability of an agonist to induce a response in a particular tissue.[50] β-Agonists and β-antagonists may share similar affinities for β-adrenoceptors but different efficacies. A full agonist will have a high efficacy whereas the pure antagonist will have low or zero efficacy. The majority of short-acting β_2-selective agonists have intermittent efficacy and potency compared to isoproterenol (see Table 12–4).

β_2-Agonist efficacy is usually assessed by examining relaxation responses in the presence of contracted preparations of airway smooth muscle. Again, one compares the maximum relaxant response with that of isoproterenol. This value is called the intrinsic activity and is a ratio of the maximum response of a given β-agonist to the maximum response of isoproterenol. Using these criteria, none of the synthetic β-agonists have higher intrinsic activity

Table 12–4 *Potency, Selectivity, and Intrinsic Activity of Commonly Used β-Adrenoceptor Agonists*

Agonist	β_1	β_2	Selectivity Ratio (β_2:β_1)	Airway Smooth Muscle Intrinsic Activity
Isoproterenol	1.0	1.0	1.0	1.0
Salbutamol	0.0004	0.48	1,375	0.91
Terbutaline	0.003	0.08	267	0.83
Fenoterol	0.005	0.9	180	0.99
Salmeterol	0.001	8.5	85,000	0.70
Formoterol	0.05	25	100	0.94

Data are relative to response to isoproterenol. Intrinsic activity is a measure of efficacy.
Data compiled from various sources.[2,35,48]

than isoproterenol. Agents with equivalent efficacy are procaterol and formoterol, whereas most saligenins and resorcinols are of moderate efficacy (65 to 85% of response of isoproterenol). The efficacy of β-agonists at extrapulmonary sites may be of clinical relevance. Fenoterol and formoterol have the same efficacy as isoproterenol at cardiac β_1-adrenoceptors, despite being less potent, whereas salbutamol and salmeterol have very low efficacy (see Table 12–4). In contrast to efficacy, lung β_2-adrenoceptor potency can be greater than that of isoproterenol. For example, salmeterol is five times more potent than isoproterenol, formoterol 25-fold more potent, and procaterol 24-fold more potent. Neither intermediate intrinsic activity (efficacy) nor intermediate potency negates the clinical value of a given β-agonist as a bronchodilator drug. Rather, the adverse consequences of prolonged use of these drugs may be influenced by whether they are partial or full agonists. The rate of desensitization is one phenomenon that could be influenced by full versus partial agonist activity (discussed later).

Pharmacokinetics of β-Adrenoceptor Agonists

Oral Administration

After administration of an oral or parenteral β-agonist, the bronchodilator effect is closely dependent on serum levels.[46] Orally administered β-agonists are incompletely absorbed and the greater proportion is metabolized by sulfate conjugation in the gut epithelium and liver. For example, oral terbutaline absorption varies from 30 to 65% and, of this, only 25% remains unconjugated in the urine.[45] Net bioavailability is thus 10 to 15%. Protein binding of terbutaline varies from 14 to 25%. Salbutamol is more completely absorbed with peak levels within 1 hour of administration when the subject is fasting.[46] Sixty percent of the absorbed dose is conjugated. Sustained-release preparations of salbutamol and terbutaline are available in various formations and may be useful in asthmatics with marked nocturnal symptoms, although long-acting inhaled β_2-agonists such as salmeterol have superseded such preparations.

Parenteral Administration

Subcutaneous or intramuscular or intravenous injection of terbutaline, salbutamol, or epinephrine provides almost immediate action and assured delivery. Following subcutaneous terbutaline 0.5 mg, significant levels are present within a few minutes and peak at 20 minutes.[51] Epinephrine has a slightly shorter duration of action, although a slow release form is available in some countries. In an intensive care setting, intravenous infusion is sometimes used when patients are moribund or responding poorly to intermittent administration of β-agonists by other routes. Both terbutaline and salbutamol have been quite widely used, with a loading dose followed by a continuous infusion of 10 to 20% of the loading dose. Intravenous isoproterenol has little advantage apart from quicker offset of action and has greater side effects including possible myocardial toxicity; its use is not recommended.

Aerosol Administration

This is the preferred method of administration of all β-agonists as there is an effect on airway caliber within seconds, with the effect of short-acting β-agonists such as salbutamol reaching 80% of maximum in 5 minutes. Compared to parenteral or oral administration, following aerosolization, a given degree of bronchodilatation is achieved with significantly fewer adverse effects such as tremor or palpitations.[52] Short-acting β_2-agonists achieve peak effects within 30 to 60 minutes, and, subsequently, bronchodilatation slowly reduces. Airway caliber is often back to baseline within 4 to 5 hours, depending on the severity of asthma. There are no important clinical differences between commonly available short-acting β_2-agonists in terms of bronchodilatation or duration of action. The effects of catecholamine aerosols such as rimiterol or epinephrine peak earlier, and bronchodilatation persists only 30 minutes to 2 hours. Serum levels are very low after inhaled administration and do not correlate with bronchodilatation.

Adverse Effects

Desensitization

The relatively large numbers of β-adrenoceptors on human airway smooth muscle or the rapid turnover of adrenoceptors may explain why this tissue is relatively resistant to desensitization.[20,53] There have been many clinical studies of desensitization following regular short-acting β-agonist use (reviewed by Nelson et al[54]). There is evidence in some studies[55] but not others[56] of a small decrease in peak bronchodilator effect and duration of action in stable mild asthma patients but not in more severe asthmatic patients.[57] The majority of positive reports have used oral β-agonists. Most investigators have examined only peak bronchodilator effects, and if changes in duration of action are more affected by desensitization, as has been suggested, then further research is required. In contrast to studies in asthmatics, normal subjects readily demonstrate densensitization both in the lung and in nonpulmonary β-adrenergic systems.[56]

Small increases in airway responsiveness have been detected following cessation of regular short-acting β-agonists. One explanation of these findings is desensitization of airway smooth muscle β-adrenoceptors (Level I).[58,59] O'Connor et al have demonstrated tolerance to nonbronchodilator effects of terbutaline (effects possibly mediated by lung mast cell β₂-adrenoceptors) in mild asthmatics.[60] The effect of desensitization of β-adrenoceptors on cell types other than smooth muscle requires further study. Overall, the importance of desensitization as a clinically relevant effect of β-agonist treatment remains unclear.

Tremor

Tremor, due to activation of β₂-adrenoceptors in skeletal muscle, occurs in up to 20% of patients at initiation of β₂-agonist therapy (Level I). Tremor usually abates with regular use due to the development of desensitization.

Cardiac Effects

Palpitations are reported by up to 5% of asthmatics at initiation of therapy, especially by patients who use agents that are full rather than partial agonists at β₂-adrenoceptors. Desensitization develops with regular therapy. Despite concern that tachyarrhythmias could develop secondary to effects of β-agonists on Q–Tc interval and potassium in hypoxemic patients, serious cardiovascular events are extremely rare when these medications are dispensed from pressurized metered-dose inhalers.[61,62] However, caution should be exercised in individuals with unstable ischemic heart disease receiving high doses of nebulized β-agonists, as angina has been precipitated in this situation.[63] Further, a recent study has shown a small increased risk of acute cardiac death in asthma patients treated with oral or nebulized short-acting β-agonists (but not when they are dispensed in metered-dose inhalers).[62] The greater systemic dose achieved with oral or nebulized short-acting β-agonists at doses commonly prescribed may explain these findings.[64]

Hypokalemia and Other Metabolic Effects

Hypokalemia is seen following both inhaled and systemic administration of β-agonists due to stimulation of Na^+/K^+-ATPase activity and stimulation of insulin secretion.[57] When high cumulative inhaled doses of salbutamol and fenoterol (1,200 μg) were given to normal subjects, decreases of 0.67 and 1.13 mmol/L, respectively, were observed.[57] Again, desensitization is observed to this effect with chronic use of β-agonists.[57] Glyconeolysis also occurs secondary to β₂-adrenoceptor activation; the changes induced are small and are of uncertain significance in patients with diabetes mellitus. Lipolysis is activated by β-agonists via β₁-, β₂-, and possibly β₃-adrenoceptors and results in the mobilization of free fatty acids from adipose tissue.

Hypoxemia

All β-agonists, including epinephrine, can reduce arterial oxygen tension. These changes are apparent 5 minutes after administration of inhaled β-agonists and return to normal values by 30 minutes. These changes are secondary to an increase in pulmonary blood flow in poorly ventilated regions of the lung, and result in ventilation perfusion inequality. The increase in blood flow may be secondary to pulmonary vasodilatation via stimulation of $β_2$-adrenoceptors on vascular smooth muscle in the lung and also to increases in cardiac output following cardiac adrenoceptor stimulation. The reduction in arterial oxygen tension is small and is unlikely to be clinically significant.

Potential Adverse Effects of Regular Use as Monotherapy

The widespread use of short-acting $β_2$-agonists over 50 years attests to their general efficacy and safety, but studies over the last 10 years have highlighted several important facts. First, there is no evidence that regular four-times-a-day treatment with short-acting $β_2$-agonists benefits patients with any degree of asthma severity, as compared with use of short-acting $β_2$-agonists only when needed for symptom relief.[65,66] The more potent $β_2$-agonists seem to have adverse effects when taken regularly; this is especially true of fenoterol for which there is clear evidence that its regular use is associated with increased morbidity and mortality due to increased severity of asthma.[67,68] Withdrawal of fenoterol in New Zealand led to a rapid decline in both mortality and in hospital admissions, strongly suggesting that adverse effects were related to increased severity rather than to cardiac toxicity.[69] A US study of regular versus as-needed salbutamol in subjects with mild asthma showed consistent trends toward more symptoms, reduced lung function, and increased airway responsiveness in the group treated four times a day regularly with salbutamol, although for all outcomes except airway responsiveness, the differences did not achieve statistically significant levels.[66] More detailed mechanistic studies have shown that regular use of salbutamol may enhance the early and late asthmatic reactions to allergens[70,71] and the degree of bronchial constriction to standardized exercise challenge.[72] Numerous studies have confirmed that stopping the regular use of short-acting $β_2$-agonists increases airway responsiveness to histamine or methacholine.[59,65,66,73–76]

The adverse effects of regularly inhaled short-acting $β_2$-agonists are not obviated by concomitant use of inhaled glucocorticosteroid.[65] No beneficial anti-inflammatory effects have been firmly attributed to short-acting inhaled $β_2$-agonists; indeed, these agents may increase rather than decrease the cellular inflammatory response in asthma.[77]

SUMMARY

The following are evidence-based recommendations for clinical use of short-acting $β_2$-agonists:

- Short-acting inhaled $β_2$-agonists are the drugs of choice for both children and adults for the relief of acute symptoms and the short-term prevention of exercise-induced bronchospasm (Level I).
- When use of short-acting inhaled $β_2$-agonists is greater than three times weekly, a controller (anti-inflammatory) medication is required (Level III).
- Regular controller medications should be used if short-acting $β_2$-agonists are used more than three times weekly, not including their use to prevent exercise-induced symptoms (Level IV).
- Patients who need a short-acting $β_2$-agonist several times daily require urgent reassessment with a view to increasing anti-inflammatory therapy (Level III).

Short-acting $β_2$-agonists are most useful as rescue medication taken on an as-needed basis. The degree of reversal of airflow obstruction achieved by inhaled $β_2$-agonist depends on the nature of the airflow obstruction and intrinsic properties of the airway wall. However, as discussed and referenced above, regular or frequent use of inhaled short-acting $β_2$-agonists may be associated with decreased control of asthma, and with increased airway responsiveness to direct and indirect provoking stimuli, including allergens (both early and late asthmatic reactions are increased), exercise challenge, and methacholine challenge.

When β₂-agonists are used as required for symptom relief, their frequency of use is a good marker of control of asthma. A pattern of escalating use of short-acting β₂-agonists is predictive of high risk of a major life-threatening episode of asthma.[75,76]

REFERENCES

1   Lands AM, Arnold A, McAuliff JP, et al. Differentiation of receptor systems activated by sympathomimetic amines. Nature 1967;214:597–8.

2.   O'Donnell SR, Wanstall JC. The use of functional antagonism to determine whether beta-adrenoceptor agonists must have a lower efficacy than isoprenaline to be trachea-atria selective in vitro in guinea-pigs. Br J Pharmacol 1977;60:255–62.

3.   Strader CD, Sigal IS, Dixon RA. Mapping the functional domains of the beta-adrenergic receptor. Am J Respir Cell Mol Biol 1989;1:81–6.

4.   Chung FZ, Lentes KU, Gocayne J, et al. Cloning and sequence analysis of the human brain beta-adrenergic receptor. Evolutionary relationship to rodent and avian beta-receptors and porcine muscarinic receptors. FEBS Lett 1987;211:200–6.

5.   Emorine LJ, Marullo S, Delavier-Klutchko C, et al. Structure of the gene for human beta 2-adrenergic receptor: expression and promoter characterization. Proc Natl Acad Sci U S A 1987;84:6995–9.

6.   Kobilka BK, Dixon RA, Frielle T, et al. cDNA for the human beta 2-adrenergic receptor: a protein with multiple membrane-spanning domains and encoded by a gene whose chromosomal location is shared with that of the receptor for platelet-derived growth factor. Proc Natl Acad Sci U S A 1987;84:46–50.

7.   Mak JC, Nishikawa M, Barnes PJ. Glucocorticosteroids increase beta 2-adrenergic receptor transcription in human lung. Am J Physiol 1995;268:L41–6.

8.   Collins S, Caron MG, Lefkowitz RJ. Beta-adrenergic receptors in hamster smooth muscle cells are transcriptionally regulated by glucocorticoids. J Biol Chem 1988;263:9067–70.

9.   Hadcock JR, Malbon CC. Down-regulation of beta-adrenergic receptors: agonist-induced reduction in receptor mRNA levels. Proc Natl Acad Sci U S A 1988;85:5021–5.

10.   Anakwe O, Zhou S, Benovic J, et al. Interleukins impair beta-adrenergic receptor adenylate cyclase (beta AR-AC) system function in human airway epithelial cells. Chest 1995;107:138–9S.

11.   Fraser CM, Venter JC. Beta-adrenergic receptors. Relationship of primary structure, receptor function, and regulation. Am Rev Respir Dis 1990;141:S22–30.

12.   Stadel JM, Lefkowitz RJ. Beta-adrenergic receptors: identification and characterization by radioligand binding studies. In: Perkins JP, editor. Beta-adrenergic receptors. Clifton (NJ): Humana Press; 1991. p. 1–41.

13.   Hausdorff WP, Caron MG, Lefkowitz RJ. Turning off the signal: desensitization of beta-adrenergic receptor function. FASEB J 1990;4:2881–9.

14.   Malbon CC. Physiological regulation of transmembrane signaling elements. Am J Respir Cell Mol Biol 1989;1:449–50.

15.   Jones TR, Charette L, Garcia ML, Kaczorowski GJ. Selective inhibition of relaxation of guinea-pig trachea by charybdotoxin, a potent Ca(++)-activated K+ channel inhibitor. J Pharmacol Exp Ther 1990;255:697–706.

16.   Kume H, Mikawa K, Takagi K, Kotlikoff MI. Role of G proteins and KCa channels in the muscarinic and beta-adrenergic regulation of airway smooth muscle. Am J Physiol 1995;268:L221–9.

17.   Watson N, Magnussen H, Rabe KF. Antagonism of beta-adrenoceptor-mediated relaxations of human bronchial smooth muscle by carbachol. Eur J Pharmacol 1995;275:307–10.

18.   Barnes PJ. Neural control of human airways in health and disease. Am Rev Respir Dis 1986;134:1289–314.

19.   Davis C, Conolly ME. Tachyphylaxis to beta-adrenoceptor agonists in human bronchial smooth muscle: studies in vitro. Br J Clin Pharmacol 1980;10:417–23.

20.   Hamid QA, Mak JC, Sheppard MN, et al. Localization of beta 2-adrenoceptor messenger RNA in human and rat lung using in situ hybridization: correlation with receptor autoradiography. Eur J Pharmacol 1991;206:133–8.

21.   Hasegawa M, Townley RG. Difference between lung and spleen susceptibility of beta-adrenergic receptors to desensitization by terbutaline. J Allergy Clin Immunol 1983;71:230–8.

22.   Whicker SD, Lummis SC, Black JL. Beta-adrenoceptors in human airway tissue: relationship between functional responsiveness and receptor number. Life Sci 1991;49:1021–9.

23.   Bai TR. Abnormalities in airway smooth muscle in fatal asthma. Am Rev Respir Dis 1990;141:552–7.

24.   Carstairs JR, Nimmo AJ, Barnes PJ. Autoradiographic visualization of beta-adrenoceptor subtypes in human lung. Am Rev Respir Dis 1985;132:541–7.

25.   Daniel EE, Kannan M, Davis C, Posey-Daniel V. Ultrastructural studies on the neuromuscular control of human tracheal and bronchial muscle. Respir Physiol 1986;63:109–28.

26.   Basbaum CB, Madison JM, Sommerhoff CP, et al. Receptors on airway gland cells. Am Rev Respir Dis 1990;141:S141–4.

27.   Kerrebijn KF. Beta agonists. In: Kaliner MA, Barnes PA, Persson CGA, editors. Asthma: its pathology and treatment. Vol. 49. Lung biology in health and disease. New York: Marcel Dekker; 1991. p. 526.

28.   Wanner A. Autonomic control of mucociliary function. In: Kaliner MA, Barnes PJ, editors: The airways: neural control in health and disease. New York: Marcel Dekker; 1988. p. 551–74.

29.   Widdicombe JG. Airway mucus. Eur Respir J 1989;2:107–15.

30.   Penn RB, Kelsen SG, Benovic JL. Regulation of beta-agonist- and prostaglandin E2-mediated adenylyl cyclase activity in human airway epithelial cells. Am J Respir Cell Mol Biol 1994;11:496–505.

31.   Mason RJ, Williams MC. Alveolar type II cells. In: Crystal RG, West JB, editors. The lung: scientific foundations. Vol. 1. New York: Raven Press; 1991. p. 235–46.

32.   Persson CGA, Svensjo E. Vascular responses and their suppression: drugs interfering with venular permeability. In: Banta IL, Bray MA, editors. Handbook of inflammation. Vol. 5. Amsterdam: Elsevier; 1985. p. 61–81.

33.   Kelly WT, Baile EM, Brancatisano A, et al. Effects of inspiratory resistance, inhaled beta-agonists and histamine on canine tracheal blood flow. Eur Respir J 1992;5:1206–14.

34.   Coupe MO, Guly U, Brown E, Barnes PJ. Nebulised adrenaline in acute severe asthma: comparison with salbutamol. Eur J Respir Dis 1987;71:227–32.

35.   Bai TR, Lam R, Prasad FY. Effects of adrenergic agonists and adenosine on cholinergic neurotransmission in human tracheal smooth muscle. Pulm Pharmacol 1989;1:193–9.

36.   Insel P. Beta-adrenergic receptors in pathophysiologic states and in clinical medicine. In: Perkins J, editor. The beta-adrenergic receptors. Clifton (NJ): Humana Press; 1991. p. 294–343.

37.   Busse WW, Sosman JM. Isoproterenol inhibition of isolated human neutrophil function. J Allergy Clin Immunol 1984;73:404–10.

38.   Yukawa T, Ukena D, Kroegel C, et al. Beta 2-adrenergic receptors on eosinophils. Binding and functional studies. Am Rev Respir Dis 1990;141:1446–52.

39.   Liggett SB. Identification and characterization of a homogeneous population of beta 2-adrenergic receptors on human alveolar macrophages. Am Rev Respir Dis 1989;139:552–5.

40.   Fuller RW, O'Malloy G, Baker AJ, MacDermot J. Human alveolar macrophage activation: inhibition by forskolin but not beta-adrenoceptor stimulation or phosphodiesterase inhibition. Pulm Pharmacol 1988;1:101–6.

41.   Butchers PR, Skidmore IF, Vardey CJ, Wheeldon A. Characterization of the receptor mediating the antianaphylactic effects of beta-adrenoceptor agonists in human lung tissue in vitro. Br J Pharmacol 1980;71:663–7.

42.   Rhoden KJ, Meldrum LA, Barnes PJ. Inhibition of cholinergic neurotransmission in human airways by beta 2-adrenoceptors. J Appl Physiol 1988;65:700–5.

43.   Grieco MH, Pierson RN Jr. Mechanism of bronchoconstriction due to beta adrenergic blockade. Studies with practolol, propranolol, and atropine. J Allergy Clin Immunol 1971;48:143–52.

44.   Chapman ID, Buchheit KH, Manley P, Morley J. Active enantiomers may cause adverse effects in asthma. Trends Pharmacol Sci 1992;13:231–2.

45.   Davies DS. The fate of inhaled terbutaline. Eur J Respir Dis 1984;134:141–7.

46.   Morgan DJ, Paull JD, Richmond BH, et al. Pharmacokinetics of intravenous and oral salbutamol and its sulphate conjugate. Br J Clin Pharmacol 1986;22:587–93.

47.   Tota MR, Candelore MR, Dixon RA, Strader CD. Biophysical and genetic analysis of the ligand-binding site of the beta-adrenoceptor. Trends Pharmacol Sci 1991;12:4–6.

48.   Johnson M, Butchers PR, Coleman RA, et al. The pharmacology of salmeterol. Life Sci 1993;52:2131–43.

49. Decker N, Quennedey MC, Rouot B, et al. Effects of N-aralkyl substitution of beta-agonists on alpha- and beta-adrenoceptor subtypes: pharmacological studies and binding assays. J Pharm Pharmacol 1982;34:107–12.

50. Stephenson RP. Modification of receptor therapy. Br J Pharmacol 1956;11:379–93.

51. van den Berg W, Leferink JG, Maes RA, et al. The effects of oral and subcutaneous administration of terbutaline in asthmatic patients. Eur J Respir Dis 1984;134:181–93.

52. Larsson S, Svedmyr N. Bronchodilating effect and side effects of beta2-adrenoceptor stimulants by different modes of administration (tablets, metered aerosol, and combinations thereof). A study with salbutamol in asthmatics. Am Rev Respir Dis 1977;116:861–9.

53. Hall IP, Daykin K, Widdop S. Beta 2-adrenoceptor desensitization in cultured human airway smooth muscle. Clin Sci 1993;84:151–7.

54. Nelson HS, Szefler SJ, Martin RJ. Regular inhaled beta-adrenergic agonists in the treatment of bronchial asthma: beneficial or detrimental? Am Rev Respir Dis 1991;144:249–50.

55. Weber RW, Smith JA, Nelson HS. Aerosolized terbutaline in asthmatics: development of subsensitivity with long-term administration. J Allergy Clin Immunol 1982;70:417–22.

56. Harvey JE, Baldwin CJ, Wood PJ, et al. Airway and metabolic responsiveness to intravenous salbutamol in asthma: effect of regular inhaled salbutamol. Clin Sci 1981;60:579–85.

57. Lipworth BJ, Struthers AD, McDevitt DG. Tachyphylaxis to systemic but not to airway responses during prolonged therapy with high dose inhaled salbutamol in asthmatics. Am Rev Respir Dis 1989;140:586–92.

58. Kraan J, Koeter GH, Vandermark TW, et al. Changes in bronchial hyperreactivity induced by 4 weeks of treatment with antiasthmatic drugs in patients with allergic asthma: a comparison between budesonide and terbutaline. J Allergy Clin Immunol 1985;76:628–36.

59. Vathenen AS, Knox AJ, Higgins BG, et al. Rebound increase in bronchial responsiveness after treatment with inhaled terbutaline. Lancet 1988;1:554–8.

60. O'Connor BJ, Aikman SL, Barnes PJ. Tolerance to the nonbronchodilator effects of inhaled beta 2-agonists in asthma. N Engl J Med 1992;327:1204–8.

61. Sears MR, Taylor DR, Print CG, et al. Regular inhaled beta-agonist treatment in bronchial asthma. Lancet 1990;336:1391–6.

62. Drazen JM, Israel E, Boushey HA, et al. Comparison of regularly scheduled with as-needed use of albuterol in mild asthma. Asthma Clinical Research Network. N Engl J Med 1996;335:841–7.

63. Taylor DR, Sears MR, Herbison GP, et al. Regular inhaled beta agonist in asthma: effects on exacerbations and lung function. Thorax 1993;48:134–8.

64. Crane J, Pearce N, Flatt A, et al. Prescribed fenoterol and death from asthma in New Zealand, 1981–83: case-control study. Lancet 1989;1:917–22.

65. Sears MR, Taylor DR. The beta 2-agonist controversy. Observations, explanations and relationship to asthma epidemiology. Drug Saf 1994;11:259–83.

66. Cockcroft DW, McParland CP, Britto SA, et al. Regular inhaled salbutamol and airway responsiveness to allergen. Lancet 1993;342:833–7.

67. Cockcroft DW, O'Byrne PM, Swystun VA, Bhagat R. Regular use of inhaled albuterol and the allergen-induced late asthmatic response. J Allergy Clin Immunol 1995;96:44–9.

68. Inman MD, O'Byrne PM. The effect of regular inhaled albuterol on exercise-induced bronchoconstriction. Am J Respir Crit Care Med 1996;153:65–9.

69. van Schayck CP, Graafsma SJ, Visch MB, et al. Increased bronchial hyperresponsiveness after inhaling salbutamol during 1 year is not caused by subsensitization to salbutamol. J Allergy Clin Immunol 1990;86:793–800.

70. Bhagat R, Swystun VA, Cockcroft DW. Salbutamol-induced increased airway responsiveness to allergen and reduced protection versus methacholine: dose response. J Allergy Clin Immunol 1996;97:47–52.

71. Taylor DR, Sears MR. Bronchodilators and bronchial hyperresponsiveness. Thorax 1994;49:190–1.

72. Wong CS, Wahedna I, Pavord ID, Tattersfield AE. Effect of regular terbutaline and budesonide on bronchial reactivity to allergen challenge. Am J Respir Crit Care Med 1994;150:1268–73.

73. Manolitsas ND, Wang J, Devalia JL, et al. Regular albuterol, nedocromil sodium, and bronchial inflammation in asthma. Am J Respir Crit Care Med 1995;151:1925–30.

74. Gauvreau GM, Jordana M, Watson RM, et al. Effect of regular inhaled albuterol on allergen-induced late responses and sputum eosinophils in asthmatic subjects. Am J Respir Crit Care Med 1997;156:1738–45.

75. Spitzer WO, Suissa S, Ernst P, et al. The use of beta-agonists and the risk of death and near death from asthma. N Engl J Med 1992;326:501–6.

76. Suissa S, Ernst P, Boivin JF, et al. A cohort analysis of excess mortality in asthma and the use of inhaled beta-agonists. Am J Respir Crit Care Med 1994;149:604–10.

77. Neilson CP, Hadjokas NE. Beta-adrenoceptor agonists block corticosteroid inhibition in eosinophils. Am J Respir Crit Care Med 1998;157:184–91.

Role of Long-Acting β_2-Adrenergic Agents

Louis-Philippe Boulet, MD, FRCPC

Ephedrine was probably the first β-adrenergic agonist to be used for the treatment of asthma, as the active ingredient of Ma Hung, a herbal medicine used for centuries in China. Since their introduction into the western world as subcutaneous adrenalin in 1930, β-adrenergic agonists have been an integral part of asthma therapy. The distinction between β_1- and β_2-adrenergic receptors made by Lands et al in 1967, led to the search for more specific β_2-adrenergic agonists, thereby avoiding the chronotropic and inotropic cardiac effects of β_1 stimulation.[1] Inhaled nonselective agents possessing β_1- and β_2-adrenergic properties, such as isoproterenol, have been followed by more selective inhaled β_2-adrenergic agonists, such as metaproterenol, salbutamol, terbutaline, fenoterol, pirbuterol, and procaterol. The most recent development in this field has been the synthesis of inhaled β_2-adrenergic agonists with a prolonged duration of action, such as salmeterol and formoterol. Oral adrenergic agonists may have a more prolonged duration of action than short-acting inhaled agents, but since they are associated with an increased incidence of side effects for a similar therapeutic effect, they are rarely indicated. This document will therefore be limited to the discussion of the long-acting inhaled β_2-adrenergic agonists formoterol and salmeterol.

PHARMACOLOGY OF LONG-ACTING β_2-ADRENERGIC AGONISTS

Salmeterol xinafoate is a saligenin derivative with a 50-fold greater affinity than salbutamol for β_2-adrenoceptors and a partial agonist effect; formoterol is a lipophilic fumarate with a high affinity for β_2-adrenoceptors and almost full agonist properties.[2,3] Both are highly selective for β_2-adrenoceptors. Their functional antagonism, as expressed by the shift to the right of the concentration-response curve of airway smooth muscle relaxation when its basal tone is increased, is similar to that of short-acting agents.[4] Although salmeterol acts as a partial β_2-adrenoceptor agonist under experimental conditions while formoterol is a full agonist, the clinical implication of these properties is uncertain.

To explain the long duration of salmeterol's action, it has been suggested that its long aliphatic side chain is anchored to a specific binding site at proximity or within the β_2-adrenoceptor binding site.[5] Other potential factors implicated in this prolonged effect are its increased lipophilicity compared with that of salbutamol and the possibility that it has access to the receptor only via the lipid membrane, therefore acting as a depot for the drug.[4] This may not be true for formoterol, whose lipophilicity is intermediate, between that of salmeterol and salbutamol. The mechanism underlying its long duration of action is still uncertain.

Bronchodilator Effects

Formoterol's onset of action is faster than that of salmeterol (Level I).[6] One minute after formoterol inhalation, specific conductance (sGaw) was found to be higher than after a 200-μg dose of salbutamol.[7] Median time to achieve a 15% increase in forced expiratory volume in 1 second (FEV$_1$) with 50 μg of salmeterol was 14 minutes for the aerosol administered with a metered-dose inhaler (MDI) and 11 minutes for the powder, compared with 7 minutes for

200 μg of salbutamol (MDI).[8] Salmeterol 50 μg has a slower onset of action than salbutamol 200 μg in reversing methacholine-induced bronchospasm.[9]

Peak bronchodilatation of these long-acting agents occurs between 2 and 4 hours.[10,11] On a μg-per-μg basis, salmeterol and formoterol are more potent bronchodilators than salbutamol, terbutaline, or fenoterol. Regarding initial peak bronchodilatation, doses of salbutamol 200 μg, salmeterol 50 μg, and formoterol 12 μg are considered equipotent.[12,13] Salmeterol and formoterol induce a prolonged bronchodilatation over 12 hours in both adults and children (Level I).[5,14–26]

Bronchoprotection

The bronchoprotective effects of formoterol and salmeterol against stimuli such as histamine, methacholine, exercise, cold-air inhalation, and hyperventilation last at least 12 hours in children and adults (Level I).[10,11,20,21,27–32] Their potency against histamine-induced bronchoconstriction is greater than that of short-acting β₂-adrenergic agonists.[29] The degree of protection these agents afford against exercise-induced asthma is of a similar magnitude to that of salbutamol but is of longer duration (Level I).[27,30] Formoterol protects against exercise-induced asthma in children and adults for more than 8 hours, compared with less than 3 hours for salbutamol.[33] Salmeterol is superior to cromoglycate in inhibiting exercise-induced asthma (Level I).[34]

Long-acting β₂-adrenergic agents reduce allergen-induced late asthmatic responses and the secondary increase in airway responsiveness (Level I).[35–37] Beclomethasone and formoterol show a similar partial inhibitory effect on late responses and increases in airway responsiveness.[37] Inhaled formoterol 12 μg has better inhibitory effects than 500 μg terbutaline when administered 4 hours before dust mite allergen provocation.[38] Finally, Taylor et al reported the inhibition of early asthmatic responses with salmeterol 50 μg and salbutamol, with salmeterol providing a more prolonged inhibitory effect.[36]

Tolerance to the Effects

As for short-acting β₂-adrenergic agents, there seems to be no clinically important tolerance to the bronchodilator effects of either salmeterol or formoterol (Level I).[18,21,39] However, a tolerance to the bronchoprotective effects of these agents against many stimuli has been reported (Level I).[40–43] Cheung et al showed that regular inhaled salmeterol 50 μg twice daily for 4 and 8 weeks resulted in a reduction in the protective effect of the drug against methacholine-induced bronchoconstriction from a 10- to a twofold concentration difference.[40] This was even more marked for adenosine monophosphate (AMP)-induced bronchoconstriction. Bronchoprotection returned to the baseline level 2 and 4 days after the end of the treatment. Reduced protection of salmeterol against exercise-induced asthma has been reported with regular use.[41]

This phenomenon of tolerance to the protective effects has also been observed after a single daily administration of long-acting β₂-adrenergic agonists.[42] The clinical significance of these observations, however, remains uncertain. We recently found that although there was a tolerance to the bronchoprotection against methacholine, even in patients on inhaled corticosteroids, it was not associated with a loss of control of asthma.[43] This suggests that, although it is a universal finding, it may not be clinically important. This is supported by the review of nine clinical trials on salmeterol by Verberne and Fuller, who concluded that reduction in the bronchoprotector effect of salmeterol occurred quickly, after the first few days of treatment, and the reduced effect was maintained afterward.[44] This degree of protection is probably sufficient in most patients to help maintain asthma control. This last report also mentioned that there was no evidence of rebound deterioration in airway responsiveness after cessation of salmeterol treatment.

Clinical Use

Effects on Asthma Control and Expiratory Flows

Inhaled formoterol and salmeterol decrease asthma symptoms and the need for short-acting β₂-adrenergic agonists (Level I); they are preferred over other bronchodilators by patients.[10,11,45,46]

Formoterol 12 µg twice a day improved asthma control and was better tolerated than salbutamol 200 µg four times a day in 301 patients with reversible airflow obstruction (Level I).[47] Inhaled formoterol 12 and 24 µg twice daily provided similar or better symptom control and pulmonary function than did the regular use of short-acting β₂-adrenergic agonists. Although formoterol has an onset of action close to that of short-acting agents, it seems preferable to use it as a maintenance treatment than as a rescue medication, to avoid overuse (Level IIID). In patients with moderate to severe reversible obstructive airway disease, 3 months of salmeterol at doses of 50 and 100 µg twice daily improved asthma control.[48] The observed improvement in pulmonary function was independent of corticosteroid use.

It seems that 50 µg is the optimal dose for salmeterol.[49] In a double-blind study in which 234 patients with mild to moderate asthma were divided into 3 subgroups receiving either 42 µg salmeterol twice a day, 180 µg salbutamol four times a day, or placebo for 12 weeks, salmeterol significantly improved morning peak expiratory flow (PEF), daytime symptoms, and, particularly, night-time symptoms.[50] Salmeterol 50 and 100 µg, as well as formoterol 12 µg, were effective in protecting against nocturnal asthma (Level I).[51,52] Muir et al found that the improvement in nocturnal asthma symptoms was associated with fewer side effects than were found with the combination of theophylline and ketotifen.[53]

A 9-month, double-blind study with parallel groups involving 667 moderate asthmatic patients compared inhaled salbutamol 200 µg four times per day to salmeterol 50 µg twice a day.[54] Morning and evening PEF were improved for the first 3 months of the study in the salmeterol group, and diurnal variation in PEF, day- and night-time symptoms, bronchodilator needs, and asthma-related events were lower with salmeterol, regardless of which inhaled/oral corticosteroids were used.[54] Furthermore, in a 12-month, open follow-up study, salmeterol 50 µg twice daily improved morning FEV₁ and was not associated with any significant cardiovascular side effects.[55] Bronchial response to salbutamol remained unchanged. Another report also found no reduced efficacy of usual or higher-than-usual doses of salbutamol when salmeterol was regularly used.[56]

Pearlman et al also showed improvements in asthma symptom scores in 234 asthmatic patients using salmeterol, whether on corticosteroids or not, as compared with those on salbutamol or placebo.[50] In a large postmarketing study, the rate of exacerbations was lower with salmeterol than with regular salbutamol.[57] Similarly, Kesten et al reported that asthma control and pulmonary function were better with formoterol than with salbutamol, and that the improvement was sustained over 1 year without evidence of tachyphylaxis.[58]

Finally, salmeterol has been shown to improve the quality of life of asthma sufferers, whether on inhaled corticosteroids or not.[59]

Association with Other Agents

Monotherapy with long-acting β₂-adrenergic agents is not generally recommended, as it is not as good as inhaled corticosteroids to maintain asthma control (Level IE).[60–62] Long-acting β₂-adrenergic agonists are therefore mostly recommended for concomitant use with inhaled corticosteroids (Level IA).[63–66] Unlike short-acting β₂-adrenergic agonists, they are not currently recommended as rescue medication (Level IIID).

In asthmatic patients whose asthma is not optimally controlled, adding formoterol or salmeterol twice daily has been found to be as effective in improving asthma symptom control as doubling the dose of inhaled corticosteroids (Level I).[67–69]

The recent Formoterol and Corticosteroids Establishing Therapy (FACET) trial showed that in patients with persistent asthma symptoms despite treatment with inhaled corticosteroids, adding formoterol to budesonide therapy improved their asthma symptoms.[70] After a 4-week run-in period of treatment with budesonide 800 μg twice daily, 852 patients being treated with glucocorticoids were randomly assigned to one of four treatments given twice daily by means of a dry-powder inhaler (Turbuhaler): 100 μg of budesonide plus placebo; 100 μg of budesonide plus 12 μg of formoterol; 400 μg of budesonide plus placebo; or 400 μg of budesonide plus 12 μg of formoterol. When formoterol was added to the lower dose of budesonide, the rates of severe and mild exacerbations were reduced by 26% and 40%, respectively. The higher dose of budesonide alone reduced the rates of severe and mild exacerbations by 49% and 37%, respectively. Patients treated with formoterol and the higher dose of budesonide had the greatest reductions, 63% and 62%, respectively. Symptoms of asthma and lung function improved with both formoterol and the higher dose of budesonide, but the improvements were greater when formoterol was added.[70]

A recent meta-analysis showed that addition of salmeterol in symptomatic patients aged 12 years and over on low to moderate doses of inhaled corticosteroid gave improved lung function and reduced numbers of days or nights without respiratory symptoms or need for rescue treatment, with no increase in asthma exacerbations.[71]

Side Effects

β_2-Adrenergic agonists may occasionally cause dose-related adverse effects, such as tremor and tachycardia, from β_2-adrenergic receptor stimulation (Level I).[72] At usual doses, however, these effects are generally mild and decrease with regular use. β_2-Adrenergic stimulation may result in a few metabolic effects, such as increases in glucose levels, lactate, pyruvates, free fatty acids, and hypokalemia, although these effects are minor and usually decrease over time. There are few β_2-type cardiac adrenergic receptors, therefore, cardiac side effects result mostly from dilatation of peripheral vessels supplying the skeletal muscles, with a resulting fall in blood pressure that triggers reflex tachycardia.

With long-acting β_2-adrenergic agents, the incidence of adverse events seems to be low and similar to what is found with short-acting bronchodilators for a given degree of bronchodilatation (Level I).[73,74] The incidence of adverse events for salmeterol 50 μg twice a day or salbutamol 200 or 400 μg four times per day was similar over 12 months, the most frequent side effects being tremor, palpitations, tachycardia, muscle cramps, and headache in up to 10% of patients.[75] The frequency of asthma exacerbations in the two groups was similar.

No clinically significant changes on electrocardiogram (ECG) or falls in potassium levels were found in asthmatic patients using formoterol.[76] When compared with a placebo, formoterol 24 μg and fenoterol 400 μg or salbutamol 400 μg slightly increased heart rate, plasma glucose, and Q–Tc interval on ECG, diastolic blood pressure, and plasma potassium (Level I).[77] Salmeterol 50 μg and salbutamol 200 μg showed similar effects on heart rate and tremor.

Castle et al compared the safety of salmeterol with that of salbutamol in 25,180 asthmatic patients over 16 weeks; 16,787 were randomly selected to take salmeterol 50 μg twice daily and 8,393 to take salbutamol 200 μg four times daily.[57] The overall mortality rate was similar to what was predicted for either group. Compared with salbutamol, however, a significant increase in asthma events, including deaths, was found with salmeterol in the group that had severe asthma on entry. Another study, which examined automated health insurance claims records, found that salmeterol was prescribed preferentially to high-risk patients and that, after adjusting for baseline risk, it was not associated with a greater risk of severe nonfatal events than those receiving theophylline.[78]

There is nevertheless a possible increased risk of side effects when subjects on long-acting β_2-adrenergic agonists also use short-acting agents as rescue medication. These short-acting agents have additive effects for plasma potassium concentration, Q–Tc interval changes, and side effects.[13] Furthermore, overuse of β_2-adrenergic agonists usually means that the anti-inflammatory treatment is insufficient and should be reassessed. Caution is therefore suggested when a patient requires more than the occasional use of short-acting β₂-agonist while using a long-acting β₂-agonist.

Other Properties

Long-acting β₂-adrenergic agonists seem to be able to inhibit eosinophil accumulation and mediator release in animal models[79] and have shown inhibitory effects on histamine and prostaglandin D_2 release from passively sensitized human lung fragments.[80] Salmeterol inhibits the allergen-induced mononuclear cell proliferation and downregulated granulo-cyte-macrophage colony–stimulating factor (GM-CSF) release and human leukocyte antigen (HLA)-DR expression by monocytes.[81,82] Salmeterol is unable to inhibit LTE_4 (leukotriene) release in humans following allergen inhalation.[36]

Bronchoalveolar lavage (BAL) differential cell counts were unchanged after salmeterol inhalation, but macrophage activation and eosinophil cationic protein levels in BAL fluid were reduced after 4 weeks of treatment. In other studies, BAL inflammatory cells and bronchial biopsy findings were unchanged after inhalation of salmeterol as compared with placebo, as were bronchial biopsy inflammatory cells.[83–85] Li et al have reported a fall in EG1 positive-cells in the lamina propria, on bronchial biopsies, following add-on therapy with solmeterol.[84] In a subanalysis of the FACET study, no significant differences in sputum mark-ers of airway inflammation were observed during a 1 year treatment with a low dose of inhaled budesonide plus formoterol compared to a large dose of budesonide.[85] In regard to the effects of long-acting β₂-adrenergic agonists (LAβ₂) during pro-inflammatory exposures, a study with formoterol showed that although it protected against late responses to allergen, it had no effect on allergen-induced increases in sputum, and that an increase in blood eosinophils and CD25+ lymphocytes suggested a bronchoprotection from functional antag-onism and not from anti-inflammatory properties.[37] It has been suggested that these agents, like short-acting ones, may allow asthmatic patients to inhale larger amounts of allergen and pollutants with a resulting increase in airway inflammation. In this regard, we found a reduc-tion in some inflammatory markers on bronchial biopsies taken 6 hours after allergen chal-lenge;[86] however, a study in a larger number of subjects with sampling at 24 hours showed instead an increased activation of certain components of cellular inflammation, such as mast cells.[87] This supports the recommendation that the LAB₂ should be used with an anti-inflam-matory agent such as I.C.. Finally, a recent study showed an increased airway inflammation for a given degree of loss of asthma control in patients using salmeterol.[88]

Additional Issues

The possibility that regular treatment by long-acting β₂-agonist could induce bronchodilator subsensitivity to repeated inhalations of short-acting β₂-agonist has been suggested.[89] This effect was partially reversed by a single dose of systemic or inhaled corticosteroid. Previous studies had not found such reduction in bronchodilator effects of drugs such as albuterol after LAβ₂-agonists.[60,90,91] These differences seem to be related to different study designs and if such effect occurs, it is unlikely to be of clinical importance in most instances.

Finally, it has been recently suggested that formoterol could be used as a "rescue" med-ication, in regard to its rapid onset of action, similar to short acting β₂-agonists.[92] However, we presently have no published study looking at this possibility, and we need to obtain more data on this matter before making recommendations on such use.

CONCLUSION

The following are concluding statements and recommendations regarding the use of long-acting β₂-adrenergic agents in the treatment of asthma:
- Long-acting β₂-adrenergic agonists are helpful in improving asthma control and air-way function when inhaled corticosteroids are insufficient (Level IA).

- Adding these agents to low/moderate doses of corticosteroids provides a similar improvement of symptoms and pulmonary function to that achieved by doubling the dose of inhaled corticosteroids and usually acts more rapidly (Level IA).
- Long-acting β_2-adrenergic agonists should always be used with concomitant anti-inflammatory therapy (Level 1A).
- Patients receiving this type of medication should be given adequate education and a clear action plan so they know what to do if their asthma worsens; in particular, they should be instructed on how to use this medication and be warned against any abuse of the medication (Level IIIA).

The author is grateful to Mariette Veillette, Lori Schubert, and Joanne Milot for their help with the preparation of this document.

REFERENCES

1. Lands AM, Arnold A, McAuliff JP, et al. Differentiation of receptor systems activated by sympathomimetic amines. Nature 1967;214:597–8.

2. Johnson M. The preclinical pharmacology of salmeterol: bronchodilator effects. Eur Respir Rev 1991;4:253–6.

3. Löfdahl CG. Basic pharmacology of new long-acting sympathomimetics. Lung 1990;168 Suppl:18–21.

4. Löfdahl CGA. Long-acting β_2-adrenoceptor agonists. In: Barnes PJ, Grunstein MM, Leff AR, Woolcock AJ, editors. Asthma. Philadelphia: Lippincott-Raven Publishers; 1997. p. 1523–34.

5. Nials AT, Sumner MJ, Johnson M, Coleman RA. Investigations into factors determining the duration of action of the beta 2-adrenoceptor agonist, salmeterol. Br J Pharmacol 1993;108:507–15.

6. Ullman A, Bergendal A, Linden A, et al. Onset of action and duration of effect of formoterol and salmeterol compared to salbutamol in isolated guinea pig trachea with or without epithelium. Allergy 1992;47:384–7.

7. Derom EY, Pauwels RA. Time course of bronchodilating effect of inhaled formoterol, a potent and long acting sympathomimetic. Thorax 1992;47:30–3.

8. Pauwels R, Derom E, Van der Straeten M. Onset of action of beta-2-agonists by comparison of inhaled formoterol vs inhaled salbutamol. Eur Respir J 1989;2:652S.

9. Beach JR, Young CL, Stenton SC, et al. A comparison of the speeds of action of salmeterol and salbutamol in reversing methacholine-induced bronchoconstriction. Pulm Pharmacol 1991;5:133–5.

10. Brogden RN, Faulds D. Salmeterol xinafoate. A review of its pharmacological properties and therapeutic potential in reversible obstructive airways disease. Drugs 1991;42:895–912.

11. Faulds D, Hollingshead LM, Goa KL. Formoterol. A review of its pharmacological properties and therapeutic efficacy in reversible obstructive airways disease. Drugs 1991;42:115–37.

12. Rabe KF, Jörres R, Nowak D, et al. Comparison of the effects of salmeterol and formoterol on airway tone and responsiveness over 24 hours in bronchial asthma. Am Rev Respir Dis 1993;147:1436–41.

13. Smyth ET, Pavord ID, Wong CS, et al. Interaction and dose equivalence of salbutamol and salmeterol in patients with asthma. Br Med J 1993;306:543–5.

14. Ullman A, Svedmyr N. Salmeterol, a new long acting β-adrenoreceptor agonist: a comparison with salbutamol in adult asthmatic patients. Thorax 1988;43:674–8.

15. Von Berg A, Berdel D. Formoterol and salbutamol metered aerosols: comparison of a new and an established beta-2 agonist for their bronchodilating efficacy in the treatment of childhood bronchial asthma. Pediatr Pulmonol 1989;7:89–93.

16. Graff-Lonnevig V, Browaldh L. Twelve hours' bronchodilating effect of inhaled formoterol in children with asthma: a double-blind cross-over study versus salbutamol. Clin Exp Allergy 1990;20:429–32.

17. Maesen FP, Smeets JJ, Gubbelmans HL, Zweers PG. Bronchodilator effect of inhaled formoterol vs salbutamol over 12 hours. Chest 1990;97:590–4.

18. Wallin A, Melander B, Rosenhall L, et al. Formoterol, a new long-acting beta-2 agonist for inhalation twice daily, compared with salbutamol in the treatment of asthma. Thorax 1990;45:259–61.

19. Foucard T, Lonnerholm G. A study with cumulative doses of formoterol in children with asthma. Eur Respir J 1991;4:1174–7.

20. Derom EY, Pauwels RA, Van Der Straeten ME. The effect of inhaled salmeterol on methacholine responsiveness in subjects with asthma up to 12 hours. J Allergy Clin Immunol 1992;89:811–5.

21. Simons FE, Soni NR, Watson WT, Becker AB. Bronchodilator and bronchoprotective effects of salmeterol in young patients with asthma. J Allergy Clin Immunol 1992;90:840–6.

22. Chetta A, Del Donno M, Maiocchi G, et al. Prolonged bronchodilating effect of formoterol versus procaterol in bronchial asthma. Ann Allergy 1993:70:171–4.

23. Verberne AA, Hop WC, Bos AB, Kerrebijn KF. Effect of a single dose of inhaled salmeterol on baseline airway caliber and methacholine-induced airway obstruction in asthmatic children. J Allergy Clin Immunol 1993;91:127–34.

24. Leblanc P, Knight A, Kreisman H, et al. A placebo-controlled, crossover comparison of salmeterol and salbutamol in patients with asthma. Am J Respir Crit Care Med 1996;154:324–8.

25. Van Noord JA, Smeets JJ, Raaijmakers JAM, et al. Salmeterol vs formoterol in patients with moderately severe asthma: onset and duration of action. Eur Respir J 1996;9:1684–88.

26. Boulet LP, Laviolette M, Boucher S, et al. A twelve-week comparison of salmeterol and salbutamol in the treatment of mild-to-moderate asthma: a Canadian multicenter study. J Allergy Clin Immunol 1997;99:13–21.

27. Ramsdale EH, Otis J, Kline PA, et al. Prolonged protection against methacholine-induced bronchoconstriction by the inhaled β₂-agonist formoterol. Am Rev Respir Dis 1991;143:998–1001.

28. Malo JL, Cartier A, Trudeau C, et al. Formoterol, a new inhaled beta-2 adrenergic agonist, has a longer blocking effect than albuterol on hyperventilation-induced bronchoconstriction. Am Rev Respir Dis 1990;142:1147–52.

29. Campos-Gongora H, Wisniewski AFZ, Tattersfield AE. A single-dose comparison of inhaled albuterol and two formulations of salmeterol on airway reactivity in asthmatic subjects. Am Rev Respir Dis 1991;144:626–9.

30. Anderson SD, Rodwell LT, Du Toit J, Young IH. Duration of protection by inhaled salmeterol in exercise-induced asthma. Chest 1991;100:1254–60.

31. Sovijarvi AR, Reinikainen K, Freudenthal Y, et al. Preventive effects of inhaled formoterol and salbutamol on histamine-induced bronchoconstriction: a placebo controlled study. Respiration 1992;59:279–82.

32. Malo JL, Ghezzo H, Trudeau C, et al. Salmeterol, a new inhaled beta 2-adrenergic agonist, has a longer blocking effect than albuterol on hyperventilation-induced bronchoconstriction. J Allergy Clin Immunol 1992;89:567–74.

33. Patessio A, Podda A, Carone M, et al. Protective effect and duration of action of formoterol aerosol on exercise-induced asthma. Eur Respir J 1991;4:296–300.

34. Guerin JC, Brambilla C, Godard P, et al. Prolonged effect against exercise-induced bronchospasm: salmeterol versus sodium cromoglycate. Rev Mal Respir 1992;9 Suppl 1:R27–30.

35. Twentyman OP, Finnerty JP, Harris A, et al. Protection against allergen-induced asthma by salmeterol. Lancet 1990;336:1338–42.

36. Taylor IK, O'Shaughnessy KM, Choudry NB, et al. A comparative study in atopic subjects with asthma of the effects of salmeterol and salbutamol on allergen-induced bronchoconstriction, increase in airway reactivity and increase in urinary leukotriene E₄ excretion. J Allergy Clin Immunol 1992;89:575–83.

37. Wong BJ, Dolovich J, Ramsdale EH, et al. Formoterol compared with beclomethasone and placebo on allergen-induced asthmatic responses. Am Rev Respir Dis 1992;146:1156–60.

38. Ferguson H, Thomas KE, Davies RJ. Comparison of single dose formoterol and terbutaline on the immediate asthmatic response to allergen provocation testing. Clin Exp Allergy 1989;19:A118.

39. Ullman A, Hedner J, Svedmyr N. Inhaled salmeterol and salbutamol in asthmatic patients. An evaluation of asthma symptoms and the possible development of tachyphylaxis. Am Rev Respir Dis 1990;142:571–5.

40. Cheung D, Timmers MC, Zwinderman AH, et al. Long-term effects of a long-acting beta 2-adrenoreceptor agonist, salmeterol, on airway hyper-responsiveness in patients with mild asthma. N Engl J Med 1992;327:1198–203.

41. Ramage L, Lipworth BJ, Ingram CG, et al. Reduced protection against exercise induced bronchoconstriction after chronic dosing with salmeterol. Respir Med 1994;88:363–8.

42. Aziz I, Tan KS. Hall IP, et al. Subsensitivity to bronchoprotection against adenosine monophosphate challenge following regular once-daily formoterol. Eur Respir J 1998;12:580–4.

43. Boulet LP, Cartier A, Milot J, et al. Tolerance to the protective effects of salmeterol on methacholine-induced bronchoconstriction: time-course, influence of corticosteroids and effects on asthma control. Eur Respir J 1998;11:1091–7.

44. Verberne AA, Fuller R. An overview of nine clinical trials of salmeterol in an asthmatic population. Respir Med 1998;92:777–82.

45. Tattersfield AE. Long-acting beta-2 agonists. Clin Exp Allergy 1992;22:600–5.

46. Boulet LP. Long- versus short-acting beta 2-agonists. Implications for drug therapy. Drugs 1994;47(2):207–222.

47. Hekking PR, Maesen F, Greefhorst A, et al. Long-term efficacy of formoterol compared to salbutamol. Lung 1990;168 Suppl:76–82.

48. Palmer JB, Stuart AM, Shepherd GL, Viskum K. Inhaled salmeterol in the treatment of patients with moderate to severe reversible obstruction airways disease, a 3 month comparison of the efficacy and safety of twice-daily salmeterol (100 micrograms) with salmeterol (50 micrograms). Respir Med 1992;86:409–17.

49. Dahl R, Earnshaw JS, Palmer JBD. Salmeterol: a four week study of a long-acting beta-adrenoreceptor agonist for the treatment of reversible airway disease. Eur Respir J 1991;4:1178–84.

50. Pearlman DS, Chervinsky P, LaForce C, et al. A comparison of salmeterol with albuterol in the treatment of mild to moderate asthma. N Engl J Med 1992;327:1420–5.

51. Fitzpatrick MF, Mackay T, Driver H, Douglas NJ. Salmeterol in nocturnal asthma: a double blind, placebo controlled trial of a long acting inhaled beta 2 agonist. Br Med J 1990;301:1365–8.

52. Maesen FP, Smeets JJ, Gubbelmans HL, Zweers PG. Formoterol in the treatment of nocturnal asthma. Chest 1990;98:866–70.

53. Muir JF, Bertin L, Georges D. Salmeterol versus slow-release theophylline combined with ketotifen in nocturnal asthma: a multicentre trial. French Multicentre Study Group. Eur Respir J 1992;5:1197–200.

54. Britton MG, Earnshaw JS, Palmer JB. A twelve month comparison of salmeterol with salbutamol in asthmatic patients: European Study Group. Eur Respir J 1992;5:1062–7.

55. Lötvall J, Lunde H, Ullman A, et al. Twelve months' treatment with inhaled salmeterol in asthmatic patients. Effects of beta 2-receptor function and inflammatory cells. Allergy 1992;47:477–83.

56. Langley SJ, Masterson CM, Batty EP, Woodcock A. Bronchodilator response to salbutamol after chronic dosing with salmeterol or placebo. Eur Respir J 1998;11:1081–5.

57. Castle W, Fuller R, Hall J, Palmer J. Serevent nationwide surveillance study: comparison of salmeterol with salbutamol in asthmatic patients who require regular bronchodilator treatment. Br Med J 1993;306:1034–7.

58. Kesten S, Chapman KR, Broder I, et al. Sustained improvement in asthma with long-term use of formoterol fumarate. Ann Allergy 1992;69:415–20.

59. Juniper EF, Johnston PR, Borkhoff CM, et al. Quality of life in asthma clinical trials: comparison of salmeterol and salbutamol. Am J Respir Crit Care Med 1995;151:66–70.

60. Arvidsson P, Larsson S, Löfdahl CG, et al. Inhaled formoterol during one year in asthma: a comparison with salbutamol. Eur Respir J 1991;4:1168–73.

61. Simons FE. A comparison of beclomethasone, salmeterol, and placebo in children with asthma. Canadian beclomethasone–salmeterol xinafoate study group. N Engl J Med 1997;337:1659–65.

62. Verberne AA, Frost C, Roorda RJ, et al. One year treatment with salmeterol compared with beclomethasone in children with asthma. The Dutch Paediatric Asthma Study Group. Am J Respir Crit Care Med 1997;156:688–95.

63. Boulet LP, Becker A, Berube D, et al. Canadian asthma consensus report 1999. Can Med Assoc J 1999;161 Suppl II:S1–52.

64. World Health Organization/National Institutes of Health. Global initiative for asthma. Bethesda (MD): National Institutes of Health; 1995.

65. Moore RH, Khan A, Dickey BF. Long-acting inhaled beta-2 agonists in asthma therapy. Chest 1998;113:1095–108.

66. Bartow RA, Brogden RN. Formoterol. An update of its pharmacological properties and therapeutic efficacy in the management of asthma. Drugs 1998;55:303–22.

67. Greening AP, Ing PW, Northfield M, Shaw G. Treatment of adult asthmatic patients symptomatic on low dose inhaled salmeterol to existing inhaled corticosteroid therapy with increasing dose of inhaled corticosteroids. Lancet 1994;344:219–24.

68. Woolcock A, Lundback B, Ringdal N, Jacques LA. Comparison of addition of salmeterol to inhaled steroids with doubling of the dose of inhaled corticosteroids. Am J Respir Crit Care Med 1996;153:1481–8.

69. Bouros D, Bachlitzanakis N, Kottakis J, et al. Formoterol and beclomethasone versus higher dose declometha-sone as maintenance therapy in adult asthma. Eur Respir J 1999;14:627–32.

70. Pauwels RA, Löfdahl C-G, Postma DS, et al. Effect of inhaled formoterol and budesonide on exacerbations of asthma. N Engl J Med 1997;337:1405–11.

71. Shrewsbury S, Pyke S, Britton M. Meta-analysis of increased dose of inhaled steroid or addition of salmeterol in symptomatic asthma. BMJ 2000;320:1368–73.

72. Lipworth BJ. Risks versus benefits of inhaled beta 2-agonists in the management of asthma. Drug Saf 1992;7:54–70.

73. Löfdahl CG, Svedmyr N. Formoterol fumarate, a new beta 2-adrenoceptor agonist. Acute studies of selectivity and duration of effect after inhaled and oral administration. Allergy 1989;44:264–71.

74. Faurschou P. Salmeterol and salbutamol: long-term efficacy and safety. Eur Respir J 1992;5 Suppl 15:A317.

75. Maesen FP, Costongs R, Smeets JJ, et al. The effect of maximal doses of formoterol and salbutamol from a metered dose inhaler on pulse rates, ECG and serum potassium concentrations. Chest 1991;99:1367–73.

76. Bremner P, Woodma K, Burgess C, et al. A comparison of the cardiovascular and metabolic effects of for-moterol, salbutamol and fenoterol. Eur Respir J 1993;2:204–10.

77. Flatt A, Crane J, Purdie G, et al. The cardiovascular effects of beta adrenergic agonist drugs administered by nebulisation. Postgrad Med 1990;66:98–101.

78. Lanes SF, Lanza LL, Wentworth CE III. Risk of emergency care, hospitalization, and ICU stays for acute asthma among recipients of salmeterol. Am J Respir Crit Care Med 1988;158:857–61.

79. Linden M. The effects of beta 2-adrenoceptor agonists and a corticosteroid budesonide on the secretion of inflammatory mediators from monocytes. Br J Pharmacol 1992;107:156–60.

80. Butcher PR, Vardey CJ, Johnson M. Salmeterol: a potent and long-acting inhibitor of inflammatory mediator release from human lung. Br J Pharmacol 1991;104:672–6.

81. Oddera S, Silvestri M, Scarso L, et al. Salmeterol inhibits the allergen-induced mononuclear cell proliferation and downregulates GM-CSF release and HLA-DR expression by monocytes. Pulm Pharmacol Ther 1997;10:43–9.

82. Weersink EJM, Aalbers R, Koëter GH, et al. Salmeterol, inhibiting or masking the late asthmatic reaction after HDM challenge. Am Rev Respir Dis 1993;147:A25.

83. Roberts JA, Bradding P, Britten KM. The long-acting β₂-agonist salmeterol xinofoate: effects on airway inflam-mation in asthma. Eur Respir J 1999;14:275–22.

84. Li A, Ward C, Thien F, et al. Anti-inflammatory effects of solmeterol, a long-acting β₂-agonist, assessed in air-way biopsy and bronchoalveolar -- in asthma. Am J Respir Crit Care Med 1999;160:1493–99.

85. Kips JC, O'Connor B, Inman M, et al. A long-term study of the anti-inflammatory effect of low-dose budes-onide plus formoterol versus high-dose budesonide in asthma. Am J Respir Crit Care Med 2000;161: 996–1001.

86. Boulet LP, Turcotte H, Boutet M, et al. Influence of salmeterol on chronic and allergen-induced airway inflam-mation in mild allergic asthma: a pilot study. Curr Ther Res 1997;58:240–59.

87. Milot J, Chakir J, Boutet M, et al. Influence of salmeterol (SM) on allergen-induced airway inflammation in mild allergic asthmatic subjects. Clin Expermin Allergy (in Press).

88. McIvor RA, Pizzichini E, Turner MO, et al. Potential masking effects of salmeterol on airway inflammation in asthma. Am J Respir Crit Care Med 1998;158:924–30.

89. Lipsworth BJ, Aziz I. Bronchodilator response to albuterol after regular formoterol and effects of acute corti-costeroid administration. Chest 2000;117:156–62.

90. Wilding P, Clark M, Coon J, et al. Effect of long term treatment with salmeterol on asthma control: a double-blind, randomised crossover study. BMJ 1997;314:1441–6.

91. Nelson HS, Berkowitz RB, Tinkelman DA, et al. Lack of subsensitivity to albuterol after treatment with salme-terol in patients with asthma. Am J Respir Crit Care Med 1999;159:1556–61.

92. Ind P, Börozörmenyi Nagy G, Pietinalho A, et al. Formoterol 4.5 µg, used as needed via turbohaler was as safe and well tolerated as terbutaline 0.5 mg. Eur Respir J 1999;14 Suppl 30:148s.

CHAPTER 14

Use of Theophylline and Anticholinergic Therapy

Brian J. O'Connor, MD,
Clive P. Page, MD

———•———

Most of the advances in asthma treatment have been founded on a background of excellent basic science. Thus, this chapter on theophyllines and anticholinergics, in addition to evaluating the clinically relevant research, will also explore the scientific background to the application of these therapies. It is axiomatic that doctors practicing evidence-based medicine will identify and apply the most efficacious interventions to maximize the quality and quantity of life for individual patients. In the context of asthma treatment, systematic reviews and meta-analyses have become the gold standard for judging whether a treatment does more good than harm.[1,2] Not surprisingly, good systematic reviews have only recently been conducted on asthma treatments. In researching the literature for this chapter, as many randomized controlled trials as possible were identified and evaluated.[3]

THEOPHYLLINE AND THE TREATMENT OF ASTHMA

Theophylline has been in clinical use for more than a century, and in the past 50 years it has been in regular use for the treatment of asthma. Methylxanthines such as theophylline remain the single most widely prescribed class of drugs for asthma in the world.[4] The mechanism of action of methylxanthines is uncertain, but it involves inhibition of phosphodiesterase with the accumulation of cyclic adenosine monophosphate (cAMP), adenosine receptor blockade, and effects on calcium flux.[5] Conventionally, the treatment benefit of xanthines in asthma has been attributed to their bronchodilator effects. However, the growing recognition that these agents modulate airway inflammation has resulted in the resurgence of their use.[6] In this chapter, the evidence for their continued use and future place in the treatment of asthma will be examined.

Theophylline was first used as an intravenous preparation in 1937 for the management of acute severe asthma. Since 1940, when it was administered in combination with ephedrine, the effects of theophylline in asthma have been well documented in numerous studies.[7] Although still widely prescribed, the number of prescriptions for theophylline has declined over the last decade, mainly due to concerns about its narrow therapeutic window.[8] Typically, when used as a bronchodilator, sufficient theophylline must be given to achieve plasma levels between 10 and 20 mg/L. Such plasma levels often result in toxic side effects.[9]

Evidence for Theophylline as Chronic Maintenance Treatment

Current asthma treatment guidelines are broadly similar across most western countries and are reflected in the simple classification drawn up by the expert panel of the National Asthma Education and Prevention Program in 1993.[10]

Step 1.   Mild intermittent asthma: recommended treatment is intermittent use of bronchodilators for symptom relief
Step 2.   Mild persistent asthma: regular low-dose anti-inflammatory therapy
Step 3.   Moderate severe persistent asthma: regular high-dose anti-inflammatory therapy plus regular bronchodilator therapy
Step 4.   Severe persistent asthma: involves a multiple-drug treatment approach incorpo-

rating several anti-inflammatory strategies, regular bronchodilators, and intermittent or regular systemic corticosteroid treatment

In their updated guidelines of 1997, the same expert panel recommends that theophylline be used as one of a range of anti-inflammatory therapies for mild persistent asthma (step 2), provided the dose used achieves a serum concentration of between 5 and 15 mg/L.[11] Thus, it is considered an alternative to either low-dose inhaled corticosteroids or chromones or leukotriene-modifying drugs.

For patients with moderate severe persistent (step 3) or severe persistent asthma (step 4), the expert panel recommends that theophylline be added to medium or high doses of inhaled corticosteroids as an alternative long-acting bronchodilator to either inhaled or oral β-agonist therapy. In effect, the guidelines recognize, with some caveats, that theophylline, although traditionally classified as a bronchodilator, has a range of other effects of potential therapeutic value in the treatment of asthma such that, theoretically, it could be used in all steps of asthma management. Let us consider the evidence for this in the ensuing sections.

Nonbronchodilator Actions

Theophylline has multiple actions that contribute to its efficacy as an antiasthma treatment. Although recognized as a bronchodilator, the degree of bronchodilatation achieved is small, and the true benefit of theophylline in asthma may result from its bronchoprotective, immunomodulatory, and anti-inflammatory actions.

Bronchoprotective effects. Several studies have demonstrated the bronchoprotective effect of theophylline with a variety of different spasmogens, including histamine, methacholine, adenosine, distilled water, sulfur dioxide, and exercise. Some of this bronchoprotection is likely due to functional antagonism of smooth muscle contraction, but it may also involve indirect mechanisms that relate to its molecular action.[5] Of the published studies on the bronchoprotective effect of theophylline, eight are blinded randomized controlled trials. The results from these studies are conflicting. For example, MacWilliams and colleagues demonstrated a 0.9 and 1.6 doubling dose protection against histamine and methacholine, respectively, following a single dose of theophylline that achieved mean plasma levels of 13 mg/L.[12] In an adult study, Magnussen et al showed that a single dose achieving comparable theophylline levels of 13 mg/L protected against histamine and methacholine by 2.6 and 1.9 doubling doses, respectively, without producing significant bronchodilatation.[13] In contrast, Tinkelman et al showed significant improvement in pulmonary function following 5 to 15 days of theophylline at two different dose levels without change in methacholine sensitivity, even in the presence of theophylline levels greater than10 mg/L.[14] This finding is supported by the study of Ibanez et al which showed that 1 week of slow-release theophylline that achieved a serum concentration of 12 mg/L did not attenuate methacholine- or exercise-induced bronchoconstriction.[15]

Crescioli et al showed that an evening dose of controlled-release theophylline for 5 days caused sustained bronchodilatation for 24 hours after the final dose but decreased airway responsiveness to methacholine for only the first 10 hours.[16] Finally, Page and colleagues showed a 1.7 doubling dose improvement in sensitivity to methacholine after 2 months of theophylline, at which time plasma levels were 11.3 mg/L.[17] This improvement in airway responsiveness was not associated with any change in forced expiratory volume in 1 second (FEV_1) or with the number or activation status of eosinophils and lymphocytes in peripheral blood.

Data from these six studies indicate that a single dose of theophylline is at least as effective in reducing airway responsiveness as chronic treatment. This suggests that the action is likely due to functional antagonisms of smooth muscle contraction. The treatment effects from these individual studies are widely disparate. Overall, these results indicate that the lower limit of the confidence interval for the treatment effect is less than the minimally clinically important benefit, which has always been regarded as a 1 doubling dose improvement in sensitivity to histamine or methacholine. Thus, the recommendation that theophylline be used as a bronchoprotective agent is based on Level IIC evidence.

Effects on exercise-induced asthma. The evidence of theophylline's protection against exercise-induced bronchospasm is more robust. Initial studies performed in the mid-1970s indicate that theophylline provides suppression of exercise-induced asthma in children.[18–20] It is, however, less effective in this regard than cromolyn in children[19] and salbutamol in adults.[21] The primacy of β_2-agonists as the treatment of choice for exercise-induced bronchospasm is well established and has been confirmed in several studies.[22] Yet, methylxanthines are effective in attenuating exercise-induced bronchoconstriction in a dose-dependent manner, with significant protection at serum concentrations as low as 6 mg/L.[23,24] If we regard a 50% inhibition of the maximum fall in FEV_1 following exercise as a clinically significant treatment effect, then we can regard the evidence for theophylline as a useful drug in exercise-induced asthma to be rated as Level IIC; the grade C results from the greater effectiveness of β_2-agonists in this role.

Effects on allergen-evoked bronchoconstriction. The inhibition of exercise-induced asthma and the attenuation of the early response to allergen imply an effect on mast cell–derived mediator release. Four studies reviewing the published randomized controlled trials on acute bronchoconstrictor and late-phase responses to inhaled allergen have specifically evaluated the early asthmatic response.[25–28] A single intravenous dose of theophylline has a small inhibitory effect on the early response, whereas dosing for up to 7 days shows contrasting results.[25] Cockcroft et al showed that 8 doses of theophylline achieving a mean plasma level of 10 mg/L resulted in a 40% attenuation of the early asthmatic response when compared to placebo, but this effect did not reach significance because of the small numbers involved.[26] Similarly, Vagaggini et al failed to show an effect on the early response after 7 days of treatment in a placebo-controlled crossover study of 6 mild asthmatics, despite achieving plasma theophylline levels of 9.8 mg/L.[27] These studies conflict with the data of Crescioli et al who showed that in 7 days of treatment of 6 mild asthmatic subjects in a placebo-controlled crossover study, there was a 65 to 70% inhibition of the early asthmatic response following active treatment that achieved plasma levels of 13 mg/L.[28] Given the paucity of the data and the conflicting results, it is difficult to make a compelling case for an effect of theophylline on mast cell function or activity.

Similarly, despite the claim that theophylline, even at low doses, has a significant impact on the late response to allergen, the evidence is not clear cut when the eight available randomized controlled trials are subjected to careful scrutiny. In one study, a single dose of theophylline caused a 50% inhibition of the late response while achieving plasma levels of 10 mg/L.[25] Three of five short-term studies using repeated doses achieved similar levels of inhibition.[28–30] Each of these studies lasted 7 to 14 days, were placebo-controlled and used adequate numbers of subjects, and achieved plasma theophylline levels in excess of 10 mg/L. Two similarly designed studies, albeit with only six enrolled subjects, failed to show a significant effect on the late response despite achieving similar plasma levels.[26,27] Two more recent studies have shown that prolonged low-dose theophylline achieving plasma levels below the "therapeutic" levels results in inhibition of the late asthmatic response. Ward and colleagues found a 75% reduction in maximal late-phase bronchoconstriction, whereas Sullivan et al showed a 40% reduction.[31,32]

The small size of many of these studies renders their interpretation difficult. The short-term studies would suggest that the inhibition of the late asthmatic response is due to functional antagonism rather than any significant immunomodulatory effect. Level II evidence provided from these data suggests that acute or short-term treatment with theophylline protects against both early and late bronchospasm occurring after exposure to allergen.

Anti-inflammatory effects. One of the more important modes of action of theophylline in asthma may be inhibition of airway inflammation. There are several in vitro studies confirming the anti-inflammatory properties of theophylline.[33-37] Although this phenomenon was recognized in the 1980s, it is only in the past decade that there has been considerable interest in the relationship between theophylline's anti-inflammatory and clinical effects. Prolonged low-dose theophylline reduces the number of activated CD4 and CD8 lymphocyte subsets seen in peripheral blood after allergen challenge; it also reduces allergen-induced airway eosinophilia and bronchoalveolar lavage (BAL)-revealed lymphocytosis following allergen challenge.[32,38] Whereas, these studies evaluated the effects of theophylline on allergen-evoked inflammation in mild asthma, the anti-inflammatory properties of theophylline may be more relevant in patients with severe disease. Withdrawal of theophylline in patients requiring high doses of inhaled corticosteroids resulted in a significant increase in symptoms and a fall in lung function accompanied by a significant fall in both activated CD4 and CD8 peripheral blood lymphocyte subsets. These findings were a mirror image of those seen on bronchial biopsy, implying that treatment with theophylline, even at low plasma concentrations, improves asthma by modulating T lymphocyte function.[39]

Theophylline not only modifies lymphocyte activity but also decreases interleukin-4 (IL-4) and IL-5 expression on cells in bronchial mucosa of moderate asthmatics[40] and reduces circulating IL-4 and IL-5 levels in mild atopic asthmatics.[41] Moreover, theophylline, which is effective in nocturnal asthma, may mediate its effect through a reduction in airway neutrophil number and activation. Kraft and colleagues showed that theophylline significantly decreased the percentage of neutrophils and eosinophils obtained from BAL at 4:00 am in patients with nocturnal asthma, implying an anti-inflammatory effect.[42] In addition, theophylline induces the production of IL-10 from asthmatic peripheral blood mononuclear cells[43] and accelerates human granulocyte apoptosis.[44]

Evidence for Clinical Use

With the development of long-acting β-agonists and inhaled corticosteroids, theophylline has been relegated to a minor role in the management of asthma. It has been supplanted by the other two classes of medication because it has relatively weak bronchodilating properties; its anti-inflammatory effects may not be clinically important; and it is difficult to use because of numerous drug interactions, the need to monitor serum levels, and a low benefit-to-risk ratio.[6,7]

Chronic Asthma

Theophylline is used widely throughout the world, and, particularly in view of the recent awareness of its anti-inflammatory actions, it has potential as an alternative to inhaled steroids in the treatment of mild to moderate asthma.[3] There have been several studies directly comparing both treatments. For example, in a 4-month crossover study of 14 children with severe perennial asthma, inhaled beclomethasone dipropionate (BDP) 400 µg daily was found to be markedly superior to a theophylline derivative.[45] Also, in an adult crossover study, 3 weeks of BDP 800 µg improved airway responsiveness and symptom control in 26 moderate to severe asthmatic patients, whereas theophylline, although achieving plasma levels of 10 mg/L or higher, did not.[46] In a parallel group study of 111 children with severe disease, 12 weeks of BDP achieved better control than theophylline alone.[47]

Two large-scale studies lasting 12 months each have been conducted in children comparing low-dose inhaled corticosteroids with sustained-release theophylline.[48,49] The first study showed a marginal benefit in favour of BDP 100 µg four times daily among 195 children as compared to a dose of theophylline adjusted to ensure adequate therapeutic blood levels.[48] The same group, 5 years later, looked at 747 patients ranging from school-aged children to adults. In a similar design using the same doses of each drug, BDP was found to be statistically more effective in reducing symptoms, supplemental β-agonist and systemic corticosteroid use, bronchial hyper-responsiveness, and eosinophilia.[49] Galant and colleagues found a marked benefit of low- and medium-dose fluticasone propionate (daily dose 100 or 200 µg) compared to a therapeutic dose of theophylline in a 12-week parallel group placebo-controlled study in moderate asthma.[50] Overall, these studies clearly show that inhaled corticosteroids are vastly superior to theophylline as single anti-inflammatory treatments. These data provide Level I evidence and a grade D recommendation against the use of theophylline in lieu of inhaled corticosteroids.

The most likely place for theophylline in the modern management of chronic asthma is as supplementary therapy to maintenance inhaled glucocorticoids. Two studies have established clinical equivalence of theophylline plus low-dose inhaled corticosteroid versus a higher dose of inhaled corticosteroid in patients with poorly controlled asthma. Ukena and colleagues enrolled 133 patients with poorly controlled asthma despite regular BDP in a daily dose of 400 µg.[51] In a parallel group study of 6 weeks' duration, patients were randomized to receive one of two treatments. The first group received BDP 400 µg daily plus theophylline at a dose adjusted to maintain plasma levels at the lower end of the therapeutic range. The second group received an increased dose of inhaled corticosteroid, BDP 800 µg daily. Both groups reported a marked improvement in asthma control. Home peak-flow recordings and clinic spirometry were significantly increased by both treatments. Also, there were significant reductions in asthma symptoms and the need for rescue medication. In a study of similar design, Evans and colleagues looked at a more severe group of patients who were poorly controlled despite doses of inhaled corticosteroids as high as 1000 µg BDP or the equivalent.[52] These patients, 62 in total, were randomized to receive either 800 µg of budesonide daily plus low-dose theophylline or 1,600 µg of budesonide. There was at least equivalent clinical improvement with abolition of peak-flow variability, reduction in symptoms, and reduction in β-agonist usage. Theophylline plus the lower dose of budesonide provided greater improvement in spirometry than the high dose of budesonide alone. Also, serum cortisol levels were significantly reduced in the group given high-dose budesonide. Otherwise, both treatments were well tolerated. The conclusion from the study was that low-dose theophylline that achieved mean plasma levels of 8.7 mg/L when added to an inhaled corticosteroid is at least equivalent to (and may be preferable, safer, and cheaper than) an increased dose of inhaled corticosteroids.

Since these studies were published, it is becoming established practice to use combination treatment of lower doses of inhaled steroids with long-acting β-agonists for the maintenance therapy of moderate asthma. The studies of Ukena et al and Evans et al suggest that theophylline may be a reasonable alternative to the long-acting β$_2$-agonists. A recent Cochrane review compared long-acting β-agonists to theophylline for maintenance treatment of asthma.[53] The study populations were primarily adult. Five of the six studies included patients who used inhaled corticosteroids. Both salmeterol and theophylline were effective in improving lung function. Salmeterol was more effective in treating nocturnal symptoms such as night-time wakening and the need for rescue medication. There were significantly increased rates of adverse events reported with theophylline when compared to salmeterol. Thus, overall, salmeterol appears to be more effective than theophylline as additive therapy to inhaled corticosteroids (Level IA).

Severe Asthma

There are few published studies on the role of theophylline in the management of severe asthma. Withdrawal of theophylline resulted in worsening of asthma in adults[39] and, even more notably, in steroid-dependent adolescents.[54] Also, an added benefit of maintenance theophylline at serum concentrations of 10 to 20 mg/L was demonstrated in a placebo-controlled randomized double-blind trial of 33 children with steroid-dependent chronic asthma.[55]

ROLE OF ANTICHOLINERGIC TREATMENT

The clinical utility of inhaled quarternary anticholinergic bronchodilators has been evaluated extensively in airways disease. They are particularly useful as inhaled bronchodilators in the management of chronic obstructive pulmonary disease. Their role in the treatment of asthma is less certain. Treatment guidelines from several countries recommend their use as adjunctive bronchodilator therapy for patients with more severe disease. The most compelling evidence for their role in asthma management is in the treatment of acute severe episodes (see Chapter 20) in which the combination of nebulized anticholinergic and β-adrenergic bronchodilators is regarded as being more effective than either of those treatments alone.[56] The evidence for the role of anticholinergic treatment in chronic asthma follows.

In the 1970s and 1980s, ipratropium bromide was regarded as an effective bronchodilator with a more sustained duration of action than β-agonists; it was considered as a possible treatment for chronic asthma.[57] In a double-blind crossover study in nine patients with stable chronic asthma, Hockley and Johnson showed that ipratropium bromide (80 μg, 200 μg, and 400 μg) produced significant bronchodilation starting as early as 15 minutes after administration of the dose and lasting up to 5 hours.[58] In a multicenter double-blind 90-day study of 144 patients with moderate asthma, ipratropium bromide, when compared to metaproterenol, produced equivalent bronchodilatation that was slower in onset but more prolonged.[59] The combination of anticholinergic and β-agonist inhaled treatment became popular and, in some studies, showed superiority over either agent alone.[60,61] Also, the combination of oxitropium bromide and salbutamol was found to be better than either drug alone, but salbutamol was superior to oxitropium.[62] Short-acting β-agonists rather than anticholinergics are the bronchodilators of choice for relief of symptoms (Level I).

Not surprisingly, in chronic maintenance treatment, anticholinergics were inferior to inhaled corticosteroids. In a 30-month randomized controlled study, combined β-agonist/corticosteroid therapy and combined β-agonist/anticholinergic therapy were compared with β-agonist/placebo therapy in 274 patients with moderately severe asthma. The group taking inhaled corticosteroids had marked improvements in lung function and reduction in symptoms and exacerbations, whereas anticholinergics were of little benefit.[63] Kerstjens et al clearly demonstrated that inhaled steroids, but not anticholinergics, reduced morbidity and improved asthma control when added to β-agonists.[64]

Do anticholinergics have any place in the maintenance treatment of asthma? They may be particularly effective in the elderly. Shioya et al examined the short-term and long-term effects of oxitropium bromide in nine elderly patients with bronchial asthma and found an immediate 28% increase in FEV_1 that was sustained and improved to 36% at 6 weeks.[65] In a study of the differential bronchodilator response to inhaled salbutamol and ipratropium in 29 asthmatic patients, all patients with a definite predominant salbutamol response were less than 40 years old.[66] The response to salbutamol declined significantly with age, whereas the response to ipratropium did not. The authors recommended that for patients aged less than 40 years, salbutamol is the drug of choice. In older patients, ipratropium, or continued therapy with both drugs, may be preferable. In a much larger study, Van Schayck and colleagues measured the acute bronchodilator response to salbutamol and to ipratropium bromide in 75 asthmatic patients and 113 patients with chronic bronchitis.[67] Patients with chronic bronchitis generally responded better to ipratropium bromide, whereas asthmatic patients responded better to salbutamol. The response pattern was also related to allergy and age. Allergic patients and patients under 60 years were more likely to respond to salbutamol than were nonallergic patients and older patients, who benefited more from ipratropium bromide. Anticholinergics may therefore serve as add-on bronchodilator therapy in older nonallergic patients with asthma (Level IIIB).

Cholinergic mechanisms may be involved in nocturnal asthma. In a double-blind placebo-controlled study in patients with nocturnal asthma, 2 consecutive nights of ipratropium did not alter the overnight fall in lung function, although the bronchodilator response to ipratropium was greater at 6:00 am than at 10:00 pm.[68] Two weeks of ipratropium bromide significantly attenuated the overnight fall in peak flow by 40%, although not all patients benefited.[69] Cox and colleagues showed an additional benefit from repeated dosing with ipratropium—reduced morning dipping, as assessed by the fall in peak flow overnight.[70] These results confirm that ipratropium improves lung function throughout the night in asthmatic patients, but they also suggest that nocturnal bronchoconstriction is not due solely to an increase in airway cholinergic activity at night. More studies with the long-acting agent tiotropium bromide are needed. Until then, the role of anticholinergic agents in asthma management remains small.

REFERENCES

1. Davidoff F, Haynes B, Sackett D, Smith R. Evidence based medicine. BMJ 1995;310:1085–6.

2. McAlister FA, Laupacis A, Wells GA, Sackett DL.Users' guides to the medical literature: XIX. Applying clinical trial results. B. Guidelines for determining whether a drug is exerting (more than) a class effect. JAMA 1999;282:1371–7.

3. Jadad AR, Moher M, Brownman GP, et al. Systematic reviews and meta-analyses on treatment of asthma: critical evaluation. BMJ 2000;320:537–40

4. Weinberger M, Hendeles L. Theophylline in asthma. N Engl J Med 1996;334:636–42.

5. Spina D, Landells LJ, Page CP. The role of theophylline and phosphodiesterase 4 isoenzyme inhibitors as anti-inflammatory drugs. Clin Exp Allergy 1998;28:24–34.

6. Barnes PJ, Pauwels RA. Theophylline in the management of asthma: time for reappraisal? Eur Respir J 1994;7:579–91.

7. Weinberger M, Riegelman S. Editorial: rational use of theophylline for bronchodilatation. New Engl J Med 1974;291:151–3.

8. Johnston IDA. Theophylline in the management of airflow obstruction. 2. Difficult drugs to use, few clinical indications. BMJ 1990;300:929–31.

9. Woodcock AA, Johnson MA, Geddes DM. Theophylline prescribing, serum concentrations, and toxicity. Lancet 1983;2:610–3.

10. Sheffer AL, Taggart VS. The National Asthma Education Program. Expert panel report guidelines for the diagnosis and management of asthma. National Heart, Lung, and Blood Institute. Med Care 1993;31:MS20–8.

11. National Institutes of Health. Expert panel report 2. Clinical practice guidelines. Guidelines for the diagnosis and management of asthma. Bethesda (MD): NIH; 1997 Publication No.: 97-4051.

12. McWilliams BC, Menendez R, Kelly HW, Howick J. Effects of theophylline on inhaled methacholine and histamine in asthmatic children. Am Rev Respir Dis 1984;130:193–7.

13. Magnussen H, Reuss G, Jorres R. Theophylline has a dose-related effect on the airway response to inhaled histamine and methacholine in asthmatics. Am Rev Respir Dis 1987;136:1163–7.

14. Tinkelman DG, Garcha BS, Lutz CN. Relationship of different serum levels of theophylline on methacholine sensitivity. J Allergy Clin Immunol 1990;85:750–5.

15. Ibanez MD, Laso MT, Alonso E, et al. Effect of theophylline on airway responsiveness to methacholine and on exercise-induced bronchoconstriction. Ann Allergy 1994;73:357–63.

16. Crescioli S, Dal Carobbo A, Maestrelli P, et al. Controlled-release theophylline inhibits early morning airway obstruction and hyperresponsiveness in asthmatic subjects. Ann Allergy Asthma Immunol 1996;77:106–10.

17. Page CP, Cotter T, Kilfeather S, et al. Effect of chronic theophylline treatment on the methacholine dose-response curve in allergic asthmatic subjects. Eur Respir J 1998;12:24–9.

18. Godfrey S, Konig P. Suppression of exercise-induced asthma by salbutamol, theophylline, atropine, cromolyn, and placebo in a group of asthmatic children. Pediatrics 1975;56:930–4.

19. Pollock J, Kiechel F, Cooper D, Weinberger M. Relationship of serum theophylline concentration to inhibition of exercise-induced bronchospasm and comparison with cromolyn. Pediatrics 1977;60:840–4.

20. Bierman CW, Shapiro GG, Pierson WE, Dorsett CS. Acute and chronic theophylline therapy in exercise-induced bronchospasm. Pediatrics 1977;60:845–9.

21. Bakran I, Vrhovac B, Plavsic F. Aminophylline vs salbutamol in exercise-induced asthma. Int J Clin Pharmacol Ther Toxicol 1980;18:442–6.

22. Virant FS. Exercise-induced bronchospasm: epidemiology, pathophysiology and therapy. Med Sci Sports Exerc 1992;24:851–5.

23. Magnussen H, Reuss G, Jorres R. Methylxanthines inhibit exercise-induced bronchoconstriction at low serum theophylline concentration and in a dose-dependent fashion. J Allergy Clin Immunol 1988;81:531–7

24. Iikura Y, Hashimoto K, Akasawa A, et al. Serum theophylline concentration levels and preventative effects on exercise-induced asthma. Clin Exp Allergy 1996;26 Suppl 2:38–41

25. Pauwels R, Van Renterghem D, Van der Straeten M, et al. The effect of theophylline and enprofylline on allergen-induced bronchoconstriction. J Allergy Clin Immunol 1985;76:583–90.

26. Cockcroft DW, Murdock KY, Gore BP, et al. Theophylline does not inhibit allergen-induced increase in airway responsiveness to methacholine. J Allergy Clin Immunol 1989;83:913–20.

27. Vagaggini B, Paggiaro PL, Bancalari L, et al. Oral slow-release theophylline does not prevent early and late asthmatic response to allergen in sensitized subjects. Monaldi Arch Chest Dis 1995;50:7–11.

28. Crescioli S, Spinazzi A, Plebani M, et al. Theophylline inhibits early and late asthmatic reactions induced by allergens in asthmatic subjects. Ann Allergy 1991;66:245–51.

29. Hendeles L, Harman E, Huang D, et al. Theophylline attenuation of airway responses to allergen: comparison with cromolyn metered-dose inhaler. J Allergy Clin Immunol 1995;95:505–14.

30. Jarjour NN, Lacouture PG, Busse WW. Theophylline inhibits the late asthmatic response to nighttime antigen challenge in patients with mild atopic asthma. Ann Allergy 1998;81:231–6.

31. Ward AJ, McKenniff M, Evans JM, et al. Theophylline—an immunomodulatory role in asthma? Am Rev Respir Dis 1993;147:518–23.

32. Sullivan P, Bekir S, Jaffar Z, et al. Anti-inflammatory effects of low-dose oral theophylline in atopic asthma. Lancet 1994;343:1006–8.

33. Kraft M, Pak J, Borish L, Martin RJ. Theophylline's effect on neutrophil function and the late asthmatic response. J Allergy Clin Immunol 1996;98:251–7.

34. Limatibul S, Shore A, Dorsch HM, Gelfard E. Theophylline modulation of E-rosette formation: an indication of T-cell maturation. Clin Exp Immunol 1987;33:503–13.

35. Pauwels R. The effects of theophylline on airway inflammation. Chest 1987;92:32–7S.

36. Scordamaglia A, Ciprandi G, Ruffoni S, et al. Theophylline and the immune response: in vitro and in vivo effects. Clin Immunol Immunopathol 1988;48:238–46.

37. Shohat B, Volovitz B, Varsano I. Induction of suppressor T cells in asthmatic children by theophylline treatment. Clin Allergy 1983;13:487–93.

38. Jaffar ZH, Sullivan P, Page C, Costello J. Low-dose theophylline modulates T-lymphocyte activation in allergen-challenged asthmatics. Eur Respir J 1996;9:456–62.

39. Kidney J, Dominguez M, Taylor PM, et al. Immunomodulation by theophylline in asthma. Demonstration by withdrawal of therapy. Am J Respir Crit Care Med 1995;151:1907–14.

40. Finnerty JP, Lee C, Wilson S, et al. Effects of theophylline on inflammatory cells and cytokines in asthmatic subjects: a placebo-controlled parallel group study. Eur Respir J 1996;9:1672–7.

41. Kosmas EN, Michaelides SA, Polychronaki A, et al. Theophylline induces a reduction in circulating interleukin-4 and interleukin-5 in atopic asthmatics. Eur Respir J 1999;13:53–8.

42. Kraft M, Torvik JA, Trudeau JB, et al. Theophylline: potential antiinflammatory effects in nocturnal asthma. J Allergy Clin Immunol 1996;97:1242–6.

43. Mascali JJ, Cvietusa P, Negri J, Borish L. Anti-inflammatory effects of theophylline: modulation of cytokine production. Ann Allergy Asthma Immunol 1996;77:34–8.

44. Yasui K, Hu B, Nakazawa T, et al. Theophylline accelerates human granulocyte apoptosis not via phosphodiesterase inhibition. J Clin Invest 1997;100:1677–84.

45. Edmunds AT, McKenzie S, Baillie E, et al. A comparison of oral choline theophyllinate and beclomethasone in severe perennial asthma in children. Br J Dis Chest 1979;73:149–56.

46. Dutoit JI, Salome CM, Woolcock AJ. Inhaled corticosteroids reduce the severity of bronchial hyperresponsiveness in asthma but oral theophylline does not. Am Rev Respir Dis 1987;136:1174–8.

47. Meltzer EO, Orgel HA, Ellis EF, et al. Long-term comparison of three combinations of albuterol, theophylline, and beclomethasone in children with chronic asthma. J Allergy Clin Immunol 1992;90:2–11.

48. Tinkelman DG, Reed CE, Nelson HS, Offord KP. Aerosol beclomethasone dipropionate compared with theophylline as primary treatment of chronic, mild to moderately severe asthma in children. Pediatrics 1993;92:64–77.

49. Reed CE, Offord KP, Nelson HS, et al. Aerosol beclomethasone dipropionate spray compared with theophylline as primary treatment for chronic mild-to-moderate asthma. The American Academy of Allergy, Asthma and Immunology Beclomethasone Dipropionate–Theophylline Study Group. J Allergy Clin Immunol 1998;101:14–23.

50. Galant SP, Lawrence M, Meltzer EO, et al. Fluticasone propionate compared with theophylline for mild-to-moderate asthma. Ann Allergy Asthma Immunol 1996;77:112–8.

51. Ukena, D, Harnest U, Sakalauskas R, et al. Comparison of addition of theophylline to inhaled steroid with doubling of the dose of inhaled steroid in asthma. Eur Respir J 1997;10:2754–60.

52. Evans DJ, Taylor DA, Zetterstrom O, et al. A comparison of low-dose inhaled budesonide plus theophylline and high-dose inhaled budesonide for moderate asthma [comments]. N Engl J Med 1997;337:1412–8.

53. Wilson AJ, Gibson PG, Coughlan J. Long acting beta-agonists versus theophylline for maintenance treatment of asthma. Cochrane Review. Oxford: The Cochrane Library; Issue 1, 2000.

54. Zairuoin BM, Ismail D, Yusuffk. Effect of adding amilophylline infusion to nebulized salbutamol in severe acute asthma. Thorax 1994;49:267–9.

55. Beveridge RC, Grunfeld AF, Hodder RV, Verbeek PR. Guidelines for the emergency management of asthma in adults. CAEP/CTS Asthma Advisory Committee. Canadian Association of Emergency Physicians and the Canadian Thoracic Society. Can Med Assoc J 1996;155:25–37.

56. diurnal variation of asthma in asthmatic children. Thorax 42:357–60.

57. Baigelman W, Chodosh S. Bronchodilator action of the anticholinergic drug, ipratropium bromide (Sch 1000), as an aerosol in chronic bronchitis and asthma. Chest 1977;71:324–8.

58. Hockley B, Johnson NM. A comparison of three high doses of ipratropium bromide in chronic asthma. Br J Dis Chest 1985;79:379–84.

59. Storms WW, Bodman SF, Nathan RA, et al. Use of ipratropium bromide in asthma. Results of a multi-clinic study. Am J Med 1986;81:61–6.

60. Flint KC, Hockley B, Johnson NM. A comparison between a combination of ipratropium bromide plus fenoterol in a single metered dose inhaler (Duovent) and salbutamol in asthma. Postgrad Med J 1983;59:724–5.

61. Crane J, Gamble S. Single dose comparison of salbutamol and a fenoterol/ipratropium combination from metered aerosols in patients with asthma. N Z Med J 1986;99:420–1.

62. Tukiainen P, Salorinne Y. Oxitropium, salbutamol and their combination in asthma. Eng J Respir Dis 1985;67:31-6.

63. Rutten-van Molken MP, Van Doorslaer EK, Jansen MC, et al. Costs and effects of inhaled corticosteroids and bronchodilators in asthma and chronic obstructive pulmonary disease. Am J Respir Crit Care Med 1995;151:975–82.

64. Kerstjens HA, Brand PL, Hughes MD, et al. A comparison of bronchodilator therapy with or without inhaled corticosteroid therapy for obstructive airways disease. Dutch Chronic Non-Specific Lung Disease Study Group. N Engl J Med 1992;327:1413–9.

65. Shioya T, Kagaya M, Onodera A, et al. Effectiveness of the anticholinergic agent oxitropium bromide in elderly patients with bronchial asthma. Arzneimittelforschung 1996;46:1130–3.

66. Ullah MI, Newman GB, Saunders KB. Influence of age on response to ipratropium and salbutamol in asthma. Thorax 1981;36:523–9.

67. van Schayck CP, Folgering H, Harbers H, et al. Effects of allergy and age on responses to salbutamol and ipratropium bromide in moderate asthma and chronic bronchitis. Thorax 1991;46:355–9.

68. Catterall JR, Rhind GB, Whyte KF, et al. Is nocturnal asthma caused by changes in airway cholinergic activity? Thorax 1988;43:720–4.

69. Coe CI, Barnes PJ. Reduction of nocturnal asthma by an inhaled anticholinergic drug. Chest 1986;90:485–8.

70. Cox ID, Hughes DT, McDonnell KA. Ipratropium bromide in patients with nocturnal asthma. Postgrad Med J 1984;60:526–8.

CHAPTER 15

Environmental Control and Immunotherapy

Allan B. Becker, MD, FRCPC

JUSTIFICATION FOR CONSIDERATION OF ENVIRONMENTAL CONTROL AND IMMUNOTHERAPY

The important relationship between asthma and allergy is now well recognized.[1–7] Environmental allergen avoidance is one of the primary goals of asthma management recommended in all asthma guidelines including those of the Canadian Asthma Consensus Conference[8] and the National Asthma Education and Prevention Program sponsored by the National Institutes of Health in the United States.[9]

The majority of children and adults with asthma are sensitized to common environmental inhalant aeroallergens.[10–13] Food allergens are not a common cause for asthma symptoms, except for those associated with anaphylaxis. Sensitization to inhalant allergens tends to occur after the second year of life, later than sensitization to food allergens.[14] Nevertheless, it appears that the risk for sensitization to inhalant allergens is increased in infancy. Sporik et al[5] found a correlation between the risk for asthma at 11 years and exposure to house dust mite allergen at 12 months; the higher the exposure, the greater the risk. In general, the worse the asthma, the more likely the patient is to have associated sensitization to aeroallergens.[10] Patients sensitized to an allergen and exposed to high concentrations of that allergen have a greater risk for acute, severe asthma (Level IIA).[15–18]

Exposure to environmental tobacco smoke (ETS) has been associated with multiple adverse effects in infants and children. Environmental tobacco smoke increases the prevalence and severity of asthma in children.[19–22] Compared to children of nonsmoking mothers, the risk of asthma in children of mothers who smoke is higher,[19,20] and asthmatic children of smoking mothers have more severe asthma.[19,20] As well, smokers have higher levels of serum IgE;[23] thus, ETS exposure may be associated with an increase in allergy, an increase in asthma, or both.

It is generally agreed that T lymphocytes play a pivotal role in the pathogenesis of asthma and allergic disorders.[24,25] The current commonly accepted paradigm is that phenotypic functional distinction occurs within the CD4+ T lymphocyte population with production of Th1 and Th2 cells. Th1 lymphocytes produce one group of cytokines, including interferon-gamma (IFN-γ), and Th2 lymphocytes produce another group of cytokines including interleukin-4 (IL-4), IL-5, and IL-13. Th2 cells promote a humoral immune allergy–associated response, whereas Th1 cells promote a cellular immune response and predominate in non-allergic individuals.[24,25] Th2 cells are essential for IgE synthesis via IL-4, and perhaps IL-13 induction of immunoglobulin gene switching. Also of note, IL-4 (along with IL-3) is a mast cell growth factor, whereas IL-5 induces proliferation, differentiation, and activation of eosinophils—cells that are critically important in asthma and other allergic disorders.[24,26]

EFFICACY OF CONTROL OF ALLERGEN EXPOSURE

There is debate as to the value of environmental control measures in the management of asthma; this is best illustrated in the case of allergy to house dust mites. A recent meta-analysis[27] was unable to find a positive effect on patients with asthma for house dust mite environmental control. The authors noted that "current chemical and physical methods aimed at reducing exposure to allergens from house dust mites seemed to be ineffective."[27] In that analysis, only 5 of 23 studies demonstrated a significant fall in house dust mite allergen concentrations; however, 4 of those 5 studies were associated with some measured improvement of asthma. There are a number of studies of the relationship between house dust mite allergen and asthma that were not considered in the meta-analysis and that have demonstrated the importance of house dust mite avoidance measures in the control of asthma.[28–31] For example, Murray and Ferguson[28] showed that a sterile bedroom environment was associated with marked improvement in children with asthma due to house dust mite allergy. In an open study of adults with asthma, Platts-Mills et al[29] showed that airway responsiveness improved over a period of months in an allergen-free hospital environment. As well, residence at high altitude where mite allergens are low has been used successfully in the treatment of asthma in house dust mite–allergic patients.[30]

One recent review[32] came to the conclusion that environmental control of allergens should be an integral part of the management of sensitized patients. These authors reviewed 31 studies, including some of those included in the meta-analysis noted above.[27] In a number of the studies, there was some evidence of clinical benefit, although the outcome parameter considered in each of the studies was somewhat different. The authors stated, "There remains an urgent need to develop a large scale trial of the widespread applicability of mite allergen avoidance and the effect on patient symptoms, exacerbation rate, use of medication, and overall health costs."[32] What appears critical and rather logical, in each of the positive studies, is the need to significantly decrease house dust mite allergen concentration if one is to have impact on the underlying asthma pathophysiology in house dust mite–allergic patients (Level IA).

ASSESSMENT OF EXPOSURE

Sensitization to specific allergens has been known for many years to be demonstrable by skin testing. However, it is only recently that we are able to measure the actual levels of exposure to allergens that may be important in asthma, particularly indoor aeroallergens. Over the past decade, studies have measured levels of house dust mite and cat allergens in dust samples collected from a variety of reservoirs in homes such as mattresses and carpeting. In the past few years, we have begun to measure allergen levels in air samples in an attempt to relate respirable exposure to asthma severity. Most particles carrying house dust mite allergen are relatively large (>10 μ) and exposure is mainly in and around the bed or carpeting (when disturbed, as with vacuuming).[33] On the other hand, animal allergens are usually carried on small, rather sticky particles (much of this material is <5 μ mean diameter) and tend to be airborne for long periods of time; therefore, they are breathable even without disturbance of the surroundings.[34] We must begin to routinely measure allergen in the indoor environment (Level IIA).

Sensitization to indoor inhalant aeroallergens is more important in asthma than sensitization to outdoor aeroallergens, although exposure to outdoor pollens and mold spores plays an important role in seasonal asthma in some patients.[35,36] We must continue to monitor outdoor inhalant allergen exposure for research and for the benefit of sensitized patients (Level IIA).

ASSESSMENT OF ALLERGEN SENSITIZATION

Testing for sensitization to specific allergens is best done in vivo with skin testing. Epicutaneous testing using the prick or puncture technique is preferred. Testing with intradermal injections is less specific and more painful and is therefore not recommended (Level IIA). In vitro testing using radioallergosorbent testing (RAST) is not routinely recommended. It is much more expensive, requires a blood sample, and the results are not immediately available. Allergy testing must be interpreted in light of the history provided by the patient. Together they should form the basis for intervention to control environmental factors that may be important for an individual's asthma (Level IA).

POLLUTANTS AND ADJUVANTS

Environmental tobacco smoke is important in development of childhood asthma and in worsening of asthma in children and adults.[37] The earlier, longer, and greater the degree of ETS exposure in early childhood, the greater the likelihood of asthma developing in children.[37–42] Environmental tobacco smoke is by far the single most important pollution exposure factor associated with asthma in infants and children and must be avoided (Level IA).

Environmental pollutants other than ETS may also be a problem.[42] These include noxious gases such as ozone, sulfur dioxide, and nitrous oxides, as well as suspended particles, especially diesel particulate. Exposure to nitrous oxides occurs from a variety of sources, such as incomplete oxidation of natural gas, and NO_X gases that are present in ETS. Most "visible" pollution that is apparent as overt discoloration of the air is not necessarily associated with increased prevalence of asthma and allergy. Changes which may be far less obvious, particularly in industrialized societies, appear to be rather more important.

EFFICACY AND PRACTICALITY OF ENVIRONMENTAL CONTROL

Given their strong relationship to asthma, avoidance of the principle indoor aeroallergens including house dust mite, companion animal(s) (particularly cat), and cockroach appears to have the greatest potential for benefit (Level IA).

House Dust Mite

Treatment to control house dust mite is actually the least disputed issue in control of aeroallergen exposure. Most house dust mite exposure can be reasonably controlled. House dust mites thrive in high humidity. Relative humidity levels less than 50% are associated with lower house dust mite concentrations (Level IIA).[43] In some environments, this may be difficult to achieve, and focused intervention on specific sites within the home become increasingly important. A summary of environmental control of house dust mites is presented in Table 15–1.

Beds

Mattresses can rapidly become infected with house dust mites and become an important source for allergen exposure in only a few months.[44] Simple encasement of mattresses and pillows in impermeable vapor barrier is effective in decreasing house dust mite exposure (Level IA).[45] Zippered vinyl encasements are effective, although they are not particularly comfortable and require covering with a fitted cotton or cotton/polyester quilted mattress cover. More comfortable encasements for bedding that are permeable to air and water vapor, but not to dust mites or the dust mite allergen, are now available but are much more expensive. Allergens will continue to accumulate on top of the encasement, and it is important that all bedding be regularly washed to remove this accumulated allergen. Laundering bed sheets in hot water (55°C) will decrease dust mite concentrations.[46] Adding benzyl benzoate or dilute essential plant oils to room temperature washes will also decrease allergen concentration and mite survival.[47]

Table 15–1 *Environmental Control of House Dust Mites*

Maintain relative humidity below 50%
Encase mattress and boxspring (and possibly pillows) in mite- and mite allergen–impermeable covers
Launder bed linen in hot (55°C) water
Remove carpeting, where possible
Air filters are not necessary as they do not effect reservoir levels of house dust mite allergen

Carpeting

The reduction of house dust mite allergen in carpeting is more difficult, but short-term decrease in house dust mites and mite allergen concentrations have been noted with various acaricides, tannic acid, liquid nitrogen (to freeze carpeting), and steam cleaning. Not all studies of acaricides have shown reduction in allergen level.[27,32] With proper application of acaricides such as benzyl benzoate, most, but not all, mites are killed. However, allergen can reaccumulate quickly and reapplication may be required every 2 months.[48] Benzyl benzoate may not be able to reduce house dust mite allergen levels below those present in Northern climates such as Scandinavia or Canada. With tannic acid there is reduction in mite allergen concentrations, but the mites themselves are not killed. At best, these benefits are temporary.[49] Placing carpets in the sun for several hours allows for decreased humidity and higher temperatures, which are effective in killing the house dust mite. Steam cleaning of carpets can kill mites and decrease house dust mite allergen concentrations, although it is not clear how long levels are decreased after steam treatment.[50] Removal of carpeting is the most effective method to decrease the concentration of house dust mite allergen on the floor (Level IA).[51]

Stuffed Toys

Mites are effectively killed and the house dust mite allergen denatured at temperatures of 55°C and above and –30°C and below. Placement of small soft toys in a regular freezer (–4°C) may result in death of the dust mite but will not denature the allergen. A standard dryer is capable of reaching temperatures of 55°C and, if it is maintained for at least 10 minutes, may effectively kill mites and denature allergen.

Vacuum Cleaners and Air Filters

Regular vacuuming is important to help decrease overall allergen load but, by itself, has not been shown to significantly reduce house dust mite allergen exposure.[52] House dust mite allergen is usually carried on moderately large particles (5 μ and larger), and most multilayer vacuum bags are capable of reasonably containing large particles.[53] Large particles do not stay airborne for long and do not circulate widely; therefore, there is little reason to consider use of air filters for house dust mite allergens. Air filters do not effect the large reservoir of house dust mite allergen, which are primarily found in the beds and carpeting (Level IE).

Pets

Removal of the pet from the home is the most effective means to reduce exposure to cat or dog allergen (Level IA).[54] However, it can take more than 6 months for cat allergen levels to return to baseline after removal of a cat.[54] Unfortunately, removal of a pet from the home is loaded with psychosocial issues, and many families will not agree to removal of the animal. In fact, although we believe it is important, there are no studies on the impact of pet removal on the disease process in cat or dog allergic patients. Nevertheless, allergen control is as important in the case of allergy to a companion animal as it is in allergy to house dust mite. As a result of the frequent reluctance to remove the pet from the home, a number of alternatives have been considered. One of the first approaches considered was washing of the animal. One early study demonstrated marked reduction of airborne Fel d I after washing a cat on a weekly basis.[55] Subsequent studies also have demonstrated that washing the cat is capable of removing a substantial amount of cat allergen and effecting a transient decrease in airborne cat allergen levels.[56] However, this approach has not resulted in sustained reduction of airborne Fel d I.[56,57] Less aggressive methods of cleaning the cat, such as wiping it with a moist cloth or the use of a commercial spray (Allerpet-C) do not appear to be effective.[57,58] Recently, a study demonstrated that the combination of a high-efficiency particulate air (HEPA) filter room air cleaner, mattress and pillow covers, and cat exclusion from the bedroom did reduce airborne cat allergen levels.[59] However, this did not effect the clinical outcome during a

3-month trial. Another study has shown long-term reduction in cat allergen with the use of HEPA filters and mattress encasements.[60] This study also demonstrated that "textile floor coverings" are an important reservoir for the allergen. A summary of environmental control of pet allergen is presented in Table 15–2.

Cat allergen exposure also occurs in public environments such as schools and hospitals, and it is presumed that pet allergen is transported to these sites on clothing, and then it settles into reservoirs such as upholstered furniture and carpeting. Children from homes with cats carry significant amounts of cat allergen on their clothing.[61] Cat has become a widespread community-based allergen. It has been suggested that "carpeting should be discouraged in environments such as schools and childcare centres where children spend considerable time."[61] Carpeting appears to be an important risk factor in allergy and asthma (Level IA).[51] Similarly, upholstered chairs in hospitals, and presumably other public places, constitute a significant reservoir of cat and dog allergen.[62] Frequent vacuuming (three times weekly using a HEPA-filtered vacuum cleaner) has been shown to significantly reduce allergen levels in upholstered furniture.[62]

Table 15–2 *Environmental Control of Pet Allergen*

Removal of the pet from the home is the most effective approach.

Where removal is not possible, the following may decrease airborne pet allergen:

• Pet exclusion from the bedroom

• HEPA room air cleaner

• Mattress and pillow covers

• Removal of carpeting

• Frequent vacuuming of upholstered furniture with a HEPA-filtered vacuum

• Washing of the pet to possibly reduce allergen load temporarily (but this must not be done by the allergic individual)

Cockroach

Cockroach allergen has been detected in up to 60 to 80% of inner city homes in the United States.[63] Extermination of cockroaches and regular vacuuming has been shown to significantly decrease levels of *Bla g* II in dormitory bedrooms and kitchens.[64] However, this decrease in cockroach allergen concentration may not be of long duration, and in home environments, it may be difficult to obtain, even with professional extermination and cleaning. Decrease in cockroach exposure in those settings will require increased awareness of this community problem. Changes in housing to impact on this problem will require not only scientific understanding but also will include social and political changes (Level IIIB).

Pollen and Outdoor Molds

Outdoor aeroallergens are generally less of a problem for patients with asthma. The only outdoor inhalant aeroallergen that has repeatedly been shown to be associated with asthma is *Alternaria*.[65–67] In agricultural, semi-arid environments around the world, *Alternaria* is a major sensitizer and has been shown to be associated with severe and often life-threatening asthma.[18] This mold spore has marked seasonality with peaks in the spring, late summer, and fall.[18,68] *Alternaria* has been found as an indoor mold spore, but this is primarily from being carried or blown in from outdoors.[69] Immunoreactive *Alternaria* allergen has been demonstrated in house dust during the winter season, suggesting that it may have some perennial activity.[69,70] Although data are not available, it would seem logical to ensure that homes are closed up as much as possible when high levels of *Alternaria* exist outside. The use of air conditioning systems with central air filters has the potential to decrease indoor exposure to outdoor allergens and, by decreasing humidity, to decrease the potential for mold growth in the home (Level IIB).

COMPLIANCE WITH ALLERGEN AVOIDANCE

Unfortunately, compliance with allergen avoidance recommendations is poor, even for a simple recommendation such as encasement of mattresses.[71–73] We believe that allergen avoidance is a critically important goal for allergic patients in any asthma management program (Level IIIA). While removal of a sensitized individual to an allergen-free environment such as a hospital or a mountain retreat can result in dramatic improvement clinically and in terms of airway function, this is neither practical nor possible in most instances. Environmental control is frequently discussed but seldom acted upon in asthma therapy. As the potential value for environmental therapy increases, we must give serious consideration to proper and effective means for environmental control. Compliance should not be a problem with house dust mite avoidance measures; however, compliance will continue to be a major issue regarding pets. Given the psychosocial issues and the widespread exposure to cat allergen, issues of ventilation and filtration in the home and work environment will be of increasing importance. We must consider carpeting a risk factor for development of allergen and asthma, and this must be reflected in our recommendations relating to home and office design. Patients at high risk for allergy and asthma should be counseled not to have carpeting in their home. Serious consideration should be given by the floor covering industry to development of textile floor covering that either prevents allergen from collecting or acts as a trap to hold, but not release, allergen. Proper and effective methods of ventilation and filtration at home and work must be the focus of increased research, particularly given the epidemic of allergy and asthma in the industrialized world over the last quarter century. We now have at our disposal effective means to rigorously assess the impact of environmental control on patients with asthma. Improved understanding of environmental control is critical to our approach to this major health problem. A summary of key points regarding allergen exposure is presented in Table 15–3.

IMMUNOTHERAPY

Given the immunologic underpinnings of the pathobiology of asthma, there has been renewed interest in the potential for immune modulation. Allergen-specific immunotherapy for allergic disease has been used extensively in the past. Extracts from aeroallergens were

Table 15–3 *Evidence-Based Data Regarding Allergen Exposure*

Increased allergen exposure increases risk for allergy and asthma (Level IA).

Allergic patients exposed to high concentrations of allergen to which they are sensitized have a greater risk for acute, severe asthma (Level IA).

Intervention must significantly decrease allergen exposure to impact on the underlying asthma (Level IA).

Carpeting is a risk factor for allergy and asthma (Level IA).

Removal of a pet from the home is the most effective means to reduce exposure to a cat or dog (Level IA).

Encasement of a mattress in impermeable vapor barrier is the single most effective method to reduce exposure to house dust mite allergen (Level IA).

used for the treatment of hayfever as early as 1911.[74] Data support the use of allergen-specific immunotherapy for the treatment of allergic rhinoconjunctivitis.[75–78] Similarly, immunotherapy has been established as potentially life-saving therapy for individuals at risk for anaphylaxis because of stinging insect venom hypersensitivity.[79] However, there is substantial debate and controversy as to the role of allergen-specific immunotherapy in the treatment of asthma.[80,81]

Impact of Immunotherapy on the Immune Response

The mechanism by which allergen-specific immunotherapy improves clinical disease is unclear. For some time, it was suggested that immunotherapy induced production of "blocking" antibody which was mostly, but not completely, IgG.[82,83] However, titers of blocking antibody did not predict clinical outcome.[84] Immunotherapy has been shown to initially increase levels of serum IgE but subsequently to prevent the seasonal increase in allergen-specific IgE antibodies and eventually to cause a decline below pretreatment levels of allergen-specific IgE.[85–87] However, again, no relationship has been found between change in IgE and clinical improvement.[87] Blocking antibody has been shown to inhibit release of histamine from basophils,[88] and immunotherapy has been shown to decrease allergen-induced histamine release from peripheral blood.[89] Studies have also demonstrated a decrease in the late phase of the allergic response following immunotherapy.[90]

Lymphocyte response appears to be extremely important in asthma with a predominance of the Th2 phenotype and production of cytokines which promote the allergic response, and mast cell and eosinophil activation and proliferation.[24–26] Immunotherapy appears to decrease lymphocyte proliferation[91] and may increase suppressor cell activity.[92] Downregulation of IL-4 production from T lymphocytes has also been demonstrated.[93] Immunotherapy with venom appears to induce a shift in the cytokine response from a Th2 to a Th1 dominant pattern.[94]

Role of Immunotherapy in Asthma

There has been a great deal of debate as to the value of immunotherapy in the treatment of asthma; this is reflected in the recommendations from various national societies and in international guidelines.[95–102] The use of immunotherapy was virtually halted in the United Kingdom several years ago following the conclusion of the British Society for Allergy and Clinical Immunology that "on the basis of uncertain efficacy and the potential for serious side-effects we recommend that allergen immunotherapy is not indicated for the treatment of asthma."[95] However, other international guidelines recommend that referral for specific allergen immunotherapy should be considered when avoidance is not possible and appropriate medication fails to control symptoms of allergic asthma.[98] All guidelines present considerations to be weighed by the individual practitioner. For example, the Canadian Society of Allergy and Clinical Immunology recommends consideration for allergen immunotherapy when optimal allergen avoidance and medication have not been effective in controlling symptoms, and there is a clear temporal association between exposure to the allergens and signs and symptoms of asthma.[96] The European Academy of Allergy and Allergology and Clinical Immunology suggests consideration where daily pharmacotherapy is required for seasonal and/or perennial disease.[97] The cost, risk, and duration of pharmacologic therapy versus allergen-specific immunotherapy must always be considered. There are data that suggest early treatment with allergen-specific immunotherapy should be considered, given that immunotherapy appears to be most effective in patients under 20 years of age.[103] This may be important since benefit from immunotherapy continues even after it has been discontinued following a 5-year course of treatment.[104,105] The potential benefit from immunotherapy is not only related to age, but also there appears to be a direct relationship between pulmonary function (percent predicted forced expiratory volume in 1 second [FEV_1]) and likelihood of clinical improvement.[103] Thus, the data suggest immunotherapy may be most effective in young patients with a normal FEV_1. This is not consonant, however, with recommendations from the various organizations.

The literature must be carefully interpreted, given the variance of recommendations from Britain,[95] Australia, and New Zealand (relating to childhood asthma)[101] against immunotherapy, compared with the Canadian,[96] European,[97] American,[98] the Global Initiative for Asthma (GINA),[99] and more recent Australasian recommendations for consideration of immunotherapy. The primary question that must be dealt with is: "Is allergen immunotherapy effective?" A recent meta-analysis of randomized controlled trials[106] reviewed data from 1966 to 1990. The authors considered 20 controlled trials of immunotherapy: 9 studied house dust mite allergen; 5, pollens; 5, animal dander; and 1, mold allergen. Twelve studies were excluded from the meta-analysis for a variety of reasons. The combined odds of symptomatic improvement in asthma from immunotherapy with any allergen were 3.2 (95% CI 2.2 to 4.9) (Table 15–4). The odds ratio for reduction in bronchial hyper-responsiveness with immunotherapy was 6.8 (95% CI 3.8 to 12.0). For house dust mite immunotherapy the reduction in bronchial hyper-responsiveness was also the greatest (odds ratio 13.7). For immunotherapy with house dust mite, there was a decrease in need for medication with an odds ratio of 4.2 (95% CI 2.2 to –7.9) for subjects receiving active therapy compared with the control group. A recent review of immunotherapy for childhood asthma has been undertaken.[107] This review considered data from 1966 to 1994 and evaluated studies for clinical efficacy but was not conducted as a meta-analysis. The authors found the most consistent evidence of benefit from those trials of house dust mite immunotherapy but found no trials that provided evidence for value of immunotherapy with dog or mold allergen. One study of children, which had been excluded from the meta-analysis because the control group received pollen immunotherapy, is of concern because in that study bronchial responsiveness actually worsened in the active immunotherapy group.[108]

There have been a number of recent studies of immunotherapy that have not been considered in the above meta-analysis or review. One multicenter study assessed the value of ragweed immunotherapy for seasonal asthma.[109] Patients' symptoms improved during the first year of treatment, but in the second year, there was no significant difference between active treatment and control. This study, as with most of the above research, was conducted using one or two allergens for immunotherapy. A more "real-world" study has recently been conducted in children with asthma.[110] In that study, up to seven allergens could be chosen per child according to the results of skin-prick tests and RAST, with preference given to perennial allergens. This prospective, randomized, controlled study of 121 children had the daily medication score as the primary outcome parameter. The median medication score declined significantly in both groups but was not different between groups. The authors concluded that "immunotherapy with injections of allergens for over 2 years was of no discernible benefit in allergic children with perennial asthma who were receiving appropriate medical treatment" (Level IE).[110] These were carefully controlled studies in which the children were selected for compliance, the children and their parents were taught about asthma management and environmental intervention control, and the children were assessed every 2 or 3 weeks by the

Table 15–4 *Efficacy of Immunotherapy*

Indicator of Efficacy	Odds Ratio (95% CI)
Symptomatic improvement	3.2 (2.2–4.9)
Reduction in bronchial hyper-responsiveness	6.8 (3.8–12.0)
Reduction in medication	4.2 (2.2– –7.9)

Adapted from Abramson HJ, Puy RM, Weiner JM. Is allergen immunotherapy effective? A meta-analysis of randomized controlled trials. Am J Respir Crit Care Med 1995;151:969–74.

investigators. In this aggressive intervention, immunotherapy with multiple allergens did not add to the asthma control during the 2 years of treatment.

There have been no controlled studies of environmental therapy directly compared to immunotherapy. Given the widespread exposure to cat allergen in the community, further studies of allergen-specific immunotherapy for cat may be extremely important. One recent study[111] of immunotherapy for cat allergen used exposure in a "cat room," a real-world environment. In that study, treatment resulted in significant protection to the upper and lower airways with less fall in peak expiratory flow and reduction in conjunctival responses.

Safety of Allergen Immunotherapy

Much of the concern raised by the British Society for Allergy and Clinical Immunology related to the potential for serious side effects from immunotherapy.[95] Both local and systemic reactions to allergen immunotherapy can occur. Systemic reactions occur in 2 to 3% of cases.[110,112–114] Fatalities are a rare, but real, risk during allergen specific immunotherapy.[95,115,116] Unfortunately, large local reactions are not predictive of a subsequent systemic reaction.[117] Patients with asthma are at greater risk for a fatal adverse reaction to immunotherapy than those individuals treated for allergic rhinitis.[115,116] Use of β-adrenergic blockers, either systemically or topically, has been associated with fatality from immunotherapy.[116] However, most systemic reactions are mild, with treatment required in as few as 0.1% of cases.[118]

Allergen immunotherapy must only be given in a setting where emergency resuscitation equipment and appropriately trained personnel are immediately available and are under the supervision of a well-trained physician (Level IIIA).

Recommendations

Specific allergen immunotherapy should be considered in patients sensitized to allergens that cannot be avoided and where optimal environmental control and pharmacotherapy do not provide acceptable control (Level IIIB). Further data are required to help us understand when best to initiate immunotherapy (eg, younger vs older patients, milder vs more severe disease) and whether multiple allergen immunotherapy can be as beneficial as the use of single well-defined allergens.

Newer approaches for immune modulation such as use of T lymphocyte–specific peptides[119] or other modified allergens,[120] use of anti-IgE,[121] and use of cytokines such as IL-12[122] or various approaches to impact on the cytokine milieu, such as inhaled solvable IL-4 receptor (SIL4r),[123] require additional research to define their potential role in our armamentarium for the treatment of asthma.

REFERENCES

1. Cockroft DW, Ruffin RE, Dolovich J, Hargrave FE. Allergen-induced increase in nonallergic bronchial reactivity. Clin Allergy 1997;8:503–13.

2. Boulet LP, Cartier A, Thomson NC, et al. Asthma and increases in nonallergic bronchial responsiveness from seasonal pollen exposure. J Allergy Clin Immunol 1983;71:399–406.

3. Peat JK, Tovey E, Mellis CM, et al. Importance of house dust mite and Alternaria allergy: an epidemiological study of children living in two climatic areas of northern New South Wales. Clin Exp Allergy 1993;23:812–20.

4. Sears MS, Hervison GP, Holdaway MD, et al. The relative risks of sensitivity to grass pollen, house dust mite, and cat dander in the development of childhood asthma. Clin Exp Allergy 1989;19:419–24.

5. Sporik R, Holgate ST, Platts-Mills TAE, Cogswell J. Exposure to house dust mite allergen (Der p 1) and the development of asthma in childhood: a prospective study. N Engl J Med 1990;323:502–7.

6. Charpin D, Birnbaum J, Haddi F, et al. Altitude and allergy to house dust mites. Ann Rev Respir Dis 1991;143:983–6.

7. Warner JO, Price JF. House dust mites sensitivity in childhood asthma. Arch Dis Child 1978;53:710–3.

8. Boulet LP, Becker A, Berube D, et al. Summary of recommendations from the Canadian Asthma Consensus Report 1999. Can Med Assoc J 1999;161:S1–12.

9. National Institutes of Health. Guidelines for the diagnosis and management of asthma. Bethesda (MD): NIH; 1997 Publication No. 97-4051.

10. Peat JK, Britton WJ, Salome CM, Woolcock AJ. Bronchial hyperresponsiveness in two populations of Australian school children. III. Effect of exposure of environmental allergens. Clin Allergy 1987;17:291–300.

11. Burrows B, Martinez FD, Halonen M, et al. Association of asthma with serum IgE levels and skin test reactivity to allergens. N Engl J Med 1989;320:271–7.

12. Bryant DH, Burns MW. Skin-prick test reactions to inhalant allergens in asthmatic patients. Med J Austr 1976;1:918–24.

13. Gerritsen J, Koeter GH, deMonchy JGR. Allergy in subjects with asthma from childhood to adulthood. J Allergy Clin Immunol 1990;85:116–25.

14. Rowntree S, Cogwell JJ, Platts-Mills TAE. Development of IgE and IgG antibodies to food and inhalant allergens in children at risk for allergic disease. Arch Dis Child 1985;60:727–35.

15. Pollart SM, Chapman MD, Fiocco GP, et al. Epidemiology of acute asthma: IgE antibodies to common inhalant allergens as a risk factor for emergency department visits. J Allergy Clin Immunol 1989;83:475–82.

16. Gelber LE, Seltzo LH, Bouzoukis JK, et al. Sensitization and exposure to indoor allergens as risk factors for asthma among patients presenting to hospital. Am Rev Respir Dis 1993;147:573–8.

17. Nelson RP Jr, DiNocolo R, Fernandez-Caldas E, et al. Allergen-specific IgE levels and mite allergen exposure in childhood with acute asthma first seen in an emergency department and in nonasthmatic control subjects. J Allergy Clin Immunol 1996;98:258–63.

18. O'Hallaren MT, Yunginger JW, Offord KP, et al. Exposure to an aeroallergen as a possible precipitating factor in respiratory arrest in young patients with asthma. N Engl J Med 1991;324:359–63.

19. Martinez F, Cline M, Burrows B. Increased incidence of asthma in children of smoking mothers. Pediatrics 1992;89:21–6.

20. Gortmarker SL, Walker DK, Jacobs FH, Ruch-Ross H. Parental smoking and the risk of childhood asthma. Am J Public Health 1982;72:574–79.

21. Murray AB, Morrison BJ. The effect of cigarette smoking from the mother on bronchial responsiveness and severity of symptoms in children with asthma. J Allergy Clin Immunol 1986;77:575–81.

22. Weitman M, Gortmacher S, Walker DK, Sobol A. Maternal smoking and childhood asthma. Pediatr 1990;85:505–11.

23. Gerrard JW, Heiner DC, Ko CG, et al. Immunoglobulin levels in smokers and non-smokers. Ann Allergy 1980;44:261–2.

24. Gelfand EW, Finkel TH. The T-lymphocyte system. In: Ed Stiehm, editor. Immunologic disorders in infants and children. 4th ed. Philadelphia (PA): WB Saunders Co; 1996. p. 14–34.

25. Umetsu DT, Dekruyff RH. Updates on cells and cytokines. J Allergy Clin Immunol 1997;100:1–6.

26. Becker AB, Moqbel R. Eosinophilic leukocytes. In: Lee GR, Foerster J, Greer J, et al, editors. Wintrobes clinical hematology. 10th ed. Baltimore (MD): Williams and Wilkins; 1999. p. 356–6.

27. Gotzsche PC, Hammarquist C, Burr M. House dust mite control measures in the management of asthma: meta-analysis. BMJ 1990;317:1105–10.

28. Murray AB, Ferguson AC. Dust-free bedrooms in the treatment of asthmatic children with house dust or dust mite allergy; a controlled trial. Pediatrics 1983;71:418–22.

29. Platts-Mills TAE, Mitchell FB, Nock P, et al. Reduction of bronchial hyper-reactivity during prolonged allergen avoidance. Lancet 1982;ii:675–8.

30. Boner AL, Nicro E, Antolini L, et al. Pulmonary function and bronchial hyperreactivity in asthmatic children with house dust mite allergy during prolonged stay in the Italian Alps (Misurina, 1756 m). Ann Allergy 1985;54:42–5.

31. Ehnert B, Lau-Schdendorf S, Weber A, et al. Reducing domestic exposure to dust mite allergen reduces bronchial hyperreactivity in sensitive children with asthma. J Allergy Clin Immunol 1992;90:135–8.

32. Custovic A, Simpson A, Chapman MD, Woodcock A. Allergen avoidance in the treatment of asthma and atopic disorders. Thorax 1998;53:63–72.

33. Tovey ER, Chapman MD, Wells CW, Platts-Mills TAE. The distribution of dust mite allergen in houses of patients with asthma. Am Rev Respir Dis 1981;124:630–5.

34. Luczynska CM, Li Y, Chapman MD, Platts-Mills TAE. Airborne concentration and particle size distribution of allergen derived from domestic cats (Felis domesticus): measurements using cascade impactor, liquid impinger and a two-site monoclonal antibody assay for Fel d I. Am Rev Respir Dis 1990;141:361–7.

35. Solomon WR, Platts-Mills TAE. Aerobiology of inhalant allergens. In: Middleton E Jr, Reed CE, Ellis EF, editors. Allergy: principles and practice. 4th ed. St. Louis: CV Mosby; 1993. p. 469–528.

36. Burge HA. Airborne allergenic fungi. Immunol Allergy Clin N Am 1989;9:307–19.

37. Weiss ST, Tager IB, Schenker M, Speizer FE. The health effects of involuntary smoking. Am Rev Respir Dis 1983;128:933–42.

38. Ehrlich RI, Du Toit D, Jordaan E, et al. Risk factors for childhood asthma and wheezing: importance of maternal and household smoking. Am J Respir Crit Care Med 1996;154:681–8.

39. Fergusson DM, Horwood LJ. Parental smoking and respiratory illness during early childhood: a six year longitudinal study. Pediatr Pulmonol 1985;1:99–106.

40. Murray AB, Morrison BJ. The effect of cigarette smoke from the mother on bronchial responsiveness and severity of symptoms in children with asthma. J Allergy Clin Immunol 1986;77:575–81.

41. Frischer T, Kuehr J, Meinert R, et al. Maternal smoking in early childhood: a risk factor for bronchial responsiveness to exercise in primary-school children. J Pediatr 1992;121:17–22.

42. Health Effects of Outdoor Air Pollution. Committee of the environmental and occupation health assembly of the American Thoracic Society. Am J Respir Crit Care Med 1996;153:3–50.

43. Chan-Yeung M, Becker A, Lam J, et al. House dust mite allergen levels in two cities in Canada: effects of season, humidity, city and home characteristics. Clin Exp Allergy 1995;25:240–6.

44. Custovic A, Green R, Smith A, et al. New mattresses: how fast do they become a significant source of exposure to house dust mite allergens? Clin Exp Allergy 1996;26:1243–5.

45. Colloff M, Ayres J, Carswell F, et al. The control of allergens of dust mites and domestic pets. Clin Exp Allergy 1992;22:1–28.

46. McDonald L, Tovey E. The role of water temperature and laundry procedures in reducing house dust mite populations and allergen content of bedding. J Allergy Clin Immunol 1992;90:599–608.

47. McDonald LG, Tovey E. The effectiveness of benzyl benzoate and some essential plant oils as laundry additives for killing house dust mites. J Allergy Clin Immunol 1993;92:771–2.

48. Hayden ML, Rose G, Diduch KB, et al. Benzyl benzoate moist powder: investigation of acaricidal activity in cultures and reduction of dust mite allergens in carpets. J Allergy Clin Immunol 1992;89:536–45.

49. Woodfolk JA, Hayden ML, Couture N, Platts-Mills TAE. Chemical treatment of carpets to reduce allergens. J Allergy Clin Immunol 1995;96:325–33.

50. Colloff MJ, Taylor C, Merrett TG. The use of domestic steam cleaning for the control of house dust mites. Clin Exp Allergy 1995;25:1061–6.

51. Becker AB, Chan-Yeung M. Environmental control: an idea whose time has come. Eur Res J 1997;10:1203–4.

52. Munir AK, Einarsson R, Dreborg SK. Vacuum cleaning decreases the levels of mite allergens in house dust. Pediatr Allergy Immunol 1993;4:136–43.

53. Woodfolk JA, Luczynska CM, de Blay F, et al. The effect of vacuum cleaners on the concentration and particle size distribution of airborne cat allergen. J Allergy Clin Immunol 1993;91:829–37.

54. Wood R, Chapman M, Adkinson NF, Eggleston P. The effect of cat removal on allergen content in household-dust samples. J Allergy Clin Immunol 1989;83:730–4.

55. De Blay F, Chapman MD, Platts-Mills TAE. Airborne cat allergen (Fel d l): environmental control with the cat in situ. Am Rev Respir Dis 1991;143:1334–9.

56. Avner DB, Perzanowski MS, Platts-Mills TAE, Woodfolk JA. Evaluation of different techniques for washing cats: quantitation of allergen removed from the cat and the effect on airborne Fel d 1. J Allergy Clin Immunol 1997;100:307–12.

57. Klucka CV, Ownby DR, Green J, Zoratti E. Cat shedding of Fel d 1 is not reduced by washings, Allerpet-C spray, or acepromazine. J Allergy Clin Immunol 1995;95:1164–71.

58. Perzanowski MS, Wheatley LM, Avner DB, et al. The effectiveness of Allerpet-C in reducing the cat allergen Feld 1. J Allergy Clin Immunol 1997;100:428–30.

59. Wood RA, Johnson EF, Van Natta ML, et al. A placebo-controlled trial of a HEPA air cleaner in the treatment of cat allergy. Am J Respir Crit Care Med 1998;158:115–20.

60. van der Heide S, Kauffman HF, Dubois AEJ, de Monchy JGR. Allergen reduction measures in houses of allergic asthmatic patients: effects of air-cleaners and allergen-impermeable mattress covers. Eur Respir J 1997;10:1217–23.

61. Patchett K, Lewis S, Crane J, Fitzharris P. Cat allergen (Fel d 1) levels on school children's clothing and in primary school classrooms in Wellington, New Zealand. J Allergy Clin Immunol 1997;100:755–9.

62. Custovic A, Fletcher A, Pickering CAC, et al. Domestic allergens in public places III: house dust mite, cat, dog and cockroach allergens in British hospitals. Clin Exp Allergy 1998;28:53–9.

63. Kang B. Study on cockroach antigen as a probable causative agent in bronchial asthma. J Allergy Clin Immunol 1976;58:357–65.

64. Sarpong SB, Wood RA, Eggleston PA. Short-term effects of extermination and cleaning on cockroach allergen Bla g 2 in settled dust. Ann Allergy Asthma Immunol 1996;76:257–60.

65. Gergen PJ, Mullally DI, Evans R. National survey of prevalence of asthma among children in the United States, 1976–1980. Pediatrics 1998;81:1–7.

66. Peat JK, Tovey CM, Mellis CM, et al. Importance of house dust mite and Alternaria allergens in childhood asthma: an epidemiological study in two climatic regions of Australia. Clin Exp Allergy 1993;23:812–20.

67. Halonen M, Stern DA, Wright AL, et al. Alternaria as a major allergen for asthma in children raised in a desert environment. Am J Respir Crit Care Med 1997;155:1356–61.

68. Watson WTA, Al-Malik SM, Lilley MK, et al. The association of aeroallergens, precipitation, and environmental pollutants with emergency department visits and hospitalizations for asthma on the Canadian prairies. J Allergy Clin Immunol 1993;91:304.

69. Verhoeff AP, van Wijnen JH, Brunekreef B, et al. Presence of viable mold propagules in indoor air in relation to house damp and outdoor air. Allergy 1992;47:83–91.

70. Becker AB, Muradia G, Vijay HM, et al. Immunoreactive Alternaria allergen in house dust: presence in prairie homes in the absence of mold spores. J Allergy Clin Immunol 1996;97:229.

71. Huss K, Squire EN Jr, Carpenter GB, et al. Effective education of adults with asthma who are allergic to dust mites. J Allergy Clin Immunol 1992;89:836–43.

72. Corsage J. Preventive measure in house-dust allergy. Am Rev Respir Dis 1982;125:80–4.

73. Eggleston PA, Wheeler B, Bollers N, et al. The effect of home environmental allergen control measures in asthmatic children enrolled in prospective clinical trial. Am Rev Respir Dis 1992;45:213.

74. Noon L. Prophylactic inoculation against hay fever. Lancet 1911;1:1572–3.

75. Coleman JW, Davies RJ, Durham SR. Allergen immunotherapy for seasonal and perennial allergic rhinitis. Clin Exp Allergy 1993;23 Suppl 3:3–6.

76. Frankland AW, Augustin R. Prophylaxis of summer hay-fever and asthma: a controlled trial comparing crude grass-pollen extracts with the isolated main protein component. Lancet 1954;1:1055–7.

77. Johnstone DE. Study of the role of antigen dosage in the treatment of pollenosis and pollen asthma. J Dis Child 1957;94:1–5.

78. Lowell FC, Franklin WA. "Double-blind" study of treatment with aqueous allergenic extracts in cases of allergic rhinitis. J Allergy 1963;34:165–82.

79. Valentine MS. Anaphylaxis and stinging insect hypersensitivity. JAMA 1992;268:2830–3.

80. Norman PS. Is there a role for immunotherapy in the treatment of asthma? YES. Am J Respir Crit Care Med 1996;154:1225–6.

81. Barnes PJ. Is there a role for immunotherapy in the treatment of asthma? NO. Am J Respir Crit Care Med 1996;154:1227–8.

82. Lichtenstein LM. A quantitative in vitro study of the chromatographic distribution and immunoglobulin characteristics of human blocking antibody. J Immunol 1968;101:317–24.

83. Norman PS, Lichtenstein LM. The clinical and immunologic specificity of immunotherapy. J Allergy Clin Immunol 1978;61:370–7.

84. Lichtenstein LM, Norman PS, Winkenwerder WL. A single year of immunotherapy for ragweed hay fever. Immunologic and clinical studies. Ann Intern Med 1971;75:663–71.

85. Lichtenstein LM, Ishizaka K, Norman PS, et al. IgE antibody measurements in ragweed hay fever. Relationship to clinical severity and the results of immunotherapy. J Clin Invest 1973;52:472–82.

86. Yunginger JW, Gleich GJ. Seasonal changes in IgE antibodies and their relationship to IgG antibodies during immunotherapy for ragweed hay fever. J Clin Invest 1973;52:1268–75.

87. Gleich GH, Jacob GL, Yunginger JW, Henderson LL. Measurement of the absolute levels of IgE antibodies in patients with ragweed hay fever: effect of immunotherapy on seasonal changes and relationship to IgG antibodies. J Allergy Clin Immunol 1977;60:188–98.

88. Lichtenstein LM, Osler AG. Studies of the mechanisms of hypersensitivity phenomena: XII. An in vitro study of reaction between ragweed pollen antigen, allergic human serum and ragweed sensitive human leukocytes. J Immunol 1966;96:169–79.

89. Van Arsdel PP Jr, Middleton E Jr. The effect of hyposensitization on the in vitro histamine release by specific antigen. J Allergy 1961;32:348–56.

90. Iliopoulos O, Proud D, Adkinson NF Jr, et al. Effects of immunotherapy on early, late and rechallenge nasal reaction to provocation with allergen: changes in inflammatory mediators and cells. J Allergy Clin Immunol 1991;87:855–66.

91. Evans R, Pence H, Kaplan H, Rocklin RE. The effect of immunotherapy on humoral and cellular responses in ragweed hay fever. J Clin Invest 1976;57:1378–85.

92. Rocklin RE, Sheffer AL, Greineder DK, Melmon KL. Generation of antigen-specific suppressor cells during allergy desensitization. N Engl J Med 1980;302:1213–9.

93. O'Brien RM, Byron KA, Varigos GA, Thomas WR. House dust mite immunotherapy results in a decrease in Der p 2-specific IFN-γ and IL-4 expression by circulating T lymphocytes. Clin Exp Allergy 1997;27:46–51.

94. McHugh SM, Deighton J, Stewart AG, et al. Bee venom immunotherapy induces a shift in cytokine responses from a Th2 to a Th1 dominant pattern: comparison of rush and conventional immunotherapy. Clin Exp Allergy 1995;25:828–38.

95. Frew AJ on behalf of a British Society for Allergy and Clinical Immunology Working Party. Injection immunotherapy. BMJ 1994;307:919–23.

96. Canadian Society of Allergy and Clinical Immunology. Guidelines for the use of allergen immunotherapy. Can Med Assoc J 1995;152:1413–9.

97. Malling H-J, Weeke B. Position paper: immunotherapy. Allergy 1993;48 Suppl 14:9–35.

98. Department of Health and Human Services, Public Health Service, National Institutes of Health. Guidelines for the diagnosis and management of asthma. Bethesda (MD): NIH; 1991 Publication No.:91-3042.

99. National Institutes of Health, National Heart, Lung and Blood Institute. Global initiative for asthma: global strategy for asthma management and prevention. NHLBI/WHO workshop report, March 1993. Bethesda (MD): NIH; 1995 Publication No.: 95-3659.

100. WHO/IUIS Working Group Report. Current status of allergen immunotherapy. Lancet 1989;1:259–61.

101. Henry RL, Landau L, Mellis C, et al. Childhood asthma: application of the international view of management in Australia and New Zealand. J Paediatr Child Health 1990:26;72–4.

102. Thoracic Society of Australia and New Zealand and Australasian Society of Clinical Immunology and Allergy. Position statement. Specific allergen immunotherapy for asthma. Med J Aust 1997;167:540–4.

103. Bousquet J, Hejjaoui A, Clauzel AM, et al. Specific immunotherapy with a standardized Dermatophagoides pteronyssinus extract. II. Prediction of efficacy of immunotherapy. J Allergy Clin Immunol 1988;82:971–7.

104. Des Roches A, Paradis L, Knani J, et al. Immunotherapy with a standardized Dermatophagoides pteronyssinus extract. V. Duration of the efficacy of immunotherapy after its cessation. Allergy 1996;51:30–3.

105. Ebner C, Kraft D, Ebner H. Booster immunotherapy (BIT). Allergy 1994;49:38–42.

106. Abramson MJ, Puy RM, Weiner JM. Is allergen immunotherapy effective in asthma? A meta-analysis of randomized controlled trials. Am J Respir Crit Care Med 1995;151:969–74.

107. Sigman K, Mazer B. Immunotherapy for childhood asthma: is there a rationale for its use? Ann Allergy Asthma Immunol 1996;76:299–309.

108. Murray AB, Ferguson AC, Morrison BJ. Nonallergic bronchial hyperreactivity in asthmatic children decreases with age and increases with mite immunotherapy. Ann Allergy 1985;54:541–4.

109. Creticos PS, Reed CE, Norman PS, et al. Ragweed immunotherapy in adult asthma. N Engl J Med 1996;334:501–6.

110. Adkinson NF Jr, Eggleston PA, Eney D, et al. A controlled trial of immunotherapy for asthma in allergic children. N Engl J Med 1997;336:324–31.

111. Varney VA, Edwards J, Tabbah K, et al. Clinical efficacy of specific immunotherapy to cat dander: a double-blind placebo-controlled trial. Clin Exp Allergy 1997;27:860–7.

112. Tinkelman DG, Cole WQ III, Tunno J. Immunotherapy: a one-year prospective study to evaluate risk factors of systemic reactions. J Allergy Clin Immunol 1995;95:8–14.

113. Matloff SM, Bailit IW, Parks P, et al. Systemic reactions to immunotherapy. Allergy Proc 1993;14:347–50.

114. Lin MS, Tanner E, Lynn E, et al. Nonfatal systemic allergic reactions induced by skin testing and immunotherapy. Ann Allergy 1993;71:557–62.

115. Lockey RF, Benedict IM, Turkeltaub PC, et al. Fatalities from immunotherapy (IT) and skin testing (ST). J Allergy Clin Immunol 1987;79:660–77.

116. Reid MJ, Lockey RF, Turkeltaub PC, et al. Survey of fatalities from skin testing and immunotherapy 1985–1989. J Allergy Clin Immunol 1993;92:6–15.

117. Nelson BL, Dupont LA, Reid MJ. Prospective survey of local and systemic reactions to immunotherapy with pollen extracts. Ann Allergy 1986;56:331–4.

118. Valyasevi MA, Yocum MW, Gosselin VA, Hunt LW. Systemic reactions to immunotherapy at the Mayo Clinic. J Allergy Clin Immunol 1997;99:S66.

119. Norman PS, Ohman JL Jr, Long AA, et al. Treatment of cat allergy with T-cell reactive peptides. Am J Respir Crit Care Med 1996;154:1623–8.

120. Lang GM, Bioh S, Becker AB, Sehon AH. Potential therapeutic efficacy of allergen-monomethoxypolyethylene glycol conjugates for in vivo inactivation of sensitized mast cells responsible for common allergies and asthma. Int Arch Allergy Immunol 1997;113:58–60.

121. Boulet LP, Chapman KR, Cote J, et al. Inhibitory effects of an anti-IgE antibody E25 on allergen-induced early asthmatic response. Am J Respir Crit Care Med 1997;155:1835–40.

122. Rempel JD, Wang MD, HayGlass KT. In vivo IL-12 administration induces profound, but transient commitment to T helper type I–associated patterns of cytokine and antibody production. J Immunol 1997;159:1490–6.

123. Borish LC, Nelson HS, Lanz MJ, et al. Interleukin-4 Receptor in Moderate Atopic Asthma. Am J Respir Crit Care Med 1999;160:1816–1823.

CHAPTER 16

Role of Inhaled Corticosteroids

Paul M. O'Byrne, MB, FRCPI, FRCPC, FCCP
Frederick E. Hargreave, MD, FRCPC, FRCP

Glucocorticosteroids have been used to treat a variety of airway diseases since an initial study in 1950 of Carryer et al[1] who reported the benefits of oral cortisone on ragweed pollen-induced hay fever and asthma. This was followed by a report by Gelfand,[2] demonstrating clinical benefit from inhaled cortisone in a small group of patients with both allergic or nonallergic asthma. Subsequently, a multicenter trial run by the Medical Research Council in the United Kingdom in 1956 demonstrated improvement in acute severe asthma in a placebo-controlled trial,[3] and reports at that time described benefit in chronic asthma.[4] This demonstrated the unequivocal benefit of corticosteroids in asthma. Subsequently, both oral and inhaled corticosteroids have evolved into the most important and useful drugs currently available to treat asthma (Level IA).

The initial studies evaluating the efficacy of inhaled corticosteroids in asthma were performed on patients with moderate to severe disease. At the time of their introduction to clinical practice in the early 1970s, and for many years after this, their use was mainly limited to patients who had persisting symptoms despite aggressive oral or inhaled bronchodilator use. The increased appreciation, in the mid-1980s, of the central role of airway inflammation in the pathogenesis of all asthma (Level I),[5-7] provided a rationale for the earlier introduction of inhaled corticosteroids, particularly as the ability of inhaled corticosteroids to reduce airway inflammation (Level I)[8] and improve some of the airway structural abnormalities associated with asthma was being identified (Level I). This has led to a reappraisal of how best to use inhaled corticosteroids in the management of asthma.

CLINICAL USE OF CORTICOSTEROIDS

Asthma is characterized by the presence of the symptoms of dyspnea, wheezing, chest tightness, and cough. These symptoms are usually caused by airflow obstruction, which is characteristically variable and by which the condition is defined. The variable airflow obstruction is associated with airway hyper-responsiveness to a variety of chemical bronchoconstrictor stimuli and physical stimuli such as exercise and hyperventilation of cold, dry air (Level I). It is now accepted that asthma symptoms, variable airflow obstruction, and airway hyper-responsiveness develop as a consequence of a characteristic form of cellular inflammation and structural changes in the airway wall (Level II).[9] The inflammation consists of the presence of activated eosinophils, lymphocytes, and an increased number of mast cells, which have been described both in bronchoalveolar lavage and airway biopsies from patients with mild stable asthma[6,7,10] as well as asthmatic subjects with more severe disease.[9] Also, there are structural changes described in asthmatic airways that appear to be characteristic of the disease and that are likely caused by persisting airway inflammation.[9] These changes include patchy desquamation of the airway epithelium,[11] thickening of the reticular collagen layer of the basement membrane,[12] and increased volume of airway smooth muscle (Level I).[9]

It has been only with this increased appreciation of the pivotal role of airway inflammation in asthma that an emphasis has been placed on treating airway inflammation rather than some of the consequences of the inflammation—airway constriction and asthma symp-

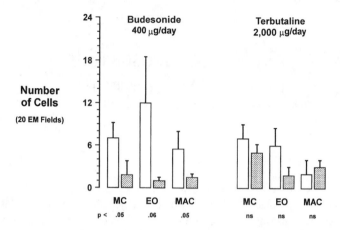

Figure 16–1 Effect of treatment with either the inhaled corticosteroid budesonide or the inhaled β₂-agonist terbutaline on the number of mast cells (MC), eosinophils (EO), or macrophages (MAC) in airway biopsies from asthmatic subjects. *Open bars* indicate pretreatment levels; *stippled bars* show levels after 6 weeks of treatment. (Reproduced with permission from Jeffrey PK, Godfrey RW, Adelroth E, et al. Effects of treatment on airway inflammation and thickening basement membrane reticular collagen in asthma. A quantitative light and electron microscopic study. Am Rev Respir Dis 1992;195:890–9.)

toms. The only antiasthma medications that have been demonstrated to improve airway inflammation (Figure 16–1) (Level I),[8,13] airway hyper-responsiveness (Figure 16–2) (Level I),[14,15] airflow obstruction, and symptoms in asthmatic patients are inhaled corticosteroids (Level IA). This evidence has been used as a rationale for using inhaled corticosteroids earlier in the treatment of asthma than was previously the case when they were suggested to be reserved for use as third- or fourth-line therapy for asthma, and only when bronchodilators were not providing asthma control.[16]

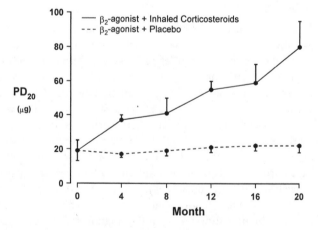

Figure 16–2 Effect of 22 months of treatment with an inhaled corticosteroid plus an inhaled β₂-agonist, or placebo plus an inhaled β₂-agonist, on methacholine airway responsiveness in asthmatic children. The inhaled corticosteroid progressively improved methacholine airway responsiveness over time. (Reproduced with permission from van Essen-Zandvliet EE, Hughes MD, Waalkens HJ, et al. Effect of 22 months of treatment with inhaled corticosteroids and/or beta2-agonists on lung function, airway responsiveness and symptoms in patients with asthma. Am Rev Respir Dis 1992;146:547–54.)

Objectives of Asthma Management

There have been many published consensus statements, from a variety of countries, on asthma management (Level IIIA).[17–19] While the consensus statements have differed in some regard, they have been remarkably consistent in identifying the objectives of asthma treatment, which are as follows:

1. To minimize or eliminate asthma symptoms
2. To achieve the best possible airway function
3. To minimize asthma exacerbations
4. To do the above with the least possible medications
5. To educate the patient about the goals and methods of management

Objectives that are implied but not explicitly stated are to reverse the causal airway inflammation and to prevent the decline in lung function and the development of fixed airflow obstruction that occurs in some asthmatic patients (and which is considered to be a result of uncontrolled inflammation).

In addition to these objectives, each of these documents has described what is meant by the term "asthma control." This includes the above objectives of minimal or no symptoms and best airway function, but it also includes minimizing the need for rescue medications such as inhaled β_2-agonists to less than daily use, minimizing the variability of flow rates that is characteristic of asthma, as well as enabling the patient to participate in normal activities of daily living. Achieving this level of asthma control should be the objective of the treating physician from the very first visit of the patient. Unfortunately, studies suggest that this does not happen.[20] This may be, in part, because the patient has learned to live with daily asthma symptoms and limitations in daily activities, and minimizes these problems to the physician. Alternatively, the idea of asthma control may not be widely accepted or understood by many physicians who see patients with asthma. This means that many (perhaps even most) patients with diagnosed asthma do not achieve optimal control.

These concepts have resulted in a much lower threshold than previously existed for intervening with inhaled corticosteroids in asthma. This "early intervention" with an effective anti-inflammatory medication in asthma has scientific rationale and is now being supported by clinical studies that have suggested that the delayed introduction of inhaled corticosteroids reduces the maximal benefit that is eventually achieved in children[21] and in adults.[22,23]

Currently Available Inhaled Corticosteroids

There are currently five topically active inhaled corticosteroids available for the treatment of asthma. These are beclomethasone dipropionate (BDP), triamcinolone, flunisolide, budesonide, and fluticasone propionate (FP) (Table 16–1). These are available in most countries in a pressurized metered-dose inhaler using chlorofluorocarbons (CFC) as propellants from the inhaler. However, BDP has, more recently, been formulated with hydrofluoroalkane (HFA) as its propellant because of the mandated phase-out of CFCs agreed to by the Montreal Protocol. This reformulation has altered the physical properties of the aerosol, which changes its lung deposition and, therefore, recommended dosage (see Table 16–1). In addition, budesonide and FP are available in dry-powder devices, the budesonide Turbuhaler and FP Diskus.

Reasons for Early Intervention with Inhaled Corticosteroids

Early intervention with inhaled corticosteroids in asthma means it is the first regular treatment used after a diagnosis is established. An argument for early intervention with inhaled corticosteroids could be made if one or more of the following conditions were met:

- Inhaled corticosteroids were *more effective* than other regular treatments to achieve optimal asthma control and meet the other treatment objectives

- Inhaled corticosteroids prevented the decline in airway function that occurs over time in asthmatic patients
- Inhaled corticosteroids were safer than an equally effective treatment modality
- Inhaled corticosteroids were more cost beneficial as an initial treatment of asthma than any other medication, as measured by a benefit to the patient or to society by reducing the morbidity of asthma

Studies using inhaled corticosteroids have addressed all of these issues and these will be considered.

Table 16–1 *Dosage Equivalence for Inhaled Corticosteroids in Adults*

Product	Low Dosage µg/d	Intermediate Dosage µg/d	High Dosage µg/d
BDP pMDI (CFC)*	< 500	500–1,000	> 1,000
BDP pMDI (HFA)†	< 250	250–500	> 500
BUD Turbuhaler‡	< 400	400–800	> 800
FP pMDI§	< 250	250–500	> 500
FP Diskus"	< 250	250–500	> 500
Flunisolide pMDI#	< 1,000	1,000–2,000	> 2,000
Triamcinolone pMDI#	< 800	800–1,600	> 1,600

*Beclomethasone dipropionate pressurized metered-dose inhaler (chlorofluorocarbon propellant).
† Beclomethasone dipropionate pressurized metered-dose inhaler (hydrofluoroalkane propellant).
‡ Budesonide Turbuhaler.
§ Fluticasone propionate pressurized metered-dose inhaler.
" Fluticasone propionate Diskus.
Dosage equivalences are less well studied for flunisolide and triamcinolone.

Efficacy of Early Intervention with Inhaled Corticosteroids

There is little debate in the literature that corticosteroids are the most effective treatment for asthma (Level IA)[24,25] and that the inhaled route is preferable to minimize unwanted effects (Level IA). There is, however, considerable debate over the early use of inhaled corticosteroids in the asthmatic patient considered to have mild asthma.[26] These patients are usually treated with inhaled β_2-agonists on demand, or with drugs considered to be clinically less effective than inhaled corticosteroids, such as cromoglycate or nedocromil sodium. In a study of newly diagnosed asthmatic patients seen in specialty clinics, early intervention with the inhaled corticosteroid budesonide was shown to be an effective first-line treatment, when compared with an inhaled β_2-agonist, as indicated by reduced symptoms, improvements in lung function, and improvements in methacholine airway hyper-responsiveness (Level IA).[27] However, many patients considered to have mild asthma are not seen in specialty clinics but are managed in primary care practices. It is possible that these patients are, in fact, ideally controlled without the use of inhaled corticosteroids. To address this issue, one study has examined the efficacy and cost benefit of inhaled corticosteroids, supplemented with bronchodilators as needed, compared to bronchodilators alone, as first-line treatment of asthma in primary care practice (Level IA).[20] This double-blind randomized controlled trial compared budesonide 400 µg/d, budesonide 800 µg/d, and placebo in patients considered by their primary care physician to have such mild asthma that they would not derive any clinical benefit from inhaled corticosteroids. In this patient population, in whom self-reported symptoms were

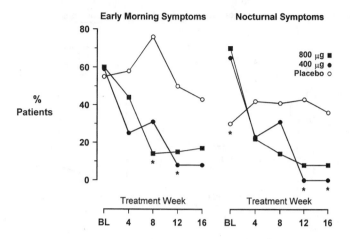

Figure 16–3 Proportion of patients considered by their family physician as having mild asthma, experiencing early morning symptoms or nocturnal symptoms in the month prior to evaluation at baseline (BL) and after treatment with inhaled budesonide at treatment weeks 4 to 16 for patients on placebo (*open circles*), budesonide 400 µg/d (*closed circles*), and budesonide 800 µg/d (*closed squares*).* $p < .05$; $p < .01$; $p < .001$. (Reproduced with permission from O'Byrne PM, Cuddy L, Taylor DW, et al. The clinical efficacy and cost benefit of inhaled corticosteroids as therapy in patients with mild asthma in primary care practice. Can Respir J 1996;3:169–75.)

mild at the start of the study, 40 to 70% of the patients were experiencing nocturnal or early morning symptoms in the month before entering the study (Figure 16–3). These symptoms suggest that asthma control was not optimal. The study demonstrated that inhaled budesonide 400 µg/d provided better asthma control and is cost beneficial when compared to bronchodilators alone in the management of these patients with mild asthma and that no differences could be demonstrated between the use of 400 µg/d and 800 µg/d of budesonide; however, the study had insufficient power to detect differences between dosages, had they been present. However, other studies with sufficient power have not been able to demonstrate a significant difference between these two dosages of inhaled budesonide.[28] The percentages of patients experiencing daily symptoms fell to less than 10% over the course of the study in the budesonide treatment groups (see Figure 16–3). Also, there was a mean 60 to 70 L/min increase in morning and evening peak expiratory flows (Figure 16–4) and an elimination of exacerbations of asthma requiring emergency department management, indicating that a clinically useful improvement was achieved in this patient population with a dosage of budesonide as low as 400 µg/d. This study supports the early intervention with inhaled corticosteroids for adult patients with regular daily symptoms of asthma, and suggests that low dosages (budesonide 400 µg/d or possibly less) are effective in the management of asthmatic patients with mild to moderate asthma. In addition, the study reinforced the need to strive for optimal control of asthma and, once control is achieved, to identify the minimum amounts of medication needed to maintain control. Last, this study demonstrated that inhaled corticosteroid treatments are more cost beneficial than asthma therapy with bronchodilators alone.

Another reason for recommending low doses of inhaled corticosteroids as first-line therapy for asthma is the recent concern about the safety of regular daily short-acting inhaled β_2-agonists. Sears et al[29] have demonstrated deterioration in a number of parameters of asthma control and reduced the time to an asthma exacerbation[30] when the short-acting inhaled β_2-agonist fenoterol was used on a regular basis rather than when needed (Level IA). A subsequent study of the regular use of the short-acting inhaled β_2-agonist salbutamol in milder asthmatic patients

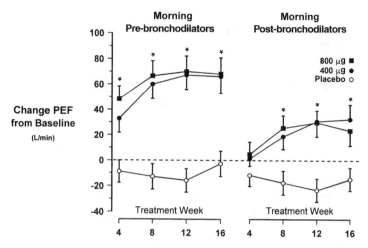

Figure 16–4 Changes in peak expiratory flow from baseline measured in the morning upon waking in patients considered by their family physician as having mild asthma, both before and after inhaled bronchodilator treatment with inhaled budesonide for treatment weeks 4 to 16 for patients on placebo (*open circles*), budesonide 400 µg/d (*closed circles*), and budesonide 800 µg/d (*closed squares*). $p < .01$; $p < .001$. (Reproduced with permission from O'Byrne PM, Cuddy L, Taylor DW, et al. The clinical efficacy and cost benefit of inhaled corticosteroids as therapy in patients with mild asthma in primary care practice. Can Respir J 1996;3:169–75.)

showed an overall trend toward deterioration in a number of asthma outcomes, although none were statistically significant.[31,32] Also, retrospective studies have associated increased risk of asthma mortality with the overuse of the β_2-agonists fenoterol[32,33] and salbutamol.[33] Regular use of inhaled β_2-agonists has been demonstrated to increase airway responsiveness in asthmatic patients (Level I)[34,35] and to result in loss of functional antagonism to the bronchoconstrictor effects of inhaled methacholine[36] and adenosine monophosphate (AMP) (Level I).[37]

Effects of Inhaled Corticosteroids on Airway Function Over Time

Asthmatic patients lose lung function more rapidly than nonasthmatic patients[38,39] but less rapidly than cigarette smokers. In occasional asthmatic patients, this leads to severe, permanent, fixed airflow obstruction, with all of the attendant disability and handicap associated with this condition. A number of recent studies in both adults and children have demonstrated that inhaled corticosteroids provide a protective effect against the deterioration in lung function seen with prolonged regular use of inhaled bronchodilator therapy alone. In one study, patients with asthma and patients with chronic obstructive pulmonary disease, previously treated with regular inhaled bronchodilators, were treated with inhaled beclomethasone 800 µg/d or placebo for 2 years.[40] Prior to the addition of inhaled corticosteroids, the forced expiratory volume in 1 second (FEV_1) had been declining at a rate of 160 mL/y. In the first 6 months of corticosteroid therapy, the FEV_1 increased by 460 mL and then continued to decline at a rate of 100 mL/y (significantly less than with bronchodilators alone). This protective effect of inhaled corticosteroids was most marked in the asthmatic patients and was associated with a significant improvement in methacholine airway hyper-responsiveness in the asthmatic patients only, and with decreased asthma symptoms and exacerbations (Level IB).

A second study[22] has addressed this issue in a different way. These investigators had previously reported that the treatment of newly diagnosed asthmatic patients with inhaled budesonide 1200 µg/d for 2 years improved asthma control as indicated by reduced symptoms, improvements in lung function, and improvements in methacholine airway hyper-responsiveness when compared to inhaled β_2-agonists.[27] The subjects receiving budesonide were subsequently randomly allocated to continuing for a third year on a lower dosage of inhaled budesonide (400 μg/d) or placebo. The improvements in all parameters were maintained on the lower dose of budesonide but were lost on placebo. The subjects who had previously been treated with inhaled β₂-agonists only were treated with the higher dosage of inhaled budesonide for the third year, and while they improved in all parameters when compared to the first 2 years of treatment, the improvement in lung function or methacholine airway hyper-responsiveness was significantly less than that achieved by the subjects treated for the first year of the study with inhaled budesonide. This suggests that these asthmatic patients had lost lung function that might have been preserved with the early use of inhaled corticosteroids (Level IB).

A study in asthmatic children has been reported by Agertoft and Pedersen[21] who studied two cohorts for up to 7 years. One cohort was treated with inhaled corticosteroids shortly after diagnosis, while the other received a variety of other antiasthma medications, including cromones, theophylline, and regular inhaled β₂-agonists, but not inhaled corticosteroids. Some children in the second cohort were converted to inhaled corticosteroids but not until an average of 5 years after initial diagnosis. These children in whom treatment with inhaled corticosteroids was started later did not achieve the level of lung function of the children who received early intervention with inhaled corticosteroids, even after 3 years of treatment with inhaled corticosteroids (Level II). The study also measured growth velocity in these children and concluded that dosages of inhaled budesonide up to 400 μg/d were not associated with a reduction in growth velocity. A subsequent study in adult asthmatic patients has confirmed these observations (Level II).[23]

These studies suggest that inhaled corticosteroids can diminish the decline in airway function that occurs in asthmatic patients, and that early intervention with inhaled corticosteroids can optimize airway function in asthmatic patients. Each of these studies, however, has limitations—mainly, that none were explicitly designed to address this issue in a prospective fashion. Therefore, while the results are consistent between the studies, they are not conclusive. This has led to the development of a large, multinational, prospective, randomized, and placebo-controlled study of the effects of early intervention with inhaled corticosteroids in both childhood and adult asthma. This study, known as the START (Steroid Therapy As Regular Treatment) trial, will evaluate the potential beneficial effects of inhaled corticosteroids treatment started within the first 2 years of the development of asthma in patients with very mild disease.

Cost Benefit of Inhaled Corticosteroids in Asthma

Until recently, few studies have examined the cost benefit of early intervention with inhaled corticosteroids. However, several recent studies have demonstrated that inhaled corticosteroids are cost beneficial when compared to other antiasthma treatments. For example, Adelroth and Thompson[41] have shown that when patients were treated with inhaled corticosteroids, the costs to the Swedish health care system declined because of a reduction in hospital use and physician visits when asthma control was optimized (Level II). Also, in the Canadian study discussed previously,[20] a cost-effectiveness analysis of the use of inhaled corticosteroids in patients thought to have mild asthma in primary care practice demonstrated an advantage with use of inhaled corticosteroids, also primarily by keeping patients out of hospital emergency departments, since asthma control was improved.

Future Trends in Inhaled Corticosteroid Use

These studies suggest that low dosages of inhaled corticosteroids should be used early in the onset of asthma and even in patients with mild disease. The impact of earlier treatment on the progression of the disease is a critical issue that needs to be evaluated in future studies. It is plausible that, by preventing the airway structural abnormalities associated with asthma, the development of fixed airflow obstruction and more severe disease can be prevented. Also, it is clear from the studies that the severity of asthma is often underappreciated by both patients and physicians. This leads to undertreatment, less than ideal asthma control, the attendant effects on patients' quality of life, and an increased cost to society. To ensure that this does not happen, optimal treatment should be offered to all patients with established asthma; this would most often be a therapeutic trial of inhaled corticosteroids.

In clinical practice, some asthma patients are overtreated with inhaled corticosteroids. Asthma can sometimes be difficult to diagnose, and diagnosis should be validated with the use of a variety of measurements that are more sensitive than symptoms and airway function, such as methacholine airway responsiveness. Clinical trials involving the reduction of inhaled corticosteroid treatment illustrate that many patients are able to discontinue treatment with inhaled steroid, or considerably reduce the dose, without a clinical exacerbation.[42] The extent of overtreatment of asthma should be investigated.

Recent studies of induced sputum cell counts suggest that it maybe difficult to optimize inhaled corticosteroid treatment in some asthmatic patients without these cell counts. Sputum eosinophils can be increased when asthma is clinically controlled.[43] When inhaled steroid or prednisone is reduced, sputum eosinophils increase before symptoms or measurements of airway function worsen.[44] Therefore, there is a need to investigate the use of induced sputum cell counts to monitor optimum corticosteroid treatment although, at present, establishing reliable sputum cell counts in practice is difficult to achieve.

Finally, there are several causes of airway inflammation and, consequently, different types of inflammation, which can overlap in clinical presentation.[45,46] While asthma is considered to be associated with an eosinophilic inflammation, it can occur with normal sputum cell counts[43] or with a neutrophilia without eosinophilia.[45] The significance of this relates to the beneficial effect of corticosteroid treatment; eosinophilic inflammation responds, whereas there is increasing evidence that noneosinophilic inflammation does not.

Systemic Side Effects

Dosages of inhaled corticosteroids (beclomethasone) of >400 μg/d in children and >1000 μg/d in adults can be demonstrated to result in unwanted systemic side effects such as changes in growth velocity in children (Level I) and biochemical changes indicating effects on bone metabolism and the adrenal glands in adults (Level I). All physicians who treat asthmatic patients should be conscious of the potential for the development of adverse effects that occur in patients who use corticosteroids to treat asthma or other diseases. These potential adverse effects of corticosteroids include an influence on the hypothalamic-pituitary-adrenal (HPA) axis; osteoporosis; posterior subcapsular cataracts; growth retardation in children; steroid psychosis; risk of lung infection; and skin bruising.

Effects on the Hypothalamic-Pituitary-Adrenal Axis

The effects of corticosteroids on the HPA axis can be measured in a number of different ways. The commonest used and easiest to obtain, but least sensitive, method has been the measurement of early morning serum cortisol levels. Much more sensitive measurements to the effects of excess corticosteroids on the HPA axis are 24-hour urinary cortisol, 2-hourly plasma cortisol measured over 24 hours, or the short tetracosactrin (ACTH) stimulation test.[47]

The different inhaled corticosteroids are not equal with regard to their effects on the HPA axis (Level I). For example, in children, a dosage-dependent effect of urinary cortisol has been demonstrated with dosages of BDP from 200 to 800 μg/d.[48] By contrast, a dosage of budesonide of 400 μg/d does not cause any effect on urinary cortisols, even when used for up to 1 year.[49] In adults, many studies have examined the effects of inhaled corticosteroids on HPA axis function, and there is no convincing evidence that dosages of BDP of $<1,500$ μg/d and budesonide $<1,600$ μg/d have any measurable effect on the HPA axis.[50] The measurable effects seen at higher doses clearly indicate systemic activity of the inhaled corticosteroid but are of questionable clinical significance. There are only two case reports of clinically evident adrenal insufficiency in patients, who have been treated with only inhaled corticosteroids, after the inhaled corticosteroid has been withdrawn (Level IIC). These occurred in an adult who was treated with a very high dosage of inhaled budesonide (6,400 μg/d)[51] and a child who was treated with a much lower dosage (250 μg/d).[52]

Osteoporosis

This is an important complication of the use of ingested corticosteroids, particularly in high-risk patients such as postmenopausal women.[53] This occurs through an increase in bone resorption and a decrease in bone formation, and results in an increased risk of fractures, especially of the hip and spine. Inhaled corticosteroids have been demonstrated to have effects on bone metabolism, although there is little evidence that, at the conventionally used dosages, they cause osteoporosis, and no evidence that they cause increased risk of fractures (Level IIC).

The effects of inhaled corticosteroids on bone metabolism have been demonstrated by measuring serum osteocalcin, which measures changes in bone formation, and urinary hydroxyproline (measured after a 12-hour fast), which is increased with increased bone resorption. Phenazopyridine hydrochloride cross-links in urine is another measure of bone resorption and has the advantage over urinary hydroxyproline of not being dietary-dependent; however, to date, the effects of inhaled corticosteroids on this measure of bone resorption have not been reported.

The effects of BDP and budesonide on serum osteocalcin and urinary hydroxyproline have been studied in adults. Both have been shown to influence serum osteocalcin levels in a dosage-dependent manner,[54] but only BDP increases urinary hydroxyproline excretion at dosages up to 2,000 μg/d. In children, dosages of budesonide of less than 800 μg/d[55] and of fluticasone of 200 μg/d[56] have no effect on any biochemical marker of bone turnover.

Bone densitometry has been measured in adult asthmatic patients taking varying doses of inhaled BDP (mean dose 630 μg/d) over 2 years.[56] This study suggested that these patients had no increase in bone loss. Also, to date, there are no studies that have demonstrated that these biochemical markers of bone turnover are associated with increased risk of bone fracture.

Posterior Subcapsular Cataracts

These occur more frequently in patients taking ingested versus inhaled corticosteroids, and this greatly complicates the issue of whether they occur with greater frequency in patients who are also using inhaled corticosteroids. Studies in adults[57] and children[58] suggest that once the confounding effect of ingested corticosteroids is removed, there is no evidence that inhaled corticosteroids increase the risk of developing posterior subcapsular cataracts (Level IIC). One recent study has, however, indicated that high inhaled dosages of BDP are associated with a slightly greater risk of posterior subcapsular cataracts[59] in older patients. This study did not, however, stratify for the confounding risk of allergy for cataract development in this population.

Growth Retardation in Children

Growth retardation in children due to the use of inhaled corticosteroids is a major reason that these drugs are used very sparingly, perhaps even underused, to treat pediatric asthma. There is little doubt that systemic corticosteroids can stunt growth in children and that this effect is usually permanent. Resolving this issue for inhaled corticosteroids in asthmatic children has been exceedingly difficult. This is partly because asthmatic children do not have the same growth patterns as nonasthmatic children. Many asthmatic children have delayed onset of puberty, and this effect appears more severe in children with severe asthma.[60] However, these

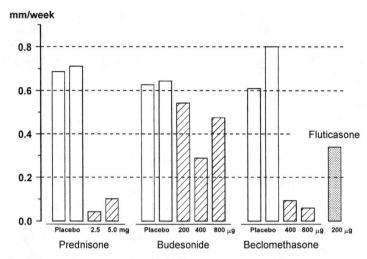

Figure 16–5 Effect of treatment with placebo, prednisone 2.5 mg/d or 5.0 mg/d for 1 week, or increasing inhaled doses of budesonide, BDP, or fluticasone on lower leg growth, measured by knemometry in children. Prednisone and BDP 400 μg/d or 800 μg/d significantly reduced lower leg growth. (Reproduced with permission from Barnes PJ, Pedersen S. Efficacy and safety of inhaled corticosteroids in asthma. Am Rev Respir Dis 1993;148:S1–26.)

children eventually do catch up with their nonasthmatic peers and achieve normal height.[61] Thus, studying asthmatic children and comparing them to nonasthmatic controls may not be appropriate. Also, studies examining growth in children need to be continued over several years, as individual children have different growth patterns.

A surrogate method for measuring growth in children is knemometry, which measures short-term linear growth in the lower leg in children. This method is extremely sensitive to the systemic effects of corticosteroids. A daily dosage of prednisone of 2.5 mg can totally inhibit lower leg growth (Figure 16–5).[62] By contrast, a dosage of inhaled budesonide of 400 μg/d has no effect on knemometry measurements,[63] whereas a daily dosage of 800 μg/d of budesonide[63] with 400 μg/d of BDP and 200 μg/d of fluticasone does significantly inhibit them (see Figure 16–5).[64] The clinical correlation of these measurements is not known; however, only BDP at an inhaled dosage of 400 μg/d has been shown, in relatively short-term studies, to reduce linear growth in children.[65–67]

Steroid Psychosis

This may occur in as high as 2% of patients treated with systemic corticosteroids and has been reported to occur occasionally in patients taking inhaled corticosteroids. A total of eight patients have been reported, thus far, who developed symptoms within days of being treated with either inhaled BDP or budesonide.[68,69] The psychosis resolved promptly after stopping the inhaled corticosteroid.

Risk of Lung Infection

Risk of lung infection is not increased in patients using inhaled corticosteroids. Also, inhaled corticosteroids do not increase the risk of reactivation of pulmonary tuberculosis, and, therefore, prophylactic isoniazid treatment is not needed when inhaled corticosteroids are used in patients with inactive pulmonary tuberculosis.

Skin Bruising

Skin bruising occurs as a dosage-dependent side effect of inhaled corticosteroid use. It is rare at daily dosages of < 1,000 μg/d, and its incidence increases with age and duration of treat-

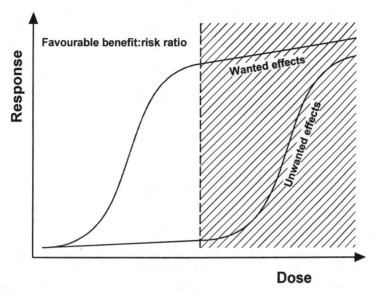

Figure 16–6 A schematic representation of the dosage-response characteristics for efficacy and side effects for inhaled corticosteroids.

ment (Level I). In one study of older patients on high doses of BDP, the prevalence of easy bruising was 47% for those on inhaled corticosteroids and 22% for those who were not.[70]

Fortunately, there has been an increased appreciation over the past 5 years that the maximal clinical benefits of inhaled corticosteroids in most patients are achieved with low to moderate dosages (see Table 16–1), thereby giving a very steep efficacy dosage-response (Figure 16–6). This has been emphasized in several studies in which a dosage-response has been evaluated (Level I).[24,25] These low to moderate dosages are not associated with systemic side effects in adults (see Figure 16–6).

Conclusion

Inhaled corticosteroids are the most effective medications currently available to treat symptomatic asthma and are, fortunately, free of clinically relevant unwanted effects when used in the dosages needed to provide optimal control in most asthmatic patients. In uncontrolled asthma, not previously treated with inhaled corticosteroids, a high dose usually is not more

Table 16–2 *Evidence-Based Data Regarding Inhaled Corticosteroids*

Inhaled corticosteroids are the most effective medications currently available to treat symptomatic asthma (Level IA).

Inhaled corticosteroids improve the physiologic abnormalities of variable airflow obstruction and airway hyper-responsiveness that characterize asthma (Level IA).

Inhaled corticosteroids are cost beneficial as compared to other treatments (Level IA).

Even low dosages of inhaled corticosteroids can cause topical unwanted effects such as oral candidiasis or dysphonia (Level IA).

Inhaled corticosteroids are free of clinically relevant systemic unwanted effects when used in the dosages needed to provide optimal control in most asthmatic patients (Level IA).

The addition of a long-acting inhaled β_2-agonist to a moderate dose of an inhaled corticosteroid provides better asthma control than increasing the dose of the inhaled corticosteroid (Level IA).

effective than a lower dose in controlling symptoms or airway function. Inhaled corticosteroids also improve the physiologic abnormalities of variable airflow obstruction and airway hyper-responsiveness that characterize asthma, as well as reduce the decline in lung function over time that occurs in asthmatic patients. Inhaled corticosteroids are cost beneficial as compared to other treatments, even in patients with milder asthma treated in primary care. For these reasons, inhaled corticosteroids are now being considered the first-line therapy for patients with daily asthma symptoms. They should be started early after a diagnosis is made, rather than delaying until all other treatment options have been found not to provide optimal control of asthma. Evidence-based data regarding inhaled corticosteroids is presented in Table 16–2.

There are, however, several issues regarding the early intervention with inhaled corticosteroids that have not yet been resolved. One such issue is whether inhaled corticosteroids should be used in asthmatic patients who have very mild and infrequent symptoms, or who develop symptoms only after being exposed to a stimulus of airway constriction, such as exercise or cold air, and who have normal airway caliber most of the time. The current consensus statements do not recommend regular treatment in such patients. These asthmatic patients do have evidence of airway inflammation and structural changes in airway biopsies; however, we do not yet know whether they lose lung function more rapidly than nonasthmatic patients, or whether the morbidity of having very mild asthma warrants the use of regular treatment. This information may be available when the results of the START trial are available. Also, not enough data is yet known about the long-term effects of even low doses of inhaled corticosteroids. Although the study by Agertoft and Pedersen[21] has provided details of some of the potential unwanted effects in children after as many as 7 years of treatment, such studies will need to be of a longer duration before the concerns and fears about using inhaled corticosteroids very early in asthma will be allayed.

REFERENCES

1. Carryer HM, Koelshe GA, Prickman LE, et al. The effect of cortisone on bronchial asthma and hay fever occurring in subjects sensitive to ragweed pollen. J Allergy 1950;21:282–7.

2. Gelfand ML. Administration of cortisone by the aerosol method in the treatment of bronchial asthma. N Engl J Med 1951;245:293–4.

3. Medical Research Council. Controlled trial of effects of cortisone acetate in status asthmaticus. Lancet 1956;2:803–6.

4. Foulds GS, Greaves DP, Herxheimer H, Kingdom LG. Hydrocortisone in treatment of allergic conjunctivitis, allergic rhinitis, and bronchial asthma. Lancet 1955;1:234–5.

5. O'Byrne PM. Airway inflammation and airway hyperresponsiveness. Chest 1986;90:575–7.

6. Kirby JG, Hargreave FE, Gleich GJ, O'Byrne PM. Bronchoalveolar cell profiles of asthmatic and nonasthmatic subjects. Am Rev Respir Dis 1987;136:379–83.

7. Beasley R, Roche WR, Roberts JA, Holgate ST. Cellular events in the bronchi in mild asthma and after bronchial provocation. Am Rev Respir Dis 1989;139:806–17.

8. Jeffery PK, Godfrey RW, Adelroth E, et al. Effects of treatment on airway inflammation and thickening of basement membrane reticular collagen in asthma. A quantitative light and electron microscopic study. Am Rev Respir Dis 1992;145:890–9.

9. Dunnill MS, Massarell GR, Anderson JA. A comparison of the quantitative anatomy of the bronchi in normal subjects, in status asthmaticus, in chronic bronchitis and in emphysema. Thorax 1969;24:176–9.

10. Jeffery PK, Wardlaw AJ, Nelson FC, et al. Bronchial biopsies in asthma. An ultrastructural, quantitative study and correlation with hyperreactivity. Am Rev Respir Dis 1989;140:1745–53.

11. Laitinen LA, Heino M, Laitinen A, et al. Damage of the airway epithelium and bronchial reactivity in patients with asthma. Am Rev Respir Dis 1985;131:599–606.

12. Roche WR, Beasley R, Williams JH, Holgate ST. Subepithelial fibrosis in the bronchi of asthmatic patients. Lancet 1989;1:520–4.

13. Adelroth E, Rosenhall L, Johansson SA, et al. Inflammatory cells and eosinophilic activity in asthmatic patients investigated by bronchoalveolar lavage. The effects of antiasthmatic treatment with budesonide or terbutaline. Am Rev Respir Dis 1990;142:91–9.

14. Juniper EF, Kline PA, Vanzieleghem MA, et al. Effect of long-term treatment with an inhaled corticosteroid (budesonide) on airway hyperresponsiveness and clinical asthma in nonsteroid-dependent asthmatic patients. Am Rev Respir Dis 1990;142:832–6.

15. van Essen-Zandvliet EE, Hughes MD, Waalkens HJ, et al. Effect of 22 months of treatment with inhaled corticosteroids and/or beta2-agonists on lung function, airway responsiveness and symptoms in patients with asthma. Am Rev Respir Dis 1992;146:547–54.

16. Rebuck AS, Chapman KR. Asthma: trends on pharmacological therapy. Can Med Assoc J 1987;136:483–8.

17. Sheffer AL, Bartal M, Bousquet J, et al. Global strategy for asthma management and prevention. Bethesda (MD): National Institutes of Health; 1995 Publication No.:95-3659. p. 70–114.

18. National Heart, Lung, Blood Institute, National Institutes of Health. Guidelines for the diagnosis and management of asthma. Bethesda (MD): US Department of Health Services; 1991 Publication No.:91-3042.

19. Boulet LP, Becker A, Berube D, et al. Summary of recommendations from the Canadian Asthma Consensus Report 1999. Can Med Assoc J 1999;161:S1–12.

20. O'Byrne PM, Cuddy L, Taylor DW, et al. The clinical efficacy and cost benefit of inhaled corticosteroids as therapy in patients with mild asthma in primary care practice. Can Respir J 1996;3:169–75.

21. Agertoft L, Pedersen S. Effects of long-term treatment with an inhaled corticosteroid on growth and pulmonary function in asthmatic children. Respir Med 1994;88:373–81.

22. Haahtela T, Jarvinen M, Kava T, et al. Effects of reducing or discontinuing inhaled budesonide in patients with mild asthma. N Engl J Med 1994;331:700–5.

23. Selroos O, Pietinalho A, Lofroos AB, Riska H. Effect of early vs late intervention with inhaled corticosteroids in asthma. Chest 1995;108:1228–34.

24. Barnes PJ, Pedersen S. Efficacy and safety of inhaled corticosteroids in asthma. Am Rev Respir Dis 1993;148:S1–26.

25. Pedersen S, O'Byrne PM. A comparison of the efficacy and safety of inhaled corticosteroids in asthma. Allergy 1997;52:1–34.

26. Drazen J, Israel E. Treating mild asthma, when are inhaled corticosteroids indicated? N Engl J Med 1994;331:737–8.

27. Haahtela T, Jarvinen M, Tuomo K, et al. Comparison of a β_2 antagonist, terbutaline, with an inhaled corticosteroid, budesonide, in newly detected asthma. N Engl J Med 1991;325:388–92.

28. Busse WW, Chervinsky P, Condemi J, et al. Budesonide delivered by Turbuhaler is effective in a dose-dependent fashion when used in the treatment of adult patients with chronic asthma. J Allergy Clin Immunol 1998;101:457–63.

29. Sears MR, Taylor DR, Print CG, et al. Regular inhaled beta-agonist treatment in bronchial asthma. Lancet 1990;336:1391–6.

30. Taylor DR, Sears MR, Herbison GP, et al. Regular inhaled β-agonists in asthma: effects on exacerbations and lung function. Thorax 1993;48:134–8.

31. Drazen JM, Israel E, Boushey HA, et al. Comparison of regularly scheduled with as-needed use of salbutamol in mild asthma. N Engl J Med 1996;335:841–7.

32. Crane J, Pearce N, Flatt A, et al. Prescribed fenoterol and death from asthma in New Zealand, 1981–83: case-control study. Lancet 1989;1:917–22.

33. Spitzer WO, Suissa S, Ernst P, et al. The use of beta-agonists and the risk of death and near death from asthma. N Engl J Med 1992;326:501–6.

34. Krahn J, Koeter GH, van der Mark TW, et al. Changes in bronchial hyperreactivity induced by 4 weeks of treatment with anti-asthmatic drugs in patients with asthma: a comparison between budesonide and terbutaline. J Allergy Clin Immunol 1985;76:628–36.

35. Vathenen AS, Knox AJ, Higgins BG, et al. Rebound increase in bronchial responsiveness after treatment with inhaled terbutaline. Lancet 1988;1:554–8.

36. Cheung D, Timmers MC, Zwinderman AH, et al. Long-term effects of a long-acting beta 2-adrenoceptor

agonist, salmeterol, on airway hyperresponsiveness in patients with mild asthma. N Engl J Med 1992;327:1198–203.

37. O'Connor BJ, Aikman SL, Barnes PJ. Tolerance to the nonbronchodilating effects of inhaled beta2-agonists in asthma. N Engl J Med 1992;327:1204–8.

38. Peat JK, Woolcock AJ, Cullen K. Rate of decline of lung function in subjects with asthma. Eur J Respir Dis 1987;70:171–9.

39. Lange P, Parner J, Vestbo J, et al. A 15-year follow-up study of ventilatory function in adults with asthma. N Engl J Med 1998;339:1194–200.

40. Dompeling E, van Schayck CP, van Grunsven PM, et al. Slowing the deterioration of asthma and chronic obstructive pulmonary disease during bronchodilator therapy by adding inhaled corticosteroids. Ann Intern Med 1993;118:770–8.

41. Adelroth E, Thompson S. Advantages of high dose budesonide. Lancet 1988;1:476.

42. Wong CS, Cooper S, Britton JR, Tattersfield AE. Steroid sparing effect of nedocromil sodium in asthmatic patients on high doses of inhaled corticosteroids. Clin Exp Allergy 1993;23:370–6.

43. Pizzichini E, Pizzichini MMM, Kidney JC, et al. Induced sputum, bronchoalveolar lavage and blood from mild asthmatic patients: inflammatory cells, lymphocyte subsets and soluble markers compared. Eur Respir J 1998;11:828–34.

44. Gibson PG, Wong BJO, Hepperle MJE, et al. A research method to induce and examine a mild exacerbation of asthma by withdrawal of inhaled corticosteroid. Clin Exp Allergy 1992;22:525–32.

45. Turner MO, Hussack P, Sears MR, et al. Exacerbations of asthma without sputum eosinophilia. Thorax 1995;50:1057–61.

46. Fahy JV, Kim KW, Liu J, Boushey HA. Prominent inflammation in sputum from subjects with asthma exacerbation. J Allergy Clin Immunol 1995;95:843–52.

47. Brown PH, Blundell G, Greening AP, Crompton GK. Screening for hypothalamo-pituitary-adrenal axis suppression in asthmatic patients taking high dose inhaled corticosteroids. Respir Med 1991;85:511–6.

48. Bisgaard H, Damkjaer Nilsen M, Andersen B. Adrenal function in children with bronchial asthma treated with beclomethasone dipropionate or budesonide. J Allergy Clin Immunol 1988;80:213–7.

49. Lofdahl C-G, Mellstrand T, Svedmyr N. Glucocorticoids and asthma. Studies of resistance and systemic effects of glucocorticoids. Eur J Respir Dis 1984;65:69–77.

50. Johansson SA, Andersson K-E, Brattsand R, et al P. Topical and systemic glucocorticoid potencies of budesonide and beclomethasone dipropionate in man. Eur J Clin Pharmacol 1982;22:523–9.

51. Wong J, Black P. Acute adrenal insufficiency associated with high dose inhaled corticosteroids. Br Med J 1992;304:1415–6.

52. Zwaan CM, Odink RJH, Delemarre-van de Waal HA, et al. Acute adrenal insufficiency after discontinuation of inhaled corticosteroid therapy. Lancet 1992;340:1289–90.

53. Reid DM, Nicholl JJ, Smith MA, et al. Corticosteroids and bone mass in asthma: comparisons with rheumatoid arthritis and polymyalgia rheumatica. Br Med J 1986;293:1463–6.

54. Puolijoki H, Liippo K, Salmi J, et al. Does high dose inhaled beclomethasone (BDP) effect calcium metabolism [abstract]? Eur Respir J 1991;4:483s.

55. Birkebaek NH, Esberg G, Andersen K, et al. Bone and collagen turnover during treatment with inhaled dry powder budesonide and beclomethasone dipropionate. Arch Dis Child 1995;73:524–7.

56. Wolthers O, Hansen M, Juul A, et al. Knemometry, urine cortisol excretion, and measures of the insulin-like growth factor axis and collagen turnover in children treated with inhaled glucocorticosteroids. Pediatr Res 1997;41:44–50.

57. Toogood JH, Markov AE, Baskerville JC, Dyson C. Association of ocular cataracts with inhaled and oral steroid therapy during long-term treatment of asthma. J Allergy Clin Immunol 1993;91:571–9.

58. Simons FE, Persaud MP, Gillespie CA, et al. Absence of posterior subcapsular cataracts in young patients treated with inhaled corticosteroids. Lancet 1993;342:776–8.

59. Cumming RG, Mitchell P, Leeder SR. Use of inhaled corticosteroids and the risk of cataracts. N Engl J Med 1997;337:8–14.

60. Balfour-Lynn L. Effect of asthma on growth and puberty. The Pediatrician 1987;24:237–41.

61. Martin AJ, Landau LI, Phelan PD. The effects on growth of childhood asthma. Acta Paediatr Scand 1981;70:683–8.

62. Wolthers OD, Pedersen S. Short term linear growth in asthmatic children during treatment with prednisolone. Br Med J 1990;301:145–8.

63. Wolthers OD, Pedersen S. Growth of asthmatic children during treatment with budesonide: a double blind trial. Br Med J 1991;303:163–5.

64. Wolthers OD, Pedersen S. Short term growth during treatment with inhaled fluticasone propionate and beclomethasone dipropionate. Arch Dis Child 1993;90:517–8.

65. Doull I, Freezer N, Holgate ST. Growth of prepubertal children with mild asthma treated with inhaled beclomethasone dipropionate. Am J Respir Crit Care Med 1995;151:1715–9.

66. Reed CE, Offord KP, Nelson HS, et al. Aerosol beclomethasone dipropionate spray compared with theophylline as primary treatment for chronic mild-to-moderate asthma. The American Academy of Allergy, Asthma and Immunology Beclomethasone Dipropionate–Theophylline Study Group. J Allergy Clin Immunol 1998;101:14–23.

67. Doull I, Freezer N, Holgate ST. Osteocalcin, growth, and inhaled corticosteroids: a prospective study. Arch Dis Child 1996;74:497–501.

68. Phelan MC. Beclomethasone mania. Br J Psychiatry 1989;155:871–2.

69. Connett G, Lenney W. Inhaled budesonide and behavioural disturbances. Lancet 1991;338:634.

70. Mak VHF, Melcor R, Spiro SG. Easy bruising as a side-effect of inhaled corticosteroids. Eur Respir J 1992; 5:1068–74.

CHAPTER 17

Leukotriene Modifiers

Elliot Israel, MD
Jeffrey M. Drazen, MD

Leukotriene modifier treatment for asthma differs from all other forms of asthma treatment in that it is truly a "designer" treatment.[1,2] That is, these drugs, targeted at the leukotrienes, are derived from basic investigation conducted over two decades ago that indicated a role for the leukotrienes in the pathogenesis of asthma. Since there is reason to believe that asthma is a heterogenous disease—that is, there are patients whose asthma is predominantly due to leukotriene excess, while, in others, leukotrienes may play a lesser role—it would seem reasonable to tailor antileukotriene therapy specifically to those individuals in whom leukotrienes have been shown to contribute importantly to the pathobiology of asthma. However, as of this time, since there is no way to identify such individuals a priori, trials are performed and treatment is dispensed without regard to the role of leukotrienes in a given person's asthma. Consequently, the evidence reviewed herein consists of trials in which all individuals with asthma, defined by standard clinical criteria, were enrolled.

Mechanism of Action

Knowledge of how to use antileukotriene drugs requires an understanding of the leukotriene pathway and its relationship to asthma. The cysteinyl leukotrienes (ie, leukotrienes containing the amino acid cysteine [Cys]) are bioactive fatty acids; their structure was elucidated in 1979 as the products of conjugation of arachidonic acid to the tripeptide glutathione and derivatives thereof.[3–5] Since leukotrienes were first structurally isolated from leukocytes, and each of the molecules contains a series of three conjugated double bonds (ie, a triene), the name leukotriene derives from "leuko" "triene."[3] These mediators are the product of metabolism of arachidonic acid, the fatty acid commonly found esterified in the sn-2 position of membrane phospholipids. Arachidonic acid (cis-5,8,11,14-eicosatetraenoic acid) is cleaved from cell membranes by the action of one of a member of a family of enzymes known as phospholipase A_2's.[6–8] These enzymes, although molecularly distinct, all share the common property of cleaving arachidonic acid from membrane phospholipids and liberating it in the microenvironment of their action. The cytosolic form of phospholipase A_2 is catalytically active in the intracellular microenvironment, and current evidence suggests its activity occurs at the perinuclear membrane.[9] In contrast, the many secretory forms of phospholipase A_2 ($sPLA_2$) operate at the external cell membrane; the arachidonic acid released by $sPLA_2$ action is thought to diffuse into the cell, where it becomes a substrate for other enzymes. Inside the cell, arachidonic acid released from membrane phospholipids is taken by the 5-lipoxygenase activating protein (also known as ALOX5-AP or FLAP) and presented to 5-lipoxygenase (5-LO).[10,11] 5-Lipoxygenase is the enzyme that adducts molecular oxygen to the arachidonic acid backbone to form leukotriene A_4. Leukotriene A_4 becomes a substrate for the enzyme leukotriene C_4 synthase (LTC$_4$-S), which adducts the tripeptide glutathione to leukotriene A_4 to form the first of the cysteinyl leukotrienes, leukotriene C_4.[12,13] Leukotriene C_4 is exported from the cells of its synthesis through the multidrug-resistance protein. In the extracellular microenvironment, the glutamic acid moiety is cleaved by γ-glutamyltransferase to yield leukotriene D_4. Leukotriene D_4 (LTD$_4$) acts at the Cys LT$_1$ receptor to mediate airway narrowing and vascular leak.[14] Leukotriene D_4 is also a substrate for a variety of dipeptidases that cleave the glycine moiety from it, leaving the 6-cysteinyl analog of leukotriene C_4, known as leukotriene E_4 (LTE$_4$). Leukotriene E_4 is diminished in biopotency by a factor of approximately 100 as compared to LTD$_4$,[15,16] and it may undergo ω-oxidation and β-elimination, or it may be N-acetylated.[17–19] In either case, there is a substantial loss of bioactivity. Interestingly, approximately 10% of LTE$_4$ is excreted unchanged in the urine.

In neutrophils, LTA$_4$ becomes a substrate for the enzyme LTA$_4$ epoxide hydrolase, which stereospecifically adducts molecular oxygen and oxygen from water to form the dihydroxy-leukotriene known as leukotriene B_4 (LTB$_4$).[20,21] In the external microenvironment, LTB$_4$ acts at what is known as the BLT receptor to transduce a variety of biologic effects, among which is chemotaxis.

Currently Available Leukotriene Modifiers

Worldwide, there are four pharmaceutic agents available by prescription that can affect the synthesis or action of the leukotrienes.[2] Zileuton (Zyflo, Abbott) inhibits the action of 5-LO and, therefore, the production of leukotriene A_4 from arachidonic acid; it is the only biosynthetic inhibitor available for clinical use. The family of "lukasts," consisting of montelukast (Singulair, Merck), pranlukast (Onon, Ono Pharmaceuticals), and zafirlukast, (Accolate, Astra-Zeneca), all inhibit the action of cysteinyl leukotrienes (ie, LTC$_4$,-D$_4$, and-E$_4$,) at the Cys LT$_1$ receptor. Studies of the capacity of each of these agents to inhibit LTD$_4$-induced bronchoconstriction indicate that zafirlukast and montelukast are similar in biopotency. Pranlukast is diminished in biopotency, compared with the other two agents, by a factor of three to five. Because there are no head-to-head comparisons of these agents currently available, the evidence for use of antileukotriene treatment in asthma will be reviewed as a class. Similarly, recommendations for the therapeutic use of these agents will be by class rather than by a specific agent.

Induced Asthma

Exercise-Induced Asthma

Almost 50 to 80% of patients with a physician's diagnosis of asthma develop bronchospasm in the peri-exercise period. Treatment of exercise-induced bronchospasm by the chronic administration of β-adrenergic agonists is complicated by a diminution of the bronchoprotective effects of this form of therapy over time (Level IB). Specifically, the degree of bronchoprotection against exercise-induced bronchospasm achieved with salbutamol when given as a single dose is more than the degree of bronchoprotection achieved when salbutamol is given on a recurring basis.[22] Since many patients cannot schedule or predict their need to exercise, there is a need for an effective treatment for exercise-induced asthma that can be administered on a recurrent and prophylactic basis without loss of bronchoprotective effect. Zileuton, montelukast, and zafirlukast have been shown in controlled clinical trials to inhibit bronchospasm following exercise.[23–26] They reduce the exercise-induced response by about a half, as indicated by an approximately 50% decrease in the magnitude of the integrated area under the FEV$_1$ (forced expiratory volume in 1 second)-curve over time following exercise.

One of the major advantages of antileukotriene treatment for exercise-induced bronchospasm is the prolonged duration of effect obtained with standard clinical dosing. For example, administration of montelukast results in significant protection against exercise-induced bronchoconstriction even 24 hours after dosing;[27] however, after 36 hours, no clinically important effect on exercise-induced asthma is noted. Prolonged treatment with montelukast, for periods as long as 12 weeks, did not result in any loss of bronchoprotective effect of this agent against exercise-induced airway narrowing.[26] Further, montelukast was shown to provide greater bronchoprotection at the end of its dosing period (24 h) than salmeterol at the end of its dosing period (12 h), when both were administered regularly. Finally, trials have been completed in children aged 6 to 14 years[25] indicating that a dosage of 5 mg daily at bedtime resulted in approximately 60% protection from exercise-induced bronchoconstriction. In summary, these data provide Level IA evidence to recommend the use of antileukotrienes in the treatment of exercise-induced bronchoconstriction.

Aspirin-Induced Asthma

The bronchoconstriction that occurs after ingestion of aspirin or other nonsteroidal anti-inflammatory agents derives predominantly from the physiologic actions of leukotrienes (Level I).[28,29] These leukotrienes are produced within a few hours of aspirin ingestion, and their effects may persist for 4 to 6 hours. Controlled clinical trials in which aspirin is administered to patients who are treated either with an active antileukotriene or placebo, using randomized, blinded trial designs, have shown statistically and clinically significant protection from the bronchoconstrictive effects observed after aspirin administration.[28,30–33] Furthermore, chronic asthma control improves in these patients. The addition of zileuton to the treatment regimen of these patients is associated with an improvement in FEV_1 as well as an improvement in nasal function.[34] In these "nonchallenge" studies, there was a return of the sense of smell, less rhinorrhea, and higher nasal inspiratory flow rates during active treatment with zileuton compared to that observed with placebo.

It is important to note that administration of an antileukotriene treatment does not totally protect against the adverse physiologic consequence of ingestion of agents inhibiting the cyclooxygenase enzyme.[35] A case has been reported in which a patient with moderately severe asthma and aspirin sensitivity, who was being treated with zafirlukast at the clinically recommended dose, developed anaphylaxis after ingestion of ibuprofen 400 mg. Since the protection noted in clinical trials has been demonstrated in the setting of administration of specific threshold doses of aspirin that may be below the clinically encountered dose, it is possible for patients to receive doses of aspirin that produce enough leukotrienes to overcome the blockade provided by these agents. Thus, even when these agents are used appropriately, patients need to remain cautious about ingestion of aspirin and related compounds.

In summary, there is Level IA evidence supporting the use of antileukotrienes in aspirin-induced asthma, with the caveat that either aspirin avoidance or aspirin desensitization must also be practiced.

CHRONIC STABLE ASTHMA

All the clinically available antileukotriene compounds have been studied in chronic stable asthma. The data, as reviewed below, indicate significant effects on physiological function, quality of life, and pharmacoeconomic outcome indicators. The interested reader is also referred to reviews on this general topic.[1,2,36,37]

Leukotriene modifiers produce improvements in patients with mild to moderate and even severe asthma who are using only short-acting β-agonists for treatment (Level IA). In double-blind, randomized, placebo-controlled trials, montelukast, pranlukast, zafirlukast, and zileuton all have been compared to placebo in the treatment of patients with mild to moderate persistent asthma.[38–53] These data indicate a significant improvement in FEV_1 compared to the improvement noted with placebo of up to 20% (baseline versus treatment) over treatment periods of 4 to 26 weeks. Furthermore, in these trials, compared to placebo, it has been shown that active treatment results in a significantly diminished need for oral corticosteroid rescue, reduced use of inhaled β-adrenergic agonists, decreased night-time awakenings, and improved asthma symptoms. Consensus panel guidelines consider leukotriene modifiers to be an alternative controller medication for patients who require a controller.

These agents also have been shown to improve pulmonary function in patients already receiving inhaled corticosteroids.[54] In patients poorly controlled on inhaled corticosteroids, the addition of montelukast improved pulmonary function and decreased night-time awakenings.[50,54] Thus, these drugs can be used as an add-on therapy with inhaled corticosteroids (Level IA).

Leukotriene modifiers have been evaluated as add-on therapy to β-agonists in comparison to other treatments. Zileuton was shown to be about equally effective as theophylline in such a design.[55] In contrast, the addition of montelukast was shown to have a weaker effect on the FEV$_1$ than inhaled beclomethasone.[49] Of note, the latter study was performed with enforced compliance measures. Considering the greater compliance with oral therapy versus inhaled therapy,[56] it is possible that some of the difference between the leukotriene modifier and inhaled corticosteroids may be less apparent in real-world clinical use.

A third type of trial has examined the ability of leukotriene modifiers to permit a reduction of the dose of inhaled corticosteroids in patients requiring moderately high doses of inhaled corticosteroids to maintain adequate asthma control. In these trials, blinded randomized treatment with antileukotriene drugs is initiated, and then inhaled corticosteroids are withdrawn; the efficacy of antileukotriene treatment is judged by the capacity of active therapy to prevent exacerbations during inhaled steroid withdrawal. For example, in the trial by Tamaoki et al, patients receiving, on average, ≈2000 μg/d of beclomethasone were able to reduce their inhaled dose of beclomethasone by a factor of 2, without a decrease in morning peak-flow rates when treated with pranlukast. In contrast, there was a reduction of over 50 L/min in morning peak-flow rates in the group not receiving therapy when the steroid dose was reduced by 50%.[57] In another study, in patients tapered to the lowest tolerable dose of inhaled corticosteroids, montelukast permitted a further 47% reduction compared to a 30% reduction with placebo.[58]

EFFICACY SUMMARY

These data provide Level IA evidence for the use of antileukotrienes in the treatment of chronic stable asthma and for the prevention of exercise-, aspirin-, and externally provoked bronchospasm. What is not clear from these clinical trials is how these agents should be placed in the stepped treatment of patients with asthma. Although the data clearly indicate that inhaled corticosteroids have greater efficacy than antileukotrienes, judging efficacy based on FEV$_1$, it is unclear how these drugs will compare in effectiveness in the context of toxicity, compliance, and patient and provider use. Indeed, long-term comparison trials have yet to be completed and, therefore, the recommendation to use antileukotriene treatment cannot be construed as an evidence-based recommendation for the use of antileukotriene versus inhaled corticosteroids. However, it is clear that antileukotrienes can have additive effects with inhaled corticosteroids.

SAFETY

As a class, these agents are safe and well tolerated. In trials performed with all the leukotriene receptor antagonists at the clinically recommended doses, there have been no differences between active treatment groups, with respect to symptoms perceived or laboratory abnormalities. With respect to zileuton, there is approximately a 3.5% incidence of elevated hepatic transaminases (ie, ALT) values.[59] This has led to the recommendation that ALT values be checked at the initiation of zileuton treatment, monthly for the first 3 months and then periodically thereafter. After 3 months of therapy, the incidence of abnormal liver function tests falls to that in the placebo group.

There are important interactions to be noted with these agents. With respect to zafirlukast, data supplied by the drug manufacturer indicates that the addition of zafirlukast to the regimen of theophylline could result in decreased theophylline clearance.[60] There has been a report of an individual in whom this combination resulted in a substantial increase in theophylline levels.[61] Although general monitoring of theophylline levels of patients on concomitant antileukotriene therapy is not specifically recommended, it is well established that monitoring serum theophylline levels in patients receiving this form of therapy is of value.

With respect to zileuton, data available from the manufacturer indicates that zileuton will increase serum theophylline levels, and monitoring of serum theophylline levels is recommended.[62] Further, zileuton can influence anticoagulation produced by warfarin. Trials conducted with zileuton indicate there is no need to change the dose of zileuton in patients with acute renal failure.[63] Data are not available on other antileukotriene agents with respect to this issue.

There have been rare reports of a systemic vasculitic syndrome, consistent with the Churg-Strauss syndrome, in patients receiving montelukast or zafirlukast therapy for asthma.[64–66] This is an exceedingly rare event, with one case occurring in approximately 25,000 patient years of treatment, and these have occurred almost exclusively in patients whose asthma control has required oral or high-dose inhaled corticosteroid therapy. Indeed, it is highly likely that these patients were developing a vasculitic syndrome that had been diagnosed as severe asthma rather than vasculitis. Thus, the use of antileukotriene treatment in patients who had previously required oral or substantial doses of inhaled corticosteroids for asthma control, and who have a substantial salutary therapeutic effect from this form of therapy, requires special attention should they develop signs or symptoms consistent with systemic vasculitis.

Summary and Recommendations

Agents active in the leukotriene pathway, known as a class as leukotriene modifier drugs, are novel, easy to administer, effective, safe, and well-tolerated antiasthma treatments for patients with mild to moderate disease. There is Level IA evidence supporting their use in exercise-induced asthma, in aspirin-induced asthma, in chronic stable asthma, and as additive therapy in patients on inhaled corticosteroids. Insufficient data are currently available to make evidence-based recommendations regarding their stepped use relative to other agents; additional comparative evidence-based trials are required.

References

1. O'Byrne PM, Israel E, Drazen JM. Antileukotrienes in the treatment of asthma. Ann Intern Med 1997;127:472–80.

2. Drazen JM, Israel E, O'Byrne PM. Treatment of asthma with drugs modifying the leukotriene pathway. N Engl J Med 1999;340:197–206.

3. Samuelsson B. Leukotrienes: mediators of immediate hypersensitivity reactions and inflammation. Science 1983;220:568–75.

4. Lewis RA, Austen KF, Soberman RJ. Leukotrienes and other products of the 5-lipoxygenase pathway. Biochemistry and relation to pathobiology in human diseases. N Engl J Med 1990;323:645–55.

5. Henderson WR. The role of leukotrienes in inflammation. Ann Intern Med 1994;121:684–97.

6. Dennis EA, Rhee SG, Billah MM, Hannun YA. Role of phospholipase in generating lipid second messengers in signal transduction. FASEB J 1991;5:2068–77.

7. Balsinde J, Dennis EA. Distinct roles in signal transduction for each of the phospholipase A2 enzymes present in P388D1 macrophages. J Biol Chem 1996;271:6758–65.

8. Dennis EA. Potential phospholipase A2s involved in inflammatory diseases. Agents Actions Suppl 1995;46:35–9.

9. Petersgolden M. Cell biology of the 5-lipoxygenase pathway. Am J Respir Crit Care Med 1998;157:S227–32.

10. Dixon RA, Diehl RE, Opas E, et al. Requirement of a 5-lipoxygenase-activating protein for leukotriene synthesis. Nature 1990;343:282–4.

11. Miller DK, Gillard JW, Vickers PJ, et al. Identification and isolation of a membrane protein necessary for leukotriene production. Nature 1990;343:78–81.

12. Lam BK, Penrose JF, Freeman GJ, Austen KF. Expression cloning of a cDNA for human leukotriene C_4 synthase, an integral membrane protein conjugating reduced glutathione to leukotriene A_4. Proc Natl Acad Sci U S A 1994;91:7663–7.

13. Penrose JF, Spector J, Baldasaro M, et al. Molecular cloning of the gene for human leukotriene C_4 synthase—organization, nucleotide sequence, and chromosomal localization to 5q35. J Biol Chem 1996;271:11356–61.

14. Coleman RA, Eglen RM, Jones RL, et al. Prostanoid and leukotriene receptors: a progress report from the IUPHAR working parties on classification and nomenclature. Prostaglandins and Related Compounds 1995;23:283–5.

15. Lewis RA, Lee CW, Levine L, et al. Biology of the C-6-sulfidopeptide leukotrienes. Adv Prostaglandin Thromboxane Leukot Res 1983;11:15–26.

16. Piper PJ. Pharmacology of leukotrienes. Br Med Bull 1983;39:255–9.

17. Stene DO, Murphy RC. Metabolism of leukotriene E_4 in isolated rat hepatocytes. Identification of beta-oxidation products of sulfidopeptide leukotrienes. J Biol Chem 1988;263:2773–8.

18. Sala A, Voelkel N, Maclouf J, Murphy RC. Leukotriene E_4 elimination and metabolism in normal human subjects. J Biol Chem 1990;265:21771–8.

19. Murphy RC, Wheelan P. Pathways of leukotriene metabolism in isolated cell models and human subjects. New York: Marcel Dekker, Inc; 1998.

20. Medina JF, Radmark O, Funk CD, Haeggstrom JZ. Molecular cloning and expression of mouse leukotriene-A_4 hydrolase cDNA. Biochem Biophys Res Commun 1991;176:516–24.

21. Serhan CN, Haeggstrom JZ, Leslie CC. Lipid mediator networks in cell signaling: update and impact of cytokines. FASEB J 1996;10:1147–58.

22. Inman MD, O'Byrne PM. The effect of regular inhaled salbutamol on exercise-induced bronchoconstriction. Am J Respir Crit Care Med 1996;153:65–9.

23. Finnerty JP, Wood-Baker R, Thomson H, Holgate ST. Role of leukotrienes in exercise-induced asthma: inhibitory effect of ICI 204219, a potent LTD4 receptor antagonist. Am Rev Respir Dis 1992;145:746–9.

24. Meltzer SS, Hasday JD, Cohn J, Bleecker ER. Inhibition of exercise-induced bronchospasm by zileuton: a 5-lipoxygenase inhibitor. Am J Respir Crit Care Med 1996;153:931–5.

25. Kemp JP, Dockhorn RJ, Shapiro GG, et al. Montelukast once daily inhibits exercise-induced bronchoconstriction in 6- to 14-year-old children with asthma. J Pediatr 1998;133:424–8.

26. Leff JA, Busse WW, Pearlman D, et al. Montelukast, a leukotriene-receptor antagonist, for the treatment of mild asthma and exercise-induced bronchoconstriction. N Engl J Med 1998;339:147–52.

27. Bronsky EA, Kemp JP, Zhang J, et al. Dose-related protection of exercise bronchoconstriction by montelukast, a cysteinyl leukotriene-receptor antagonist, at the end of a once-daily dosing interval. Clin Pharmacol Ther 1997;62:556–61.

28. Israel E, Fischer AR, Rosenberg MA, et al. The pivotal role of 5-lipoxygenase products in the reaction of aspirin-sensitive asthmatic patients to aspirin. Am Rev Respir Dis 1993;148:1447–51.

29. Nasser SMS, Lee TH. Aspirin-induced early and late asthmatic responses. Clin Exp Allergy 1995;25:1–3.

30. Dahlen B, Margolskee DJ, Zetterstrom O, Dahlen SE. Effect of the leukotriene receptor antagonist MK-0679 on baseline pulmonary function in aspirin sensitive asthmatic subjects. Thorax 1993;48:1205–10.

31. Nasser SM, Bell GS, Hawksworth RJ, et al. Effect of the 5-lipoxygenase inhibitor ZD2138 on allergen-induced early and late asthmatic responses. Thorax 1994;49:743–8.

32. Fischer AR, Rosenberg MA, Lilly CM, et al. Direct evidence for a role of the mast cell in the nasal response to aspirin in aspirin-sensitive asthma. J Allergy Clin Immunol 1994;94:1046–56.

33. O'Sullivan S, Dahlen B, Dahlen SE, Kumlin M. Increased urinary excretion of the prostaglandin D_2 metabolite 9 alpha,11 beta-prostaglandin F_{2a} after aspirin challenge supports mast cell activation in aspirin-induced airway obstruction. J Allergy Clin Immunol 1996;98:421–32.

34. Dahlen B, Nizankowska E, Szczeklik A, et al. Benefits from adding the 5-lipoxygenase inhibitor zileuton to conventional therapy in aspirin-intolerant asthmatic patients. Am J Respir Crit Care Med 1998;157:1187–94.

35. Menendez R, Venzor J, Ortiz G. Failure of zafirlukast to prevent ibuprofen-induced anaphylaxis. Ann Allergy Asthma Immunol 1998;80:25–6.

36. Adkins JC, Brogden RN. Zafirlukast: a review of its pharmacology and therapeutic potential in the management of asthma. Drugs 1998;55:121–44.

37. Calhoun WJ. Summary of clinical trials with zafirlukast. Am J Respir Crit Care Med 1998;157:S238–45.

38. Israel E, Cohn J, Dube L, Drazen JM. Effect of treatment with zileuton, a 5-lipoxygenase inhibitor, in patients with asthma: a randomized controlled trial. JAMA 1996;275:931–6.

39. Grossman J, Faiferman I, Dubb JW, et al. Results of the first U.S. double-blind, placebo-controlled, multicenter clinical study in asthma with pranlukast, a novel leukotriene receptor antagonist. J Asthma 1997;34:321–8.

40. Israel E, Rubin P, Kemp JP, et al. The effect of inhibition of 5-lipoxygenase by zileuton in mild to moderate asthma. Ann Intern Med 1993;119:1059–66.

41. Spector SL, Smith LJ, Glass M, et al. Effects of 6 weeks of therapy with oral doses of ICI 204, 219, a leukotriene D_4 receptor antagonist, in subjects with bronchial asthma. Am J Respir Crit Care Med 1994;150:618–23.

42. Liu MC, Dube LM, Lancaster J. Acute and chronic effects of a 5-lipoxygenase inhibitor in asthma: a 6-month randomized multicenter trial. J Allergy Clin Immunol 1996;98:859–71.

43. Reiss TF, Altman LC, Chervinsky P, et al. Effects of montelukast (MK-0476), a new potent cysteinyl leukotriene (LTD_4) receptor antagonist, in patients with chronic asthma. J Allergy Clin Immunol 1996;98:528–34.

44. Barnes NC, Pujet JC. Pranlukast, a novel leukotriene receptor antagonist: results of the first European, placebo controlled, multicentre clinical study in asthma. Thorax 1997;52:523–7.

45. Suissa S, Dennis R, Ernst P, et al. Effectiveness of the leukotriene receptor antagonist zafirlukast for mild-to-moderate asthma—a randomized, double-blind, placebo-controlled trial. Ann Intern Med 1997;126:177–83.

46. Knorr B, Matz J, Bernstein JA, et al. Montelukast for chronic asthma in 6- to 14-year-old children: a randomized, double-blind trial. Pediatric Montelukast Study Group. JAMA 1998;279:1181–6.

47. Altman LC, Munk Z, Seltzer J, et al. A placebo-controlled, dose-ranging study of montelukast, a cysteinyl leukotriene-receptor antagonist. Montelukast Asthma Study Group. J Allergy Clin Immunol 1998;102:50–6.

48. Noonan MJ, Chervinsky P, Brandon M, et al. Montelukast, a potent leukotriene receptor antagonist, causes dose-related improvements in chronic asthma. Eur Respir J 1998;11:232–9.

49. Malmstrom K, Rodriguez-Gomez G, Guerra J, et al. Oral montelukast, inhaled beclomethasone, and placebo for chronic asthma. A randomized controlled trial. Ann Intern Med 1999;130:487–95.

50. Laviolette M, Malmstrom K, Lu S, et al. Montelukast added to inhaled beclomethasone in treatment of asthma. Am J Respir Crit Care Med 1999;160:1862–8.

51. Kemp JP, Minkwitz MC, Bonuccelli CM, Warren MS. Therapeutic effect of zafirlukast as monotherapy in steroid-naive patients with severe persistent asthma. Chest 1999;115:336–42.

52. Reiss TF, Chervinsky P, Dockhorn RJ, et al. Montelukast a once daily leukotriene receptor antagonist in the treatment of chronic asthma. Arch Intern Med 1998;158:1213–20.

53. Fish JE, Kemp JP, Lockey RF, et al. Zafirlukast for symptomatic mild-to-moderate asthma: a 13-week multicenter study. The Zafirlukast Trialists Group. Clin Ther 1997;19:675–90.

54. Reiss TF, Sorkness CA, Stricker W, et al. Effects of montelukast (MK-0476), a potent cysteinyl leukotriene receptor antagonist, on bronchodilation in asthmatic subjects treated with and without inhaled corticosteroids. Thorax 1997;52:45–8.

55. Schwartz HJ, Petty T, Dube LM, et al. A randomized controlled trial comparing zileuton with theophylline in moderate asthma. Arch Intern Med 1998;158:141–8.

56. Kelloway JS, Wyatt RA, Adlis SA. Comparison of patient's compliance with prescribed oral and inhaled asthma medications. Arch Intern Med 1994;154:1349–52.

57. Tamaoki J, Kondo M, Sakai N, et al. Leukotriene antagonist prevents exacerbation of asthma during reduction of high-dose inhaled corticosteroid. Am J Respir Crit Care Med 1997;155:1235–40.

58. Lofdahl CG, Reiss TF, Leff JA, et al. Randomised, placebo controlled trial of effect of a leukotriene receptor antagonist, montelukast, on tapering inhaled corticosteroids in asthmatic patients. Br Med J 1999;319:87–90.

59. Lazarus SC, Lee T, Kemp JP, et al. Safety and clinical efficacy of zileuton in patients with chronic asthma. Am J Manag Care 1998;4:841–8.

60. Zafirlukast Research and Marketing Team. Zafirlukast package insert [pamphlet]. Rahway (NJ): Merck; 1998.

61. Katial RK, Stelzle RC, Bonner MW, et al. A drug interaction between zafirlukast and theophylline. Arch Intern Med 1998;158:1713–5.

62. Mcgill KA, Busse WW. Zileuton. Lancet 1996;348:19–24.

63. Awni WM, Wong S, Chu SY, et al. Pharmacokinetics of zileuton and its metabolites in patients with renal impairment. J Clin Pharmacol 1997;37:395–404.

64. Wechsler ME, Garpestad E, Flier SR, et al. Pulmonary infiltrates, eosinophilia, and cardiomyopathy following corticosteroid withdrawal in patients with asthma receiving zafirlukast. JAMA 1998;279:455–7.

65. Knoell DL, Lucas J, Allen JN. Churg-Strauss syndrome associated with zafirlukast. Chest 1998;114:332–4.

66. Holloway J, Ferriss J, Groff J, et al. Churg-Strauss syndrome associated with zafirlukast. J Am Osteopath Assoc 1998;98:275–8.

CHAPTER 18

Alternative Anti-inflammatory Therapies

Christopher J. Corrigan, MA, MSc, PhD, FRCP

THE CLINICAL NEED

Inhaled glucocorticoids form the mainstay of asthma therapy for the majority of patients. Topical glucocorticoids are relatively free of unwanted effects and offer a very favourable benefit:risk ratio. There remains, however, a group of chronic, severe asthmatic patients whose disease is inadequately controlled by inhaled glucocorticoid therapy, even when optimal delivery has been assured, compliance has been verified, and the effects of other exacerbating factors have been minimized.[1] In these patients, oral glucocorticoids are often required to control symptoms. Patients taking oral glucocorticoids are at risk of developing unwanted effects of these drugs, particularly with long-term administration, and may remain symptomatic despite this therapy. In addition, an important minority of patients appear to be resistant to the clinical antiasthma effects of glucocorticoids; this may be related, at least in part, to a relative resistance of their T cells to glucocorticoid inhibition.[2] For all these patients, alternative modalities of therapy are urgently required. This chapter contains a critical appraisal of trials of alternative "anti-inflammatory" agents for asthma therapy, followed by a brief look at emerging therapies resulting from our increasing understanding of disease pathogenesis.

TRIALS OF IMMUNOSUPPRESSIVE THERAPY

Background

It is increasingly recognized that asthma is associated with chronic, cell-mediated inflammation of the bronchial mucosa in which eosinophil-active cytokine products of activated T cells play a prominent role. Evidence suggests that glucocorticoids ameliorate asthma at least partly through inhibition of T cells and elaboration of their asthma-relevant cytokine products, particularly interleukin-5 (IL-5).[3–5] For this reason, there has been interest in the investigation of other "anti-inflammatory" or "immunosuppressive" agents for their possible therapeutic effects in asthma. Since many of these agents have potentially serious unwanted effects, attention has generally been focused on their use for those asthmatic patients who continue to have severe disease despite properly administered, maximal topical glucocorticoid therapy and additional continuous systemic therapy. With such patients, it is perceived that the benefits of amelioration of the disease and/or reduction or abolition of systemic glucocorticoid therapy, with its associated hazards, might outweigh the risks.

Azathioprine, Methotrexate, and Gold Salts

Evaluation of these drugs in asthma has been based on empiric observation of their "anti-inflammatory" effects in diseases such as rheumatoid arthritis, rather than cogent hypotheses regarding their possible mechanisms of action.

Azathioprine is used in a range of inflammatory diseases for its "glucocorticoid-sparing" effect. It is a pro-drug that is metabolized to 6-mercaptopurine (6-MP) and 6-thioinosinic acid, both of which inhibit deoxyribonucleic acid (DNA) synthesis. Aside from the theoretic possibility that azathioprine may impair T and B cell proliferation in vivo, and demonstration of an inhibitory effect of azathioprine on granulocyte trafficking, in some studies,[6] the mechanism of its anti-inflammatory action is unclear. There is no evidence that it inhibits the production of asthma-relevant cytokines or the effects of these cytokines on eosinophils. One trial of azathioprine[7] and two trials of its metabolite 6-MP[8,9] failed to demonstrate any therapeutic benefit in glucocorticoid-dependent asthmatic patients, although in retrospect it seems likely that these trials were too short and involved too few patients to have the power to address these questions reliably. Thus, whereas a possible glucocorticoid-sparing effect of azathioprine in glucocorticoid-dependent asthma cannot be ruled out, its use for this purpose cannot be recommended on the basis of current clinical trial data (Level IC).

Both parenteral and oral gold salt preparations have been evaluated for their possible therapeutic benefits in chronic asthma. Mechanisms of action of gold salts that may be relevant to a glucocorticoid-sparing effect in asthma are ill defined, although these drugs do inhibit T cell proliferation in vitro and have recently been shown to inhibit IL-5-mediated prolongation of eosinophil survival, albeit at high concentrations.[10] In addition, gold salts have been reported to inhibit immunoglobulin E (IgE)-mediated degranulation of mast cells and basophils,[11] and leukotriene production by granulocytes.[12] In one blinded trial,[13] 79 asthma patients not taking oral glucocorticoids were treated with intramuscular gold salts or placebo over a 30-week period. Patients treated with gold showed increased benefit over those treated with placebo in terms of reduction of symptoms and concomitant medication, although unwanted effects (dermatitis, stomatitis, and proteinuria) were common and frequently severe. Similarly, a small, blinded, crossover study of parenteral gold therapy in severe glucocorticoid-dependent asthmatic patients[14] revealed some marginal benefits of active therapy as compared with placebo in terms of reduction of glucocorticoid therapy, but the authors concluded that the unwanted effects of the therapy were likely to preclude its routine use. Oral gold salts have also been evaluated for therapy of severe asthma in two double-blind placebo-controlled parallel group studies. In the first study,[15] 28 severe asthmatic patients taking small dosages of oral glucocorticoids were treated with oral gold salts (3 mg twice daily) or placebo for 26 weeks in a parallel group design, and progressive oral glucocorticoid dose reduction was attempted. Those patients treated with gold salts achieved a significantly higher reduction in oral glucocorticoid dosage (mean 4 mg daily prednisone or equivalent) as compared with those taking placebo (mean 0.3 mg daily) with little change in lung function, although the frequency of disease exacerbations requiring increased oral glucocorticoids was somewhat lower in those patients receiving active therapy. In the second study,[16] 279 patients requiring at least 10 mg prednisone (or equivalent) daily were treated for 6 months with oral gold salts (3 mg twice daily) or placebo in a parallel group design. Sixty percent of patients receiving active therapy were able to reduce their daily dosages of oral glucocorticoids by at least 50%; dosages were reduced by 32% in those receiving placebo. Lung function and concomitant medication were not significantly altered.

In summary, several placebo-controlled clinical trials (Level IA) have confirmed that oral gold salts allow significant reduction of oral glucocorticoid therapy in glucocorticoid-dependent asthmatic patients, although not all patients appeared to show a significant response. The minimum duration of a valid trial of therapy is not clear, but this should probably be 6 months. The unwanted effects associated with oral gold salt therapy have been the subject of a recent review[17] and include dermatitis, hepatic dysfunction, proteinuria, and interstitial pneumonitis. Blood dyscrasias are rarely seen. Patients must be monitored carefully for these effects. Finally, in a comparative analysis of the glucocorticoid-sparing effects of gold salts, methotrexate, and cyclosporine in severe asthma,[18] it was concluded that gold salts provided the optimal risk:benefit ratio in terms of efficacy and tolerability of unwanted effects.

Methotrexate is a folic acid analogue used at low dosage for its anti-inflammatory activity in an increasing variety of chronic diseases. Surprisingly, the precise mechanisms by which methotrexate exerts this activity remain uncertain, although it has been shown to inhibit cytokine secretion and granulocyte chemotaxis.[19] In addition, because methotrexate is an antimetabolite suppressing DNA synthesis, it inhibits T cell proliferation.[20] It exerts a delayed but sustained therapeutic effect even with intermittent, weekly dosage regimens. This probably reflects methotrexate accumulation in cells as active polyglutamate complexes, resulting in accumulation of S-adenosyl methionine and adenosine, both of which are inhibitory to T cell function.[21] Following an initial open study[22] in which 25 chronic severe asthmatic patients who were apparently dependent on very large dosages of oral prednisone were able to reduce them considerably (mean dosages 6 to 27 mg daily) in association with methotrexate therapy (15 to 50 mg weekly for at least 18 months) without significant alteration of lung function, several placebo-controlled studies were subsequently performed. In a randomized, double-blind parallel group study,[23] 69 patients with oral glucocorticoid-dependent asthma (mean daily prednisolone dosage 14.2 mg) were treated with methotrexate (15 mg weekly) or placebo for 24 weeks, and daily prednisolone dosages were reduced by 2.5 mg every 4 weeks if symptoms or lung function were unchanged or improved. Little benefit was seen after 12 weeks of therapy, but after 24 weeks, 50% of those patients treated with methotrexate, compared with 14% of those taking placebo, were able to reduce their oral prednisolone, although this reduction was not maintained when the study medication was discontinued. Methotrexate therapy produced no significant alteration of lung function but was associated with a reduction in disease exacerbations requiring elevation of glucocorticoid dosages. Three further placebo-controlled trials[24-26] have confirmed a small but significant glucocorticoid-sparing effect of methotrexate in glucocorticoid-dependent asthma, without significant effect on lung function.

In contrast, three placebo-controlled trials of oral methotrexate therapy[27-29] and one trial of intramuscular[30] methotrexate therapy in glucocorticoid-dependent asthmatic patients failed to confirm any significant glucocorticoid-sparing effect. The negative studies of oral methotrexate therapy all employed a randomized, crossover design. The reasons for these negative studies may perhaps be understood in the light of two subsequent meta-analyses of trials of methotrexate therapy in glucocorticoid-dependent asthma.[31,32] Both have confirmed that concomitant weekly methotrexate therapy for a minimum of 3 to 6 months enables a significant (approximately 20%) overall reduction in oral glucocorticoid requirements in glucocorticoid-dependent asthmatic patients, but that only approximately 60% of patients show a significant response, whereas the remainder show little or no response. Response to therapy is more evident in those studies in which attempts have been made to minimize oral glucocorticoid therapy prior to initiation of methotrexate (otherwise a large placebo effect is observed), and those in which parallel group, as opposed to crossover, designs are employed (possibly reflecting significant "carry-over" effects of methotrexate therapy in crossover trials).

The most serious potential unwanted effect of methotrexate therapy is cumulative hepatic toxicity and hepatic fibrosis. Despite much clinical experience of this problem gleaned from treating other diseases such as rheumatoid arthritis, views about its seriousness vary. Originally, liver biopsy of all patients treated with methotrexate was advocated after each cumulative dosage of 1.5 g or after every 3 years of therapy.[33] More recently, consensus guidelines from the American College of Rheumatologists stipulated that liver biopsy is not required unless there is sustained, progressive elevation of liver function tests or concomitant alcohol abuse.[34] In addition to hepatic toxicity, there have been isolated reports of deaths from opportunistic infections,[35,36] pneumonitis,[37] and paradoxical increases in bronchial hyper-reactivity[38] in oral glucocorticoid-dependent asthmatic patients treated with methotrexate.

In summary, there is adequate evidence from several controlled trials that methotrexate therapy allows reduction of systemic glucocorticoid therapy in chronic, severe asthmatic patients without significant change in lung function (Level IA). Therapy should be assessed for a minimum of 3 to 6 months, after which it may be continued if effective. Blood counts and liver function must be monitored, and rare but potentially fatal opportunistic infections should be anticipated and treated promptly.

Cyclosporine

Cyclosporine is a lipophilic, cyclic undecapeptide derived from the fungus *Tolypocladium inflatum*. Like glucocorticoids, cyclosporine is thought to exert its immunosuppressive effects predominantly through inhibition of T cell proliferation and cytokine secretion,[39] although it does have potential anti-inflammatory effects on other cells (eg, it rapidly inhibits degranulation of mast cells and basophils[40,41] and reduces cytokine production by eosinophils[42]). Cyclosporine is not myelotoxic and is now widely used for the suppression of allograft rejection. It has also been shown to be effective at a relatively low dosage in many "autoimmune" diseases such as rheumatoid arthritis, psoriasis, and Crohn's disease.

Cyclosporine inhibits early T cell signaling mechanisms following ligation of the T cell antigen receptor[39] by binding to a ubiquitous cytoplasmic protein called cyclophilin. The complex inhibits the activity of calcineurin, a calcium- and calmodulin-dependent serine/threonine phosphatase required for the dephosphorylation of the cytoplasmic subunit of the T cell–specific transcriptional activator nuclear factor of activated T cells (NF-AT). Without dephosphorylation, this subunit cannot traverse the nuclear membrane and combine with its nuclear subunit. The end result of NF-AT inhibition is reduced transcription of IL-2, the autocrine T cell growth factor, and other cytokines, and arrest of T cellular proliferation in the G0/G1 phase. The fact that T cells are particularly dependent on NF-AT for activation of transcription of IL-2 may explain why cyclosporine is particularly inhibitory for T cells, rather than proliferating cells in general. Its mechanism of action in inhibiting mast cell and basophil degranulation is not yet clear but may reflect the fact that cyclosporine/cyclophilin complexes also inhibit the activity of the enzyme peptidyl-prolyl *cis-trans* isomerase (PPIase), which is required for conformational changes in proteins involved in extracellular transport.

In view of the increasing evidence for a role for activated T cells in pathogenesis of asthma, and the predominant inhibitory effects of cyclosporine on T cell proliferation and cytokine production, the appraisal of cyclosporine for a possible antiasthma effect would appear to be soundly based in theory. This has recently been undertaken in three double-blind, placebo-controlled trials. In the first trial,[43] 33 chronic, severe glucocorticoid-dependent asthmatic patients were treated for 12 weeks with cyclosporine (initial dosage 5 mg/kg/d, subsequently adjusted according to whole blood trough concentrations) and identical placebo in random order, with a 2-week washout period. Oral glucocorticoid therapy was maintained at a constant level throughout the entire trial period unless it was required to be increased because of disease exacerbation. Cyclosporine, as compared with placebo therapy, was associated with moderate and statistically significant increases in morning peak expiratory flow (PEF) and forced expiratory volume in 1 second (FEV_1) in these patients (12% and 17.6%, respectively). The frequency of disease exacerbations requiring increased dosages of prednisolone was also significantly reduced. A second trial[44] addressed the possible glucocorticoid-sparing effects of concomitant cyclosporine therapy in 39 oral glucocorticoid-dependent asthmatic patients established on maintenance dosages of glucocorticoid at the minimum level required to maintain disease stability. After a run-in period, patients were then randomized to receive cyclosporine (5 mg/kg/d initially) or identical placebo for 36 weeks in a parallel group design. Attempts were made to reduce prednisolone dosages at 14-day intervals if the patients' asthma had been stable or had improved as judged by diary card symptom scores and measurement of lung function. Concomitant therapy with cyclosporine allowed a reduction in the median dosage of prednisolone of 62% (10 to 3.5 mg) as compared with only a 25% reduction (10 to 7.5 mg) in the patients treated with placebo. Despite this reduction in oral prednisolone dosage, mean morning PEF values significantly increased in the patients treated with cyclosporine by a mean of 9.4%, compared with no significant change in the group taking placebo. A third study[45] of similar design and duration to this second study showed only a trend for reduction of oral glucocorticoid dosages that was not significantly different from placebo, without change in lung function.

In addition to the results of these trials, cyclosporine has been shown in a double-blind, placebo-controlled study[46] to reduce the late-phase bronchoconstrictor response to bronchial allergen challenge of atopic asthmatic patients, which is widely regarded as a clinical model of asthma, and in an open study,[47] to reduce bronchial hyper-responsiveness and peripheral blood T cell activation in asthmatic patients. Further evidence supporting the hypothesis that cyclosporine exerts these effects in asthmatic patients through inhibition of T cell activation and cytokine production has been provided by the observations[48,49] that cyclosporine therapy of these patients is accompanied by a reduction in serum concentrations of soluble CD25 (a product of proliferating T cells) in vivo, and that cyclosporine inhibits IL-5 production by activated T cells from asthmatic patients in vitro. Nevertheless, it remains possible that some of the additional described activities of cyclosporine, such as its ability to inhibit mast cell degranulation, may also be relevant to an antiasthma effect.

Well-described unwanted effects of low-dosage cyclosporine therapy, evident in the aforementioned trials, include hypertension and renal impairment, although, in contrast to higher-dosage therapy used for prevention of allograft rejection, the risks of these effects are now considered to be very low.[50] Other minor unwanted effects, which may nevertheless not be trivial in individual patients, include hepatic dysfunction, hypertrichosis, tremor, gingival hyperplasia, and paresthesia. Lymphoproliferative disorders and serious opportunistic infections appear to be very uncommon.

In summary, these studies suggest that cyclosporine therapy is effective in only a proportion of chronic, severe, oral glucocorticoid–sensitive asthmatic patients, where it may improve disease severity and/or enable reductions in dosages of maintenance oral glucocorticoids (Level IB). It may be particularly beneficial in glucocorticoid-resistant asthmatic patients,[2] since T cells from these patients have been shown to be relatively resistant to the inhibitory effects of glucocorticoids at therapeutic concentrations in vitro, whereas cyclosporine inhibits T cells from both glucocorticoid-sensitive and -resistant asthmatic patients with equivalent potency at therapeutic concentrations.[51,52] Cyclosporine therapy should probably be assessed for at least 3 months, after which it maybe continued if effective. Regular monitoring of renal function, blood pressure, and whole blood trough concentrations of cyclosporine is currently required, although recent trials in dermatologic diseases suggest that cyclosporine may be effective at even lower dosages, and, for these, routine monitoring of whole blood concentrations may not be necessary.

Intravenous Immunoglobulin Therapy

Therapy with pooled intravenous immunoglobulin (IVIG), originally designed to restore immune deficiency, also appears to have therapeutic effects in diseases involving immune effector mechanisms, most notably "autoimmune" diseases such as thrombocytopenia. Intravenous immunoglobulin therapy is currently being evaluated for a possible therapeutic benefit in many other such diseases, including rheumatoid arthritis, systemic lupus erythematosus, systemic vasculitis, and myasthenia gravis.

The possible efficacy of IVIG therapy for asthma has been investigated in open-label, uncontrolled studies. In one of these,[53] eight children who required continuous systemic glucocorticoid therapy for asthma control were treated with IVIG 1 g/kg as a 6% solution on 2 consecutive days monthly for a total of 6 months (7 infusions). Therapy allowed mean alternate-day prednisone dosages, which were claimed to be the lowest possible for stable maintenance, to be reduced from 32.5 mg to 11.5 mg. Lung function and provocative concentration of methacholine required to reduce baseline FEV_1 by 20% (PC_{20}) did not change significantly, although diary symptom scores and β_2-agonist use were significantly reduced. A second open study of similar design[54] involving 11 adolescents and adults with severe, glucocorticoid-dependent asthma also suggested a glucocorticoid-sparing effect of IVIG therapy along with improvement in lung function and symptoms. Less favorable conclusions were reached in a third study[55] involving 14 adolescents requiring inhaled glucocorticoids (400 to 2,000 µg daily) to keep them "almost free from symptoms" (ie, requiring no more than two dosages of inhaled β_2-agonist daily). Owing to ethical constraints, the children were offered IVIG therapy or entry to an untreated "reference" group in an open fashion. Nine patients choosing therapy were commenced on IVIG at an intended dosage of 1 g/kg on a single day monthly for 5 months. In the event, this dosage had to be decreased to 0.5 g/kg after the first infusion, because it caused severe headache, and then progressively increased (mean dosage 0.8 g/kg). Even at these lower dosages, infusions were frequently accompanied by fever and rigors. During the infusion period, 6 patients were able to reduce dosages of inhaled glucocorticoid (mean 720 to 400 µg daily), whereas 3 were not. Histamine bronchial reactivity was also reduced (mean PC_{20} 0.33 to 1.23 mg/mL), as were total symptom scores. These differences, by comparison with the "reference" group, were not maintained after 10 additional months of follow-up. Two double-blind, placebo-controlled studies of IVIG therapy in severe childhood asthma[56,57] failed to show any benefit of IVIG over placebo in terms of changes in symptoms and lung function, although both trials involved therapy of relatively short duration, and in neither study was a possible glucocorticoid-sparing effect of therapy addressed.

The possible mechanisms by which IVIG therapy could exert a beneficial effect in asthma are not clear. Some of the benefits may result from immunoglobulin replacement itself, since a proportion of chronic asthmatic patients have depressed serum IgG concentrations, possibly at least partly as a result of protracted systemic glucocorticoid therapy,[58] although there is little evidence that this results in defective humoral immunity.[59] Additionally, it has been postulated[53] that IVIG therapy might represent a form of passive immunotherapy, interfering with IgE-mediated reactions. In support of this, IVIG therapy of atopic asthmatic patients was associated with reduced immediate skin-prick test reactivity to a variety of allergens,[53] although this was not accompanied by RAST inhibition in vitro. The mechanism of this phenomenon, as well as its possible relevance to amelioration of asthma, remains therefore obscure. Intravenous immunoglobulin has been shown to abrogate activation of both T and B cells in vitro.[60,61] Furthermore, soluble CD4, CD8, and human leukocyte antigen (HLA) molecules have been identified in IVIG preparations,[62] and may act to inhibit presentation of antigen to T cells.

In summary, although several open studies have suggested that IVIG therapy may improve symptoms in glucocorticoid-dependent asthmatic patients, this has not been verified in controlled studies, which unfortunately have been of short duration and have not addressed a possible glucocorticoid-sparing effect of therapy. Intravenous immunoglobulin therapy is expensive and is associated with a high incidence of unpleasant urticarial and anaphylactic reactions, as well as fever and aseptic meningitis. It is difficult to recommend its usage for asthma on the basis of existing clinical trial evidence, although it is fair to say that such trials have not entirely ruled out a possible beneficial effect (Level ID).

Summary

Although immunosuppressive therapy appears to be of some benefit to a subgroup of chronic, severe, glucocorticoid-dependent asthmatic patients, many reservations remain about the use of currently available drugs in this clinical situation. The unwanted effects of specific drugs, while potentially acceptable in certain patients, are certainly not trivial. In view of these unwanted effects, it is not yet clear whether treatment of patients with any of these drugs will afford them a better overall benefit:risk ratio for therapy of their asthma in the long term, even if they are able to reduce their dosages of oral glucocorticoids.

Another problem is related to the fact that only a proportion of asthmatic patients appear to show a clinically favorable response to additional immunosuppressive therapy. This inevitably means that patients must be given a trial of therapy of sufficient dosage and duration to clearly confirm or exclude a beneficial clinical effect. So far, it has not been possible to identify cyclosporine-responsive patients a priori by clinical and demographic data[43] or by laboratory tests.[63] In patients who do not respond to immunosuppressive therapy, the benefit:risk ratio associated with its addition must inevitably be poorer.

Further to these problems, there is a clear risk of opportunistic infection in asthmatic patients treated with oral glucocorticoids and additional immunosuppressive agents. There remains also a small but definite increased risk of neoplasia. Patients who are pregnant or at risk of pregnancy may not be treated with immunosuppressive therapy, and there are specific contraindications to therapy according to the particular immunosuppressive drug employed.

In view of all these observations, it is clear that any further investigation of immunosuppressive therapy for asthma should be performed within the confines of a controlled trial. There is an urgent need to produce a global definition of precisely which patients are suitable for such trials and what constitutes an appropriate trial of therapy. Finally, nothing is known about the long-term efficacy of immunosuppressive therapy in asthma. Alterations in such efficacy could change the benefit:risk ratio for individual patients with time.

The possibility of topical immunosuppressive therapy for asthma remains an intriguing one. For example, it would appear highly desirable for cyclosporine therapy to be administered topically, and indeed preliminary studies investigating this possibility in patients having received lung transplants have appeared in the literature. There are considerable technical problems associated with this technology, since cyclosporine is highly insoluble in aqueous media, but it may be possible to overcome this problem.[64]

NEWER IMMUNOSUPPRESSIVE AGENTS

FK506 (tacrolimus) is a macrolide derived from the soil organism *Streptomyces tsukudaiensis* that, despite having a different structure to cyclosporine, has similar immunosuppressive properties, although it is more potent. Like cyclosporine, tacrolimus binds to a ubiquitous cytoplasmic protein called FK binding protein (FKBP), which has PPIase activity.[39] The tacrolimus-FKBP complex also binds to calcineurin, inhibiting its serine/threonine phosphatase activity and thus NF-AT translocation. Therefore, like cyclosporine, it inhibits the production of asthma-relevant cytokines such as IL-5[49] as well as IgE-mediated release of mediators from mast cells and basophils. Tacrolimus is being evaluated for prevention of rejection of allografts, but its increased potency may be outweighed by similarly increased toxicity.

Rapamycin (sirolimus) is also a macrolide derived from *Streptomyces hygroscopicus*. It competes with tacrolimus for binding to FKBP. Despite this, sirolimus has a fundamentally different mechanism of action from cyclosporine and tacrolimus[65] and, unlike cyclosporine, is effective even when added late after T cellular activation. Sirolimus inhibits calcium-independent cell signaling pathways that result from binding of cytokine receptors on the surface of T cells to their specific ligands. In particular, sirolimus inhibits the T cell signal transduction pathway following binding of IL-2 to its surface receptor. It probably acts by inhibiting phosphorylation/activation of the kinase p70 S6 (p70S6k) and by inhibiting the enzymatic activity of the cyclin-dependent kinase cdk2–cyclin E complex. Thus, sirolimus impedes progression through the G1/S transition of the T cell proliferation cycle, resulting in a mid-to-late G1 arrest.[65]

Other new immunosuppressive drugs, the antiproliferative actions of which are relatively specific for T cells, continue to appear. Brequinar sodium and mycophenolate mofetil are inhibitors of de novo synthesis of pyrimidines and purines, respectively, and their actions are particularly marked on T cells. Mycophenolate mofetil has already undergone promising assessment as a therapy for allograft rejection. Like cyclosporine, pharmacologic concentrations of both rapamycin and mycophenolate mofetil have been shown to inhibit the proliferation of T cells from glucocorticoid-resistant asthmatic patients whose T cells are resistant to inhibition by therapeutic concentrations of glucocorticoids in vitro,[52,66] although it remains to be seen whether these drugs will inhibit the local production of asthma-relevant cytokines. Other drugs with T cell antiproliferative activity include leflunomide and the napthopyrans.

HUMANIZED ANTIBODIES

Modern genetic manipulation techniques have facilitated the construction and bulk production of chimeric antibodies composed of constant regions similar or identical in structure to that of human IgG and variable regions raised in animals against specific ligands. Such antibodies offer the opportunity for highly targeted therapeutic intervention and are generally well tolerated since their immunogenicity is low. Chimeric mouse/human anti-IgE antibodies, which inhibit binding of IgE to its high-affinity receptor (FcεRI) on mast cells and basophils without cross-linking bound IgE, are now undergoing clinical trials. Parenteral administration of these antibodies results in medium term (3 to 30 days) falls in circulating IgE concentrations in atopic subjects along with reduced sensitivity of the nose and bronchus to allergen provocation.[67] It remains to be seen whether this approach will be effective for the therapy of chronic asthma.

Another recent approach has been the development of a humanized primate/human anti-CD4 chimeric antibody that, in a preliminary controlled trial, has been shown transiently and specifically to reduce circulating numbers of peripheral blood CD4 T cells and to improve lung function and reduce symptoms in a group of chronic, severe asthmatic patients.[68] It seems likely that a range of such monoclonal antibodies with more restricted target specificity (eg, anti-IL-5 antibodies) will appear and undergo assessment in the near future for their possible benefits in asthma therapy.

CONCLUSION

In view of the evidence that activated T cells and their cytokine products play a fundamental role in asthma pathogenesis, it is likely that T cell inhibition will continue to form one fundamental basis of antiasthma therapy. Glucocorticoids appear to act at least partly through this mechanism and are effective for the therapy of a majority of asthmatic patients with a favourable benefit:risk ratio. New approaches to therapy are still urgently required for those patients who continue to have severe disease despite optimized delivery of inhaled and systemic glucocorticoid and minimization of exacerbating factors. In these patients, the potential hazards of continuous oral glucocorticoid therapy remain a cause for grave concern.

Unfortunately, none of the alternative therapies so far assessed in this category of patients has yet emerged as clearly beneficial in terms of improving the long-term benefit:risk ratio of therapy. Systematized approaches to the assessment of the possible value of these drugs are required. Other, possibly more promising, approaches for the future include topical delivery of immunosuppressive drugs, the use of humanized monoclonal antibodies directed against T cells and key cytokines or their receptors, and small-molecule antagonists of cytokines or other key steps in the asthma inflammatory process.

REFERENCES

1.   Woolcock AJ. Steroid resistant asthma: what is the clinical definition? Eur Respir J 1993;6:743–7.

2.   Corrigan CJ, Brown P, Barnes NC, et al. Glucocorticoid resistance in chronic asthma. Glucocorticoid pharmacokinetics, receptor characteristics, and inhibition of peripheral blood T cell proliferation by glucocorticoids in vitro. Am Rev Respir Dis 1991;144:1016–25.

3.   Corrigan CJ, Haczku A, Gemou-Engesaeth V, et al. CD4 T lymphocyte activation in asthma is accompanied by increased serum concentrations of interleukin-5: effect of glucocorticoid therapy. Am Rev Respir Dis 1993;147:540–7.

4. Doi S, Gemou-Engesaeth V, Kay AB, Corrigan CJ. Polymerase chain reaction quantification of cytokine messenger RNA expression in peripheral blood mononuclear cells of patients with severe asthma: effect of glucocorticoid therapy. Clin Exp Allergy 1994;24:854–67.

5. Corrigan CJ, Hamid Q, North J, et al. Peripheral blood CD4, but not CD8 T lymphocytes in patients with exacerbation of asthma transcribe and translate messenger RNA encoding cytokines which prolong eosinophil survival in the context of a Th2-type pattern: effect of glucocorticoid therapy. Am J Respir Cell Mol Biol 1995;12:567–78.

6. Lynch JP, McCune WJ. Immunosuppressive and cytotoxic pharmacotherapy for pulmonary disorders. Am J Respir Crit Care Med 1997;155:395–420.

7. Hodges NG, Brewis RAL, Howell JBL. An evaluation of azathioprine in severe chronic asthma. Thorax 1971;26:734–9.

8. Arkins JA, Hirsch SR. Clinical effectiveness of 6-mercaptopurine in bronchial asthma. J Allergy 1966;37:90–5.

9. Asmundsson T, Kilburn KH, Laszlo J, Krock CJ. Immunosuppressive therapy of asthma. J Allergy 1971;47:136–47.

10. Suzuki S, Okubo M, Kaise S, et al. Gold sodium thiomalate selectively inhibits interleukin-5 mediated eosinophil survival. J Allergy Clin Immunol 1995;96:251–6.

11. Marone G, Columbo M, Galeone D, et al. Modulation of the release of histamine and arachidonic acid metabolites from human basophils and mast cells by auranofin. Agents Actions 1986;18:100–2.

12. Parente JE, Wong K, Davis P, et al. Effects of gold compounds on leukotriene B_4, leukotriene C_4 and prostaglandin E_2 production by polymorphonuclear leukocytes. J Rheumatol 1986;13:47–51.

13. Muranaka M, Miyamoto T, Shida T, et al. Gold salt in the treatment of bronchial asthma: a double blind study. Ann Allergy 1978;40:132–7.

14. Klaustermeyer WB, Noritake DT, Kwong FK. Chrysotherapy in the treatment of corticosteroid-dependent asthma. J Allergy Clin Immunol 1987;79:720–5.

15. Nierop G, Gijzel WP, Bel EH, et al. Auranofin in the treatment of steroid dependent asthma: a double blind study. Thorax 1992;47:349–54.

16. Bernstein IL, Bernstein DI, Dubb JW, et al. A placebo-controlled multicenter study of auranofin in the treatment of patients with corticosteroid-dependent asthma. Auranofin Multicenter Drug Trial. J Allergy Clin Immunol 1996;98:317–24.

17. Tomioka H, King TE. Gold-induced pulmonary disease: clinical features, outcome, and differentiation from rheumatoid lung disease. Am J Respir Crit Care Med 1997;155:1011–20.

18. Bernstein IL, Bernstein DI, Bernstein JA. How does auranofin compare with methotrexate and cyclosporin as a corticosteroid-sparing agent in severe asthma? Biodrugs 1997;8:205–15.

19. Kremer JM. The mechanism of action of methotrexate in rheumatoid arthritis: the search continues. J Rheumatol 1994;21:1–5.

20. Olsen NJ, Murray LM. Anti-proliferative effect of methotrexate on peripheral blood mononuclear cells. Arthritis Rheum 1989;32:378–85.

21. Cronstein BN. Methotrexate and its mechanism of action. Arthritis Rheum 1996;39:1951–60.

22. Mullarkey MF, Lammert JK, Blumenstein BA. Long-term methotrexate treatment in corticosteroid-dependent asthma. Ann Intern Med 1990;112:577–81.

23. Shiner RJ, Nunn AJ, Chung KF, Geddes DM. Randomised, double-blind, placebo-controlled trial of methotrexate in steroid-dependent asthma. Lancet 1990;336:137–40.

24. Dyer PD, Vaughan TR, Weber RW. Methotrexate in the treatment of steroid-dependent asthma. J Allergy Clin Immunol 1991;88:208–12.

25. Stewart GE, Diaz JD, Lockey RF, et al. Comparison of oral pulse methotrexate with placebo in the treatment of severe glucocorticosteroid-dependent asthma. J Allergy Clin Immunol 1994;94:482–9.

26. Hedman J, Seideman P, Albertioni F, Stenius-Aarniala B. Controlled trial of methotrexate in patients with severe chronic asthma. Eur J Clin Pharmacol 1996;49:347–9.

27. Coffey MJ, Sanders G, Eschenbacher WL, et al. The role of methotrexate in the management of steroid-dependent asthma. Chest 1994;105:117–21.

28. Trigg CJ, Davies RJ. Comparison of methotrexate 30 mg per week with placebo in chronic steroid-dependent asthma: a 12 week double-blind, cross-over study. Respir Med 1993;87:211–6.

29. Taylor DR, Flannery EM, Herbison GP. Methotrexate in the management of severe steroid dependent asthma. N Z Med J 1993;106:409–11.

30. Erzurum SC, Leff JA, Cochran JE, et al. Lack of benefit of methotrexate in severe, steroid-dependent asthma. A double-blind, placebo-controlled study. Ann Intern Med 1991;114:353–60.

31. Aaron SD, Dales RE, Pham B. Management of steroid-dependent asthma with methotrexate: a meta-analysis of randomised clinical trials. Respir Med 1998;92:1059–65.

32. Marin MG. Low-dose methotrexate spares steroid usage in steroid-dependent chronic asthmatic patients: a meta-analysis. Chest 1997;112:29–33.

33. Lewis JH, Schiff E. Methotrexate-induced chronic liver injury: guidelines for detection and prevention. The ACG Committee on FDA-related matters. Am J Gastroenterol 1988;83:1337–45.

34. Kremer JM, Alarcon GS, Lightfoot RW, et al. Methotrexate for rheumatoid arthritis. Suggested guidelines for monitoring liver toxicity. Arthritis Rheum 1994;37:316–28.

35. Morice AH, Lai WK. Fatal varicella zoster infection in a severe steroid dependent asthmatic patient receiving methotrexate. Thorax 1995;50:1221–2.

36. Gatnash AA, Connolly CK. Fatal chickenpox pneumonia in an asthmatic patient on oral corticosteroids and methotrexate. Thorax 1995;50:422–3.

37. Tsai JJ, Shin JF, Chen CH, Wang SR. Methotrexate pneumonitis in bronchial asthma. Int Arch Allergy Immunol 1993;100:287–90.

38. Jones G, Mierins E, Karsh J. Methotrexate-induced asthma. Am Rev Respir Dis 1991;143:179–81.

39. Schreiber SL, Crabtree GR. The mechanism of action of cyclosporin A and FK506. Immunol Today 1992;13:136–42.

40. Triggiani M, Cirillo R, Lichtenstein LM, Marone G. Inhibition of histamine and prostaglandin D_2 release from human lung mast cells by cyclosporin A. Int Arch Allergy Appl Immunol 1989;88:253–5.

41. Cirillo R, Triggiani M, Siri L, et al. Cyclosporin A rapidly inhibits mediator release from human basophils presumably by interacting with cyclophilin. J Immunol 1990;144:3891–7.

42. Kita H, Ohnishi T, Okubo Y, et al. Granulocyte/macrophage colony stimulating factor and interleukin 3 release from human peripheral blood eosinophils and neutrophils. J Exp Med 1991;174:745–8.

43. Alexander AG, Barnes NC, Kay AB. Trial of cyclosporin in corticosteroid-dependent chronic severe asthma. Lancet 1992;339:324–8.

44. Lock SH, Kay AB, Barnes NC. Double-blind, placebo-controlled study of cyclosporin A as a corticosteroid-sparing agent in corticosteroid-dependent asthma. Am J Respir Crit Care Med 1993;153:509–14.

45. Nizankowska E, Soja J, Pinis G, et al. Treatment of steroid-dependent bronchial asthma with cyclosporin. Eur Respir J 1995;8:1091–9.

46. Sihra BS, Kon OM, Durham SR, et al. Effect of cyclosporin A on the allergen-induced late asthmatic reaction. Thorax 1997;52:447–52.

47. Fukuda T, Asakawa J, Motojima S, Makino S. Cyclosporin A reduces T lymphocyte activity and improves airway hyperresponsiveness in corticosteroid-dependent chronic severe asthma. Ann Allergy Asthma Immunol 1995;75:65–72.

48. Alexander AG, Barnes NC, Kay AB, Corrigan CJ. Clinical response to cyclosporin in chronic severe asthma is associated with reduction in serum soluble interleukin-2 receptor concentrations. Eur Respir J 1995;8:574–8.

49. Mori A, Suko M, Nishizaki Y, et al. IL-5 production by CD4+ T cells of asthmatic patients is suppressed by glucocorticoids and the immunosuppressants FK506 and cyclosporin A. Int Immunol 1995;7:449–57.

50. Rodriguez F, Krayenbuhl JC, Harrison WB, et al. Renal biopsy findings and follow up of renal function in rheumatoid arthritis patients treated with cyclosporin A. Arthritis Rheum 1996;39:1491–8.

51. Corrigan CJ, Brown PH, Barnes NC, et al. Glucocorticoid resistance in chronic asthma. Peripheral blood T lymphocyte activation and comparison of the T lymphocyte inhibitory effects of glucocorticoids and cyclosporin A. Am Rev Respir Dis 1991;144:1026–32.

52. Haczku A, Alexander A, Brown P, et al. The effect of dexamethasone, cyclosporin and rapamycin on T lymphocyte proliferation in vitro: comparison of cells from patients with glucocorticoid-sensitive and glucocorticoid-resistant chronic asthma. J Allergy Clin Immunol 1994;93:510–9.

53. Mazer BD, Gelfand EW. An open-label study of high-dose intravenous immunoglobulin in severe childhood asthma. J Allergy Clin Immunol 1991;87:976–83.

54. Landwehr LP, Jeppson JD, Katlan MG, et al. Benefits of high-dose IV immunoglobulin in patients with severe steroid-dependent asthma. Chest 1998;114:1349–56.

55. Jakobsson T, Croner S, Kjellman N-IM, et al. Slight steroid-sparing effect of intravenous immunoglobulin in children and adolescents with moderately severe bronchial asthma. Allergy 1994;49:413–20.

56. Niggemann B, Leupold W, Schuster A, et al. Prospective, double-blind, placebo-controlled, multicentre study on the effect of high-dose intravenous immunoglobulin in children and adolescents with severe bronchial asthma. Clin Exp Allergy 1998;28:205–10.

57. Abernathy RS, Strem EL, Good RA. Chronic asthma in childhood: double-blind controlled study of treatment with gamma-globulin. Pediatrics 1958;21:980–93.

58. Ayres JG, Thompson RA. Low IgG subclass levels in brittle asthma and patients with exacerbations of asthma associated with respiratory infection. Respir Med 1997;91:464–9.

59. Lack G, Ochs HD, Gelfand EW. Humoral immunity in steroid-dependent children with asthma and hypogammaglobulinaemia. J Pediatr 1996;129:898–903.

60. Stohl W. Cellular mechanisms in the in vitro inhibition of pokeweed mitogen-induced B cell differentiation by immunoglobulin for intravenous use. J Immunol 1986;126:4407–13.

61. Kawada K, Terasaki PI. Evidence for immunosuppression by high-dose gamma globulin. Exp Hematol 1987;15:133–6.

62. Blasczyk R, Westhoff U, Grosse-Wilde M. Soluble CD4, CD8 and HLA molecules in commercial immunoglobulin preparations. Lancet 1993;341:789–90.

63. Alexander AG, Barnes NC, Kay AB, Corrigan CJ. Can clinical response to cyclosporin in chronic severe asthma be predicted by an in vitro T-lymphocyte proliferation assay? Eur Respir J 1996;9:1421–6.

64. Waldrep JC. New aerosol drug delivery systems for the treatment of immune-mediated pulmonary diseases. Drugs Today 1998;34:549–61.

65. Dumont FJ, Su Q. Mechanism of action of the immunosuppressant rapamycin. Life Science 1995;58:373–95.

66. Corrigan CJ, Bungre JK, Assoufi B, et al. Intracellular steroid metabolism and relative sensitivity to glucocorticoids and immunosuppressive agents of T lymphocytes from glucocorticoid sensitive and resistant asthmatic patients. Eur Respir J 1996;9:2077–86.

67. Fahy JV, Fleming HE, Wong HH, et al. The effect of an anti-IgE monoclonal antibody on the early- and late-phase responses to allergen inhalation in asthmatic subjects. Am J Respir Crit Care Med 1997;155:1828–34.

68. Kon OM, Sihra BS, Compton CH, et al. Randomised, dose-ranging, placebo-controlled study of chimeric anti-CD4 (keliximab) in chronic severe asthma. Lancet 1998;352:1109–13.

CHAPTER 19

Exercise-Induced Bronchoconstriction

Mark D. Inman, MD, PhD

Exercise-induced bronchoconstriction (EIB) is a common clinical manifestation of asthma, occurring in 70 to 80% of asthmatic patients. The bronchoconstriction associated with exercise is often referred to as "exercise-induced asthma"; however, this is a misnomer, as exercise, unlike allergen inhalation, does not cause asthma, but rather causes bronchoconstriction in patients with asthma. The term "exercise-induced asthma" should be avoided to reduce the belief, often held by parents of asthmatic children, that exercise will worsen their child's asthma. Moreover, with correct management, exercise-induced bronchoconstriction can be prevented or markedly reduced in almost all cases. This means that exercise should not be avoided by asthmatic patients.

DOES EXERCISE MAKE ASTHMA WORSE?

One of the major developments in the understanding of asthma in the past 20 years is the recognition that differences in disease severity between patients, as well fluctuations in the severity of the disease within individual patients, are associated with varying degrees of airway inflammation, typically involving increases in airway eosinophils, neutrophils, mast cells, lymphocytes, and several inflammatory mediators including interleukin-5 (IL-5) and granulocyte-macrophage colony–stimulating factor (GM-CSF).[1,2] It has further been observed that structural changes in the airway including increased numbers of myofibroblasts, collagen deposition, and subepithelial fibrosis are a prominent feature of the asthmatic airway.[3] There is concern that these structural changes represent a permanent remodeling of the airway in response to repeated inflammatory and repair processes, and may result in permanent physiologic dysfunction of the airway.[4] As a result of this increased understanding, it is now clear that the management of asthma should be aimed at minimizing even minor inflammatory insults to the airway, both through effective anti-inflammatory treatment and, more importantly, through the avoidance of exacerbating events. This approach should not only reduce symptoms but may also favorably influence the natural progression of the disease.

Whether exercise produces inflammatory changes in the asthmatic airway has been a matter of debate for several years. Given the recent advances in our understanding of the pathophysiology of asthma, the answer to this question could have major implications in the management of the asthmatic patient with EIB. Clearly, if exercise produces repeated inflammatory and repair processes in the airway, then it may ultimately worsen the natural progression of the disease. If, on the other hand, exercise is simply an indirect means of stimulating bronchoconstriction, then it should be safe for asthmatic patients to exercise regularly, provided adequate symptomatic relief is available and the underlying inflammatory component of their disease is optimally managed. This issue has been addressed in studies in which exercise challenges have been performed in association with direct evaluation of inflammation, late asthmatic responses, and changes in airway responsiveness.

Is EIB Associated with Worsened Airway Inflammation?

There have been a few investigations of changes in inflammatory indices in the airway in response to exercise. Several of these studies are flawed due to a lack of relevant controls. As it is known that asthmatic patients can display diurnal variation in several inflammatory indices,[5] it is crucial that control measurements be made at the same time of day as those following exercise. Crimi et al have performed bronchoalveolar lavage (BAL) 3 hours following exercise challenge and at the same time following a methacholine challenge. The mean percent of fall in forced expiratory volume in 1 second (FEV_1) was 28.0 following both challenges. These authors observed a small but significantly higher percentage of eosinophils following exercise (median values 1.0% vs 2.5%) (Level I).[6] Tateishi et al have compared inflammatory indices before and following both allergen and exercise challenges without measurements on a control day.[7] In this study, allergen but not exercise was associated with increases in sputum epithelial cells, eosinophils, and eosinophilic cationic protein (ECP). In the most extensive and well-controlled investigation of airway inflammation following exercise, Jarjour and Calhoun performed BAL at 1 and 24 hours after exercise challenges where there was a mean fall in FEV_1 of 41%.[8] Control lavages were performed on a separate day at the same times. In this study with marked bronchoconstriction following exercise, there were no associated changes in BAL levels of eosinophils, neutrophils, macrophages, lymphocytes (CD4+, CD8+, and total), or in oxygen radical levels either immediately following, or the day after, exercise (Level I).

Is EIB Associated with a Late Response?

When sensitized asthmatic patients are challenged with allergen, there is usually an immediate bronchoconstrictor response, which is often followed 4 to 8 hours later by a late bronchoconstrictor response. This late response is associated with airway inflammation, including increases in eosinophils, neutrophils, lymphocytes, and several inflammatory mediators.[2,9] Several studies have reported that exercise challenge of asthmatic patients can also result in a late asthmatic response.[6,10] The association between allergen-induced late responses and airway inflammation could be interpreted as evidence that exercise is also a trigger of airway inflammation. However, as with measures of inflammation, it is crucial that studies of late responses following exercise be appropriately controlled. For example, in one of the studies reporting a late response following exercise, the late fall in FEV_1 was actually no different than the late fall following a methacholine challenge in the same subjects and, therefore, likely reflected diurnal variation.[6] Recent well-controlled studies have found no evidence of late responses following exercise in children[11] or adults,[12] and, therefore, do not provide evidence for inflammatory changes in the airway following exercise (Level I).

Is EIB Associated with Worsened Airway Hyper-responsiveness?

While a large component of airway hyper-responsiveness in asthma appears to be irreversible, there is a component that fluctuates in response to acute changes in airway inflammation. One would expect, therefore, that putative inflammatory changes associated with exercise would be reflected by increased airway responsiveness to nonspecific bronchoconstricting mediators. Tateishi et al have recently shown that an increase in airway hyper-responsiveness to methacholine occurs following allergen challenge but not following exercise challenge, although the degree of bronchoconstriction associated with each challenge was similar (Level II).[7] In a similar study, EIB did not result in a change in airway responsiveness to histamine in 26 asthmatic children (Level II).[13]

Taken together, these studies indicate that there is no strong evidence to suggest that exercise-induced bronchoconstriction is associated with significant changes in airway inflammation or worsening of asthma. These findings support the concept that exercise is a nonspecific means for triggering bronchoconstriction in the asthmatic airway when there is a background of inflammation and airway hyper-responsiveness. A schematic representation of this view is presented in Figure 19–1. Thus, there is no basis for recommending exercise avoidance by patients suffering from EIB (Level IE).

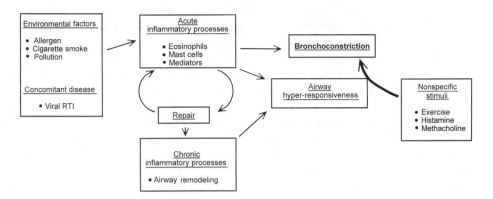

Figure 19–1 Schematic illustration of the role of exercise in asthma. Available evidence suggests that acute and chronic inflammatory processes in the asthmatic airway produce a level of hyper-responsiveness, such that nonspecific challenges including exercise result in a degree of broncho-constriction not seen in normal individuals. Exercise itself does not appear to worsen airway inflammation or airway responsiveness.

TREATMENT OPTIONS

The first treatment options considered in the management of a patient with EIB as a manifestation of their asthma should be the same as in any other asthmatic patient. As is reflected in most treatment guidelines, management of asthma should be aimed at reducing the degree of airway inflammation, with resulting decreases in the morbidity associated with the disease. This recommendation also should apply to the management of EIB. It is quite common, however, for EIB to persist despite otherwise good control of asthma symptoms in patients treated with anti-inflammatory agents. For this reason, the use of bronchodilating or bronchoprotecting agents is common in asthmatic patients with EIB. Discussion in the following sections will focus on the effects of inhaled corticosteroids, which can substantially attenuate EIB when used to control asthma; the additional benefit that can be obtained from agents including inhaled β_2-agonists, antileukotrienes, inhaled cromones, anticholinergic compounds, and antihistamines; and, finally, benefits that can result from nonpharmacologic interventions. Fortunately, well-controlled trials have been performed using all of these treatment options.

Corticosteroids

When treating patients with EIB, the primary concern should be appropriate management of the underlying asthma, rather than simply relief from the symptoms of EIB. Almost all patients with EIB will have moderate to severe airway hyper-responsiveness,[14] and the severity of EIB has recently been significantly correlated with the extent of eosinophilia measured in induced sputum.[15] Therefore, it is not surprising that inhaled corticosteroids, which reduce airway inflammation[16] and airway hyper-responsiveness,[17] will reduce, although usually not eliminate, symptoms associated with exercise.

The first investigation of the effects of inhaled corticosteroids on the magnitude of EIB did not observe any benefit from this treatment.[18] However, in this study, 11 subjects were treated with single inhalations of beclomethasone (100 μg) only 20 minutes before exercise. A further study was performed with 6 subjects after treatment with beclomethasone for periods ranging from 1 to 4 weeks, with no difference detected between placebo and treatment arms (Level IC).[18] Since these initial studies, it has been demonstrated that, to have an effect on airway inflammation or airway hyper-responsiveness, treatment with inhaled corticosteroids must persist over a period of weeks to months. Studies with longer treatment periods have demonstrated that the severity of EIB can be reduced by corticosteroid therapy.

Henriksen and Dahl[19] treated 14 children with inhaled budesonide (400 μg/d) for 4 weeks and attenuated the exercise-induced fall in FEV$_1$ by 51% (Level IA). Vathenen et al[20] treated 40 adults with inhaled budesonide (800 μg twice daily) for 6 weeks and attenuated the postexercise fall in FEV$_1$ by 71% (Level IA). In this study, the attenuation of EIB correlated significantly with reductions in histamine airway responsiveness. Henriksen[21] subsequently treated 14 children with budesonide (200 μg twice daily) for 2 weeks and attenuated the postexercise fall in FEV$_1$ by 62% (Level IA). The need for persisting treatment with inhaled corticosteroids was highlighted by Molema et al,[22] who treated 22 young adults with inhaled budesonide (100 μg four times daily) for a total of 6 weeks, performing exercise challenges during an initial placebo treatment period and at 3 and 6 weeks of active treatment. There was significant attenuation of the postexercise fall in FEV$_1$ after 3 weeks of treatment (33% attenuated), with further reduction after 6 weeks of treatment (52% attenuated) (Level IIA). Farrero et al[23] have recently treated 20 children and young adults with inhaled budesonide for 2 months and observed a 75% reduction in the postexercise fall in FEV$_1$ (Level IA). Perhaps the most compelling support for inhaled corticosteroids in the management of EIB was that shown by Pedersen and Hansen,[24] who observed a dose-response effect to increasing doses of budesonide delivered to asthmatic children for 4 weeks prior to exercise. The greatest attenuation relative to placebo in this study was 83%, following 4 weeks of 400 μg/d treatment.

Thus, while single- or short-course treatments with inhaled or oral corticosteroids are not effective in the management of EIB, prolonged treatment of asthmatic patients of all ages with inhaled corticosteroids produces significant and substantial reduction in the magnitude of EIB. In all of these studies in which a range of steroid doses were employed, the attenuation of the postexercise fall in FEV$_1$ exceeded 50% (Figure 19–2). Thus, this compelling evidence points to the early introduction of low doses of inhaled corticosteroids in the management of asthmatic patients affected by symptoms of EIB (Level IA). However, these studies also demonstrated that, in many patients, a component of EIB will persist despite inhaled corticosteroid treatment. Depending on the magnitude of this steroid-resistant bronchoconstriction following exercise, patients may require treatment with one or more of the following agents shown to be effective in attenuating EIB.

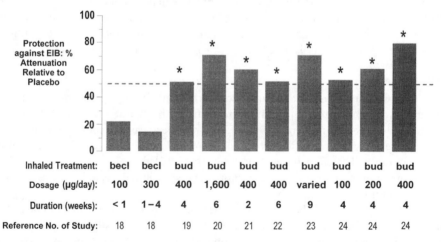

Figure 19–2 The degree of protection afforded against EIB in a number of trials of inhaled corticosteroids. (*Attenuation of postexercise fall in FEV$_1$ exceeds 50%. becl = beclomethasone; bud = budesonide.)

Bronchodilator Therapy: Inhaled β$_2$-Agonists

Inhaled β$_2$-agonists remain the most widely used form of treatment for the prevention of, or relief from, EIB. Rather than acting on specific mediators, these agents act directly on airway smooth muscle, either protecting against bronchoconstriction or reversing existing bronchoconstriction. Recently, the use of the newer long-acting β_2-agonists has been recommended for the treatment of EIB. While both short- and long-acting agents provide excellent protection against EIB, there is currently controversy regarding their use on a regular basis.

Short-Acting β_2-Agonists

When inhaled in the hour before exercise, β_2-agonists produce both bronchodilation before exercise as well as marked attenuation of EIB. In numerous clinical trials with both adult and pediatric populations, the degree of attenuation of the postexercise fall in FEV_1 has ranged from 50 to 100% for inhaled salbutamol (200 µg),[25] terbutaline (500 µg),[26] and fenoterol (50 to 800 µg) (Level I).[27] Another important feature of inhaled β_2-agonist treatment is its ability to reverse EIB when administered after exercise. When eight adults in each of three parallel treatment groups were treated with either inhaled placebo, salbutamol (200 µg on two occasions separated by 5 minutes), or terbutaline (500 µg twice) 10 minutes after exercise, there was 100% reversal of the postexercise fall in peak expiratory flow within 5 minutes of treatment in the salbutamol and terbutaline groups (Level I).[28]

While oral delivery of β_2-agonists is frequently employed in the management of pediatric asthma, this delivery route provides questionable protection against EIB. In doses sufficient to provide significant bronchodilation, oral salbutamol has been shown to provide protection against EIB in some studies[29] but not in others.[25] While an early study of oral terbutaline (5 mg) demonstrated effectiveness compared to placebo for up to 6 hours in the prevention of EIB in 5 adult asthmatic patients,[30] a subsequent study has found no effect relative to placebo of doses ranging from 4 to 12 mg[31] in 17 asthmatic children. Thus, oral β_2-agonists do not provide reliable protection against EIB (Level ID).

The duration of action of inhaled short-acting β_2-agonists is an important concern for the patient, especially in the pediatric population. While the protection from inhaled salbutamol (200 µg),[32] terbutaline (500 µg),[26] and fenoterol (400 to 800 µg)[33] persists for at least 2 hours, this protection is completely lost compared to placebo as early as 3 hours after dosing.[26,32,33] Thus, although short-acting inhaled β_2-agonists provide excellent relief from EIB, this protection cannot be expected to last for more than 2 to 3 hours (Level I). Clearly multiple doses throughout the day would be required by children or individuals who are expected to exercise frequently during a single day. However, this type of repeated dose treatment with inhaled β_2-agonists cannot be recommended for management of EIB. Two studies have observed the effect of regular short-acting β_2-agonists on EIB. Gibson et al[29] demonstrated that treatment of 6 adults with oral salbutamol for 4 to 20 weeks resulted in significant loss of the protective effect from inhaled salbutamol (200 µg) against EIB. In this same study, however, 6 adolescents were treated for similar periods with regular inhaled salbutamol (200 µg four times per day) with no observed loss of protection. We have subsequently demonstrated significant loss of protection against EIB at the end of only 1 week of regular treatment with inhaled salbutamol (200 µg four times daily). In this study, the postexercise FEV_1, both with and without pre-exercise salbutamol, was significantly lower following 1 week of regular inhaled salbutamol (Figure 19–3).[34] Thus, while inhaled β_2-agonists provide excellent protection against EIB, the degree of protection may be attenuated following periods of regular or frequent use (Level ID). If patients who are treated with inhaled corticosteroids are still requiring frequent β_2-agonist use to protect against EIB, a trial with another agent should be considered.

Long-Acting β_2-Agonists

As discussed above, protection against EIB can only be expected to last for 2 to 3 hours after treatment with inhaled short-acting β_2-agonists. In response to this short effective duration, new classes of longer-acting inhaled β_2-agonists have been developed. Treatment with the

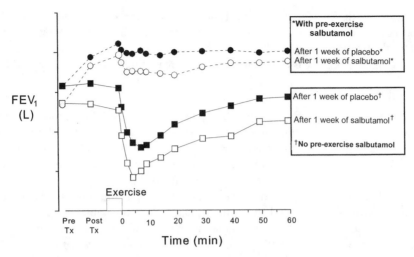

Figure 19–3 Effects of salbutamol treatment on response of FEV₁ following exercise. Regular treatment was with inhaled salbutamol (200 μg four times daily) or placebo for the week before the exercise challenge. Pre-exercise treatment was with inhaled salbutamol (200 μg) or placebo, inhaled
5 minutes before exercise. Postexercise FEV₁ responses with or without pre-exercise salbutamol were
significantly lower when regular salbutamol had been taken during the previous week. (Reproduced
with permission from Inman MD, O'Byrne PM. The effect of regular inhaled salbutamol on exercise-
induced bronchoconstriction. Am J Respir Crit Care Med 1996;153:65–9.)

inhaled long-acting β_2-agonist salmeterol (50 μg) provides almost complete attenuation of EIB
when taken 30 minutes before exercise.[35] Moreover, the degree of attenuation of the postexercise fall in FEV₁ at this dose remains greater than 50% compared to placebo or short-acting
β_2-agonists for at least 12 hours.[35] Also, inhaled formoterol almost completely prevents EIB
when taken 30 minutes before exercise[36] and attenuates at least 50% of the postexercise fall in
FEV₁ compared to placebo or short-acting β_2-agonists at 4 to 12 hours following treatment.[36]
Clearly, these longer-acting agents solve the problem of the short duration of protection
afforded by single doses of salbutamol, terbutaline, or fenoterol (Level I).

However, there is compelling evidence that regular treatment with long-acting β_2-ago-
nists will result in loss of protection. Ramage et al[37] observed the protective effects of a single
dose of salmeterol (50 μg inhaled) on exercise challenges performed 6 and 12 hours later, both
before and at the end of a 4-week period of regular treatment with salmeterol (50 μg twice
daily) in 12 adult asthmatic patients. Before the period of regular treatment, salmeterol attenuated 65% of the postexercise fall in FEV₁, 6 hours after treatment, and 40%, 12 hours after
treatment; both results were significantly different than those with placebo treatment. When
the same treatment and challenges were performed following 4 weeks of regular treatment,
attenuation of both challenges was less than 30% and was not significantly different than
those with placebo treatment. In a similar study, 14 asthmatic children were treated for
4 7weeks with once-daily salmeterol (50 μg inhaled).[38] In this study, following 4 weeks of
treatment, the protective effect of salmeterol was reduced from 67 to 33% and was no longer
different from that of placebo. Furthermore, it has recently been shown that the duration of
protection against EIB afforded by salmeterol inhalation is less at the end of a period of
chronic treatment than after a single dose.[39] While no studies have reported a loss of protective effect against EIB following regular formoterol treatment, diminished protection against
methacholine-induced bronchoconstriction has been reported.[40]

Thus, while long-acting β_2-agonists provide excellent and lasting protection against EIB,
this effect may be reduced following periods of regular treatment. Care must be taken when
using these agents frequently for prevention of symptoms, particularly given that the dose,
frequency, and treatment duration required for loss of protection is not known (Level IB).

Treatment Directed at Bronchoconstrictor Mediators

Cromolyn Sodium

It has been known since 1972 that cromolyn sodium inhaled before exercise substantially attenuates the degree of bronchoconstriction in asthmatic patients.[41,42] While the mechanism of action of cromolyn is not understood, it may involve prevention of bronchoconstricting mediator release from mast cells. Silverman and Turner-Warwick,[42] in the first randomized, placebo-controlled trial, showed that cromolyn (20 mg spinhaler inhaled 10 to 15 minutes before exercise) attenuated the postexercise fall in FEV_1 by 62% (Level I). Since these first studies, the effects of cromolyn, inhaled in various forms, have been studied extensively. In a dose-response study of 11 young adults, it was shown that the maximum degree of protection was 70% attenuation of the postexercise fall in FEV_1 (Level I).[43] This protection was achieved with a dose of 20 mg (aerosolized metered-dose inhaler); less protection (55% attenuation) was achieved at the lower dose of 10 mg. The duration of protection afforded by different doses of cromolyn have also been studied (Level IA).[44] Maximum protection was 75% attenuation of the postexercise fall in FEV_1 and was afforded by 20 mg (metered-dose aerosol) inhaled 15 minutes before exercise. In the same study, there was still 64% attenuation of the postexercise fall in FEV_1 when 20 mg of cromolyn was inhaled 4 hours before exercise. Smaller degrees and durations of protection against EIB were afforded by lower doses. Thus, there is strong evidence that cromolyn provides considerable protection against EIB, provided it is taken shortly prior to exercise (Level I).

It is quite common to treat patients with combinations of cromolyn and β_2-agonists in the management of EIB. Support for this practice can be found in a study in which terbutaline sulfate (1,000 μg) and cromolyn (20 mg aerosol) were inhaled either alone or in combination 20 minutes prior to isocapnic hyperventilation and were found to have additive protective properties.[45] In an attempt to reproduce these findings during exercise, Woolley et al[26] treated patients with terbutaline sulfate (500 μg) and cromolyn (2 mg aerosol) alone or in combination at several times before exercise. These authors did not observe any additive protection from the combination of the two agents. However, the dose of cromolyn in this study was only 2 mg which is suboptimal,[43,44] as is demonstrated by the attenuation of only 24% of the postexercise fall in FEV_1 when 2 mg cromolyn was used alone in this study.[26] Thus, available evidence does not support this form of combination therapy, although there may be patients who would derive some benefit (Level IC).

Nedocromil

Nedocromil, inhaled before exercise, has been shown to attenuate the magnitude and duration of EIB. Inhalation of a range of concentrations of nebulized nedocromil (0.5 to 20 mg/mL) as well as 4 mg of aerosolized nedocromil offered similar degrees of attenuation of the postexercise fall in FEV_1 (50 to 62%) (Level I).[46] While nedocromil offers protection against EIB, there is no evidence that this protection is any greater than that provided by cromolyn. In direct comparisons of these agents, there has been no advantage in terms of the degree of protection against EIB (Level IC).[47] In this study, however, cromolyn still afforded protection against EIB 2 hours after treatment, whereas nedocromil did not.[47]

Antileukotriene Agents

The first demonstration that treatment with specific cysteinyl leukotriene$_1$ receptor antagonists are effective in attenuating EIB was by Manning et al.[48] In this study, a single treatment with MK-571 (160 mg intravenously 20 minutes before exercise) was effective in attenuating the postexercise fall in FEV_1 by 69%. Several other antileukotriene agents have been evaluated in exercise challenge studies and afforded significant attenuation of EIB (Level IA).[49–51]

We addressed the issue of the duration of effectiveness of one leukotriene receptor antagonist in protection against EIB.[50] In this study, subjects were given either placebo or one of three doses of the long-acting cysteinyl leukotriene$_1$ receptor antagonist cinalukast (10, 50, or 200 mg orally). Exercise challenges were performed at both 2 and 8 hours following treatment. All three doses were effective in attenuating the postexercise fall in FEV$_1$, and this protection was still present to the same extent 8 hours following treatment. Interestingly, in this same study, the protective effect afforded by the 10-mg dose was lost after 1 week regular treatment (10 mg orally three times daily). However, this loss of protection did not occur following the same treatment regimen at either of the higher doses. We concluded from this study that leukotriene receptor blockade may provide protection against EIB for periods greater than 8 hours, but that loss of protection, possibly through receptor upregulation, may occur with regular treatment at lower doses. Recently, Leff et al[51] have observed the degree of protection afforded by montelukast (10 mg nightly) on exercise challenges performed 20 to 24 hours following treatment. In this study, there was approximately 47% protection against EIB, and this protection was maintained throughout a 12-week period of regular therapy.

While the degree of protection afforded with antileukotriene treatment does not appear to match that for inhaled β_2-agonists, the duration of effectiveness (up to 24 hours) suggests a useful role in the management of EIB (Level IA). This is particularly true for children and elite athletes, who often exercise frequently throughout the day. In this group, for whom regular treatment with inhaled β_2-agonists may have diminishing effectiveness,[34,37] antileukotriene treatment may prove to be valuable.

Anticholinergics

Treatment with the inhaled anticholinergic agent ipratropium bromide has been effective in reducing EIB in some studies but not in others. Poppius et al[52] found no protective effect against EIB from inhalation of ipratropium (0.2 to 2 mg) 1 hour before exercise (Level I). However, Boulet et al[53] and Finnerty and Holgate[54] have reported protective effects of 54% and 34%, respectively. While it appears that anticholinergic treatment may offer only modest protection and not be effective in all patients, it may be useful in some (Level IB).

Antihistamines

Pretreatment with the oral antihistamine terfenadine offers some protection against EIB. In two separate studies, Finnerty and Holgate demonstrated that terfenadine treatment (180 mg) attenuated the postexercise fall in FEV$_1$ by 18 to 36%.[54,55] MacFarlane and Heaf observed that terfenadine treatment attenuated the postexercise fall in FEV$_1$ by 32% in 20 asthmatic children.[56] This degree of protection is modest compared with other agents. However, the combination of terfenadine with other treatments may provide additive effects. For example, it has been shown that the combination of terfenadine and ipratropium bromide treatment results in attenuation of the postexercise fall in FEV$_1$ by 55%, significantly greater than the protection afforded by either agent alone.[54] With growing concern over the use of frequent or regular treatment with inhaled β_2-agonists, treatment with drug combinations such as this may become more common in the management of EIB (Level IB).

Nonpharmacologic Attenuation of EIB

Conditioning of Inspired Air

Exercise-induced bronchoconstriction is caused by respiratory heat loss, brought about by both the heating and humidification of inspired air. This concept is supported by studies demonstrating that virtually no bronchoconstriction occurs with warm humid air breathed during exercise by individuals who experience bronchoconstriction following the same exercise with cold or dry air.[57] Several investigators have tried to capitalize on these findings by attempting to reduce the severity of EIB by conditioning the inspired air of asthmatic patients. In the simplest of these manipulations, 10 asthmatic children experienced significantly less bronchoconstriction following exercise during nasal breathing (8% fall in FEV$_1$)

than during either spontaneous (16%) or mouth breathing (22%) (Level IIB).[58] In another study, nasal breathing appeared to protect asthmatic children following exercise of uncontrolled intensity (Level IIB).[59] Expanding on these observations, other investigators have observed in controlled but unblinded trials that warming masks attenuate EIB due to exercise in cold air by up to 80% (Level IIIB).[60,61]

Exercise Training

The respiratory heat and water loss that causes EIB is a function of the volume of air inhaled during exercise, rather than the exercise itself. Thus, if patients were able to exercise at a lower ventilation rate at the same level of exercise (as would be expected with increased cardiovascular fitness), they should experience less bronchoconstriction. To determine whether this is the case, several investigators have observed the effect of training on EIB. In several of these studies, results are different to interpret due to lack of a control group,[62] failure to demonstrate improved cardiovascular fitness after training,[63,64] or failure to ensure that pretraining and post-training exercise challenges were at the same absolute work rate.[65] In a parallel group controlled study, 22 adult asthmatic patients receiving training experienced a 15% increase in peak O_2 consumption.[66] This study was further controlled in that patients were challenged with the same magnitude of exercise before and after training. In this study, the training resulted in a 64% attenuation of the postexercise fall in FEV_1 (Level IA). In a similar study of asthmatic children, exercise training produced a smaller (27%) but still significant attenuation of EIB.[67] Obviously, these benefits from training would be beneficial only when patients continued to exercise at their pretraining intensity. When patients are allowed to exercise freely following training, the degree of bronchoconstriction remains unchanged.[65] Thus, while training should not be discouraged in asthmatic patients, it may not reduce their symptoms or treatment requirements associated with exercise (Level IB).

Pattern of Exercise

In most patients, following an episode of EIB, there is a period where further exercise is followed by a smaller episode of bronchoconstriction.[68] This "refractory period" can be prevented by prior treatment with indomethacin[69] and is likely due to the release of prostaglandin (PG) E_2, which has been shown to protect against EIB.[70]

Several investigators have attempted to design exercise programs that use the refractory period to reduce the severity of EIB experienced by patients during exercise. The simplest of these modifications involves the introduction of a warm-up period of exercise before a bout of exercise known to produce EIB. The first investigation of the effect of warm-up showed that inclusion of a 3-minute bout of moderate exercise prior to 5 minutes of higher-intensity exercise had no influence on the subsequent magnitude of EIB.[71] However, in this study, there was no break between the warm-up and the challenge exercise. Current understanding of the refractory period following EIB would predict that some separation between the warm-up and the challenge should be allowed in order for a small degree of bronchoconstriction to occur and result in the production of protective prostaglandins. In another study, 10 adult asthmatic patients were required to exercise for a 30-minute warm-up at a moderate work rate followed 21 minutes later by a 6-minute exercise challenge at a higher work rate.[72] The postexercise fall in FEV_1 following these two bouts of exercise was 17% and 26% below baseline, respectively. When the 6-minute exercise bout was performed without warm-up, the fall in FEV_1 was 46% below baseline. Thus, in this case, the period of warm-up resulting in a modest degree of bronchoconstriction resulted in a 43% attenuation of the magnitude of EIB following a subsequent period of more intense exercise (Level II). Other investigators have observed that similar protection is afforded by performing 7 repeated 30-second sprints approximately 30 minutes before an exercise challenge.[73] While the nature of these interventions precludes a completely blinded, controlled study, these findings support a prolonged period of modest exercise 20 to 30 minutes prior to vigorous exercise for both elite and recreational athletes (Level IIA).

In an alternate approach, Morton et al[74] have shown that separating a standard 6-minute exercise challenge into progressively smaller components separated by periods of rest can result in increasingly greater attenuation of subsequent EIB. In this study, the greatest degree of protection was found when the exercise was performed as 36 repetitions of 10-second bouts with 30 seconds of rest between each bout. In this case, the postexercise fall in FEV_1 was attenuated by 74% (Level IIA). Certainly these findings suggest a pattern of exercise that could easily be adopted by patients to reduce their symptoms associated with exercise.

SUMMARY

Evidenced-based data regarding EIB are summarized in Table 19–1. The initial management of asthmatic patients with EIB should be to optimally manage their asthma, which in most cases will involve the use of inhaled corticosteroids. This treatment over a period of weeks will, in most cases, reduce the magnitude of EIB by at least 50%. There will, however, be patients who continue to have symptoms associated with exercise that require further treatment. When the occurrence of these symptoms is infrequent, then control with short-acting inhaled β_2-agonists provides almost complete attenuation of symptoms. Care should be taken, however, because this protective effect can be diminished with frequent β_2-agonist use. This may also occur with long-acting β_2-agonists. In patients requiring frequent protection from EIB despite appropriate steroid use, additional treatment with cromolyn or leukotriene-blocking agents should prove beneficial. When daily prolonged protection is required, particularly in school-aged children, leukotriene-blocking agents may be a valuable treatment option. Further protection may be obtained by the addition of antihistamines and anticholinergic agents, although the additional benefits to be obtained by all the possible drug combinations remain to be studied. Finally, nonpharmacologic interventions are possible and may reduce or eliminate the need for one or more drugs in some patients.

Table 19–1 *Evidence-Based Data Regarding Exercise-Induced Bronchoconstriction*

Although exercise can result in bronchoconstriction in many asthmatic patients, it does not cause asthma or worsen existing asthma (Level IA).

Regular treatment with inhaled corticosteroids may reduce the severity of EIB by more than 50% (Level IA).

Pretreatment with inhaled β_2-agonists can almost completely prevent EIB (Level IA).

Prolonged regular treatment with short- or long-acting β_2-agonists can reduce their ability to prevent EIB (Level IA).

Antileukotriene drugs provide long-lasting partial protection against EIB that does not appear to be lost with regular treatment (Level IA).

REFERENCES

1. Pizzichini MM, Pizzichini E, Clelland L, et al. Sputum in severe exacerbations of asthma: kinetics of inflammatory indices after prednisone treatment. Am J Respir Crit Care Med 1997;155:1501–8.
2. Woolley KL, Adelroth E, Woolley MJ, et al. Effects of allergen challenge on eosinophils, eosinophil cationic protein and granulocyte-macrophage colony stimulating factor in mild asthma. Am J Respir Crit Care Med 1995;151:1915–24.
3. Jeffery PK, Wardlaw AJ, Nelson FC, et al. Bronchial biopsies in asthma. An ultrastructural, quantitative study and correlation with hyperreactivity. Am Rev Respir Dis 1989;140:1745–53.

4. Boulet LP, Chakir J, Dubé J, et al. Airway inflammation and structural changes in airway hyperresponsiveness and asthma: an overview. Can Respir J 1998;5:16–21.

5. Oosterhoff Y, Timens W, Postma DS. The role of airway inflammation in the pathophysiology of nocturnal asthma [review]. Clin Exp Allergy 1995;25:915–21.

6. Crimi E, Balbo A, Milanese M, et al. Airway inflammation and occurrence of delayed bronchoconstriction in exercise-induced asthma. Am Rev Respir Dis 1992;146:507–12.

7. Tateishi K, Motojima S, Kushima A, et al. Comparison between allergen-induced and exercise-induced asthma with respect to the late asthmatic response, airway responsiveness, and Creola bodies in sputum. Ann Allergy Asthma Immunol 1996;77:229–37.

8. Jarjour NN, Calhoun WJ. Exercise-induced asthma is not associated with mast cell activation or airway inflammation. J Allergy Clin Immunol 1992;89:60–8.

9. Gratziou C, Carroll M, Montefort S, et al. Inflammatory and T-cell profile of asthmatic airways 6 hours after local allergen provocation. Am J Respir Crit Care Med 1996;153:515–20.

10. Bierman CW. A comparison of late reactions to antigen and exercise. J Allergy Clin Immunol 1984;73:654–9.

11. Hofstra WB, Sterk PJ, Neijens HJ, et al. Occurrence of a late response to exercise in asthmatic children: multiple regression approach using time-matched baseline and histamine control days. Eur Respir J 1996;9:1348–55.

12. Rubinstein I, Levison H, Slutsky AS, et al. Immediate and delayed bronchoconstriction after exercise in patients with asthma. N Engl J Med 1987;317:482–5.

13. Boner AL, Vallone G, Chiesa M, et al. Reproducibility of late phase pulmonary response to exercise and its relationship to bronchial hyperreactivity in children with chronic asthma. Pediatr Pulmonol 1992;14:156–9.

14. Anderson SD, Silverman M, Konig P, Godfrey S. Exercise-induced asthma. Br J Dis Chest 1975;69:1–39.

15. Yoshikawa T, Shoji S, Fujii T, et al. Severity of exercise-induced bronchoconstriction is related to airway eosinophilic inflammation in patients with asthma. Eur Respir J 1998;12:879–84.

16. Woolley KL, Gibson PG, Carty K, et al. Eosinophil apoptosis and the resolution of airway inflammation in asthma. Am J Respir Crit Care Med 1996;154:237–43.

17. Juniper EF, Kline PA, Vanzieleghem MA, et al. Effect of long-term treatment with an inhaled corticosteroid (budesonide) on airway hyperresponsiveness and clinical asthma in non steroid-dependent asthmatic patients. Am Rev Respir Dis 1990;142:832–6.

18. Konig P, Jaffe P, Godfrey S. Effect of corticosteroids on exercise-induced asthma. J Allergy Clin Immunol 1974;54:14–9.

19. Henriksen JM, Dahl R. Effects of inhaled budesonide alone and in combination with low-dose terbutaline in children with exercise-induced asthma. Am Rev Respir Dis 1983;128:993–7.

20. Vathenen AS, Knox AJ, Wisniewski A, Tattersfield AE. Effect of inhaled budesonide on bronchial reactivity to histamine, exercise, and eucapnic dry air hyperventilation in patients with asthma. Thorax 1991;46:811–6.

21. Henriksen JM. Effect of inhalation of corticosteroids on exercise-induced asthma: randomized double blind crossover study of budesonide in asthmatic children. Br Med J 1985;291:248–9.

22. Molema J, van Herwaarden CL, Folgering HT. Effects of long-term treatment with inhaled cromoglycate and budesonide on bronchial hyperresponsiveness in patients with allergic asthma. Eur Respir J 1989;2:308–16.

23. Farrero E, Llunell A, Canete C, et al. Inhaled corticosteroids treatment and withdrawal in asthmatic children. Allergol Immunopathol 1995;23:182–8.

24. Pedersen S, Hansen OR. Budesonide treatment of moderate and severe asthma in children: a dose-response study. J Allergy Clin Immunol 1995;95:29–33.

25. Anderson SD, Seale JP, Rozea P, et al. Inhaled and oral salbutamol in exercise-induced asthma. Am Rev Respir Dis 1976;114:493–500.

26. Woolley M, Anderson SD, Quigley BM. Duration of protective effect of terbutaline sulfate and cromolyn sodium alone and in combination on exercise-induced asthma. Chest 1990;97:39–45.

27. Rabe KF, Jorres R, Magnussen H. The effect of 10, 50 and 200 micrograms inhaled fenoterol on exercise induced asthma. Clin Exp Allergy 1993;23:440–5.

28. Vilsvik J, Schaanning J, Stahl E, Holthe S. Comparison between Bricanyl Turbuhaler and Ventolin metered dose inhaler in the treatment of exercise-induced asthma in adults. Ann Allergy 1991;67:315–8.

29. Gibson GJ, Greenacre JK, Konig P, et al. Use of exercise challenge to investigate possible tolerance to beta-adrenoceptor stimulation in asthma. Br J Dis Chest 1978;72:199–206.

30. Morse JL, Jones NL, Anderson GD. The effect of terbutaline in exercise-induced asthma. Am Rev Respir Dis 1976;113:89–92.

31. Fuglsang G, Hertz B, Holm EB. No protection by oral terbutaline against exercise-induced asthma in children: a dose-response study. Eur Respir J 1993;6:527–30.

32. McAlpine LG, Thomson NC. Prophylaxis of exercise-induced asthma with inhaled formoterol, a long-acting beta 2-adrenergic agonist. Respir Med 1990;84:293–5.

33. Konig P, Hordvik NL, Serby CW. Fenoterol in exercise-induced asthma. Effect of dose on efficacy and duration of action. Chest 1984;85:462–4.

34. Inman MD, O'Byrne PM. The effect of regular inhaled salbutamol on exercise-induced bronchoconstriction. Am J Respir Crit Care Med 1996;153:65–9.

35. Anderson SD, Rodwell LT, Du Toit J, Young IH. Duration of protection by inhaled salmeterol in exercise-induced asthma. Chest 1991;100:1254–60.

36. Boner AL, Spezia E, Piovesan P, et al. Inhaled formoterol in the prevention of exercise-induced bronchoconstriction in asthmatic children. Am J Respir Crit Care Med 1994;149:935–9.

37. Ramage L, Lipworth BJ, Ingram CG, et al. Reduced protection against exercise induced bronchoconstriction after chronic dosing with salmeterol. Respir Med 1994;88:363–8.

38. Simons FE, Gerstner TV, Cheang MS. Tolerance to the bronchoprotective effect of salmeterol in adolescents with exercise-induced asthma using concurrent inhaled glucocorticoid treatment. Pediatrics 1997;99:655–9.

39. Nelson JA, Strauss L, Skowronski M, et al. Effect of long-term salmeterol treatment on exercise-induced asthma. N Engl J Med 1998;339:141–6.

40. Yates DH, Sussman HS, Shaw MJ, et al. Regular formoterol treatment in mild asthma. Effect on bronchial responsiveness during and after treatment. Am J Respir Crit Care Med 1995;152:1170–4.

41. Anderson SD, McEvoy JDS, Bianco S. Changes in lung volumes and airway resistance after exercise in asthmatic subjects. Am Rev Respir Dis 1972;106:30–7.

42. Silverman M, Turner-Warwick M. Exercise induced asthma: response to disodium cromoglycate in skin-test positive and skin-test negative subjects. Clin Allergy 1972;2:137–42.

43. Tullett WM, Tan KM, Wall RT, Patel KR. Dose-response effect of sodium cromoglycate pressurised aerosol in exercise induced asthma. Thorax 1985;40:41–4.

44. Patel KR, Wall RT. Dose-duration effect of sodium cromoglycate aerosol in exercise-induced asthma. Eur J Respir Dis 1986;69:256–60.

45. Latimer KM, O'Byrne PM, Morris MM, et al. Bronchoconstriction stimulated by airway cooling. Better protection with combined inhalation of terbutaline sulphate and cromolyn sodium than with either alone. Am Rev Respir Dis 1983;128:440–3.

46. Albazzaz MK, Neale MG, Patel KR. Dose-response study of nebulised nedocromil sodium in exercise induced asthma. Thorax 1989;44:816–9.

47. Konig P, Hordvik NL, Kreutz C. The preventive effect and duration of action of nedocromil sodium and cromolyn sodium on exercise-induced asthma (EIA) in adults. J Allergy Clin Immunol 1987;79:64–8.

48. Manning PJ, Watson RM, Margolskee DJ, et al. Inhibition of exercise-induced bronchoconstriction by MK-571, a potent leukotriene D4-receptor antagonist. N Engl J Med 1990;323:1736–9.

49. Meltzer SS, Hasday JD, Cohn J, Bleecker ER. Inhibition of exercise-induced bronchospasm by zileuton: a 5-lipoxygenase inhibitor. Am J Respir Crit Care Med 1996;153:931–5.

50. Adelroth E, Inman MD, Summers E, et al. Prolonged protection against exercise-induced bronchoconstriction by the leukotriene D4-receptor antagonist cinalukast. J Allergy Clin Immunol 1997;99:210–5.

51. Leff JA, Busse WW, Pearlman D, et al. Montelukast, a leukotriene-receptor antagonist, for the treatment of mild asthma and exercise-induced bronchoconstriction. N Engl J Med 1998;339:147–52.

52. Poppius H, Sovijarvi AR, Tammilento L. Lack of protective effect of high-dose ipratropium on bronchoconstriction following exercise with cold air breathing in patients with mild asthma. Eur J Respir Dis 1986;68:3199–25.

53. Boulet LP, Turcotte H, Tennina S. Comparative efficacy of salbutamol, ipratropium, and cromoglycate in the prevention of bronchospasm induced by exercise and hyperosmolar challenges. J Allergy Clin Immunol 1989;83:882–7.

54. Finnerty JP, Holgate ST. The contribution of histamine release and vagal reflexes, alone and in combination, to exercise-induced asthma. Eur Respir J 1993;6:1132–7.

55. Finnerty JP, Holgate ST. Evidence for the roles of histamine and prostaglandins as mediators in exercise-induced asthma: the inhibitory effect of terfenadine and flurbiprofen alone and in combination. Eur Respir J 1990;3:540–7.

56. MacFarlane PI, Heaf DP. Selective histamine blockade in childhood asthma; the effect of terfenadine on resting bronchial tone and exercise induced bronchoconstriction. Respir Med 1989;83:19–24.

57. Strauss RH, McFadden ER, Ingram RH, Chandler E. Influence of heat and humidity on airway obstruction induced by exercise in asthma. J Clin Invest 1978;61:433–40.

58. Mangla PK, Menon MP. Effect of nasal and oral breathing on exercise-induced asthma. Clin Allergy 1981;11:433–9.

59. Shturman-Ellstein R, Zeballos RJ, Buckley JM, Souhrada JF. The beneficial effect of nasal breathing on exercise-induced bronchoconstriction. Am Rev Respir Dis 1978;118:65–73.

60. Schachter EN, Lach E, Lee M. The protective effect of a cold weather mask on exercise-induced asthma. Ann Allergy 1981;46:12–6.

61. Brenner AM, Weiser PC, Krogh LA, Loren ML. Effectiveness of a portable face mask in attenuating exercise-induced asthma. JAMA 1980;244:2196–8.

62. Fitch KD, Blitvich JD, Morton AR. The effect of running training on exercise-induced asthma. Ann Allergy 1986;57:90–4.

63. Nickerson BG, Bautista DB, Namey MA, et al. Distance running improves fitness in asthmatic children without pulmonary complications or changes in exercise-induced bronchospasm. Pediatrics 1983;71:147–52.

64. Fitch KD, Morton AR, Blanksby BA. Effects of swimming training on children with asthma. Arch Dis Child 1976;51:190–4.

65. Bundgaard A, Ingemann-Hansen T, Schmidt A, Halkjaer-Kristensen J. Effect of physical training on peak oxygen consumption rate and exercise-induced asthma in adult asthmatic patients. Scand J Clin Lab Invest 1982;42:9–13.

66. Haas F, Pasierski S, Levine N, et al. Effect of aerobic training on forced expiratory airflow in exercising asthmatic humans. J Appl Physiol 1987;63:1230–5.

67. Henriksen JM, Nielsen TT. Effect of physical training on exercise-induced bronchoconstriction. Acta Paediatr Scand 1983;72:31–6.

68. Edmunds AT, Tooley M, Godfrey S. The refractory period after exercise-induced asthma: its duration and relation to the severity of exercise. Am Rev Respir Dis 1978;117:247–54.

69. O'Byrne PM, Jones GL. The effect of indomethacin on exercise-induced bronchoconstriction and refractoriness after exercise. Am Rev Respir Dis 1986;134:69–72.

70. Melillo E, Woolley KL, Manning PJ, et al. Effect of inhaled PGE_2 on exercise-induced bronchoconstriction in asthmatic subjects. Am J Respir Crit Care Med 1994;149:1138–41.

71. Morton AR, Fitch KD, Davis T. The effect of "warm-up" on exercise-induced asthma. Ann Allergy 1979;42:257–60.

72. Reiff DB, Choudry NB, Pride NB, Ind PW. The effect of prolonged submaximal warm-up exercise on exercise-induced asthma. Am Rev Respir Dis 1989;139:479–84.

73. Schnall RP, Landau LI. Protective effects of repeated short sprints in exercise-induced asthma. Thorax 1980;35:828–32.

74. Morton AR, Hahn AG, Fitch KD. Continuous and intermittent running in the provocation of asthma. Ann Allergy 1982;48:123–9.

CHAPTER 20

Acute Life-Threatening Asthma

J. Mark FitzGerald, MD, FRCPC, FRCP(I)
Anton Grunfeld, MD, FRCPC

Acute life-threatening asthma is a common medical emergency[1] that in the past, has been poorly managed (Level II).[2] Although we have recently shown improvement in asthma management based on self-reported care, it remains suboptimal.[3] The immediate optimal management of an attack is important, but it is also important to recognize that subjects who visit the emergency department are at risk for further life-threatening attacks.[4] Therefore, the opportunity should be taken not only to manage the current attack optimally but also to initiate appropriate specialist referral. This has been shown at follow-up to reduce the subsequent risk for life-threatening events (Level IA).[5]

In this chapter, we have reviewed critically the literature focusing on randomized controlled trials. In keeping with the principles of the textbook, levels of evidence are explicitly stated. A formal meta-analysis was not completed, but a comprehensive search of the literature was made using MEDLINE, and the authors' extensive article files were also reviewed. The recently published evidence-based Canadian guidelines for the management of acute asthma were also used extensively.[6]

ASSESSMENT

Patient Evaluation

Certain historic features[4] should alert the physician to be especially careful when evaluating a patient having an acute asthma attack; risk factors for asthma death are listed in Table 20–1. Monosyllabic speech and difficulty completing a full sentence represent clear evidence of a severe attack. The patient's response as well as caregivers' response are important to document, particularly with a view to preventing subsequent life-threatening events. For example, Was the patient on appropriate anti-inflammatory treatment? Was treatment increased upon the first sign of deteriorating asthma? Did the patient use a greater than usual dose of a β-agonist?

Table 20–1 *Risk Factors for Asthma Death*

Prior near fatal episode of asthma
Prior sudden precipitous attack
Prior emergency department visit
Frequent hospitalization
Recent use of or dependence on systemic corticosteroids
Recent attack of prolonged duration
Poor compliance or lack of knowledge about asthma
Return to locations with environmental triggers
Excessive or increasing reliance on β_2-agonists, especially in the absence of inhaled corticosteroids

A previous history of a life-threatening episode (Level II)[7] or clinical deterioration despite the current use of prednisone should alert the examining physician to be cautious, particularly with regard to discharging the patient. In a prospective study, we found that patients with a history of previous mechanical ventilation (OR 27.5, 95% CI 6.6 to 113.7) and admission to the intensive care unit (OR 9.9, 95% CI 3.0 to 32.9) were at a higher risk for near-fatal asthma when compared to hospitalized control patients.[7]

Clinical Examination

Signs of severe life-threatening attacks of asthma include tachycardia, tachypnea, hyperinflation, wheeze, accessory muscle use, and pulsus paradoxus. Various attempts have been made to formulate a scoring index for severity of the attack, based on clinical parameters and level of airflow obstruction,[8,9] but all have generally been unsuccessful in subsequent prospective validation studies.[10] The poor correlation between these indices and the subsequent need for admission highlight the fact that the assessment of the patient in the emergency department must take many factors into account.

Investigations

Next to the patient's history, the most important investigation is the objective assessment of airflow obstruction. It not only gives the clinician information regarding the severity of the attack at presentation, but it also allows response to therapy to be monitored. Failure to use objective measurements will lead to patients with suboptimal management being discharged from the emergency department. Many patients and physicians[11,12] poorly perceive the level of airflow obstruction, and therapeutic discussions based on clinical examination or a patient's perception of symptoms may lead to an unacceptable risk of relapse (Level II). Males appear to have a diminished perception of dyspnea as compared to females, and they tend to present with more severe airflow obstruction.[13]

Arterial Blood Gases

Routine uses of arterial blood gases is not warranted, particularly with the ready availability of oximetry. Where patients have very severe airflow obstruction, and in particular if the forced expiratory volume in 1 second (FEV_1) is less than 40% of that predicted, arterial blood gases are indicated (Level II).[14] In addition, arterial blood gases should be measured if there is concern that a patient's clinical status is deteriorating. A normal or rising PCO_2 should alert the physician to the possible need for intubation and mechanical ventilation.

Chest Radiography

As with arterial blood gases, routine chest radiography is not required, particularly if the patient is having a moderately severe attack and is responding appropriately to bronchodilator therapy. Chest radiography should be performed if there is a failure to respond, so that an unrecognized pneumothorax or pneumomediastinum may be detected (Level II).[15] Patients with airflow obstruction severe enough to require hospitalization should undergo chest radiography.[16,17]

Electrocardiography

In general, routine use of electrocardiography is not required unless the patient is of an age for which ischemic heart disease is a possible differential diagnosis, particularly if there is some question of chest tightness that is suggestive of ischemia. Previous studies have shown that during an acute attack of asthma, signs of right ventricular strain including T wave inversion may be present on an electrocardiogram, but these promptly revert in a matter of hours once the acute attack is under control (Level II).[17]

Sputum Examination

The routine use of sputum examination for Gram's stain, culture, and sensitivity is not warranted. Viral infections are the usual cause of exacerbations due to an infection.[18] More recently sputum induction has been used in the emergency department to characterize the degree of inflammation in the sputum of patients presenting with an acute asthma attack.[19] Induced sputum showed a significant increase in eosinophils and increased levels in fluid-phase eosinophil cationic protein (ECP).

DECISIONS WITH REGARD TO ADMISSION OR DISCHARGE

The decision to admit or discharge a patient having an acute asthma attack depends on the level of airflow obstruction. Generally, patients who present with an FEV_1 or peak flow less than 25 to 30% of their predicted require hospitalization.[20] It is clear from prospective studies that patients who achieve an FEV_1 of 60% of predicted or greater can be discharged safely (Level IIA).[21] Between these two levels of lung function is a grey zone in which there is considerable overlap between patients discharged without further relapse and patients discharged requiring re-evaluation in the emergency department and subsequent hospitalization. The decision to admit or discharge a patient whose degree of airflow obstruction is in this range will need to be based on the examining physician's knowledge of the patient's previous ability to manage an attack (ie, the likelihood of him/her being compliant) and the usual time course for response to an acute flare up of this patient's asthma. When there are concerns with regard to compliance, and, in particular, if there is, for example, a previous history of mechanical ventilation or frequent emergency department visits, a cautious approach may be reasonable, and a short 24- to 48-hour admission may be indicated. Appropriate therapeutic strategies at the time of discharge, as outlined below, should ensure that close to 90% of patients can be discharged from the emergency department safely, without risk of relapse.

THERAPY

Treatment of patients suffering from a severe asthma attack must be initiated early and aggressively and should continue while the assessment of the patient is in progress.

First-Line Therapy

Initial treatment consists of routine supplemental oxygen, aggressive use of bronchodilators, and corticosteroids.[22]

Oxygen

Oxygen should be given to all patients with acute life-threatening asthma (Level IIIA). In severely ill patients, extreme hypoxia and hypercapnia, demonstrating asphyxia, are frequently seen and must be addressed urgently. Oxygen can be delivered by nasal prongs, a mask, or an endotracheal tube to maintain a $SaO_2 > 92$ to 95% (Table 20–2). Oxygen will not suppress the respiratory drive in acute asthma.

Bronchodilators

Sympathomimetic drugs have been used in the management of life-threatening asthma since the 1950s. Adrenaline, the original agent,[23] has been replaced by selective β_2-agonists (Level IA).[22] There is little disagreement that, in the aerosol form, β_2-agonists are the agents of first choice to relieve bronchoconstriction in acute asthma. Compared to other agents, they provide more significant bronchodilatation and the most prompt relief, are cheaper, and have fewer side effects. Aerosolized β_2-agonists have also been shown to be at least equal to and often superior to parenteral therapy with the same agent, providing equal bronchodilatation with fewer side effects (Level IB).[24,25] β_2-Agonists have also been convincingly shown to be effective even for those patients who have pretreated themselves unsuccessfully with the same medications prior to their arrival to the emergency department (ED) (as is commonly seen) (Level IIB).[26] The reason for self-administered β_2-agonists not being effective prior to arrival may be underdosing or improper use of metered-dose inhalers (MDIs).

Equally effective delivery of aerosolized β_2-agonists can be achieved by using nebulized medication or MDIs, preferably with a spacer device (Level IA).[27] In a recently published meta-analysis, we have shown that MDI therapy was at least as effective as nebulized therapy. Most physicians are accustomed to using wet nebulizers for treatment of severe asthma. These devices are well accepted by patients. Metered-dose inhalers, however, have several advantages: medication given this way can be administered and repeated very quickly (2 minutes vs 10 to 20 minutes for the wet nebulizers); using MDIs is cheaper; because they are inexpensive to use, and physicians can educate patients in their proper use by way of a demonstration. Although cheaper, the difference in cost between metered-dose therapy versus nebulized therapy has probably been exaggerated in previous studies.[28]

The dosage of β_2-agonists is empiric and is titrated to patient response (see Table 20–2). If one uses aerosolized therapy aggressively, intravenous forms of β_2-agonists are usually not needed. Because of the increased risk of arrhythmias with parenteral therapy, these drugs should be administered in a monitored area.[25]

Table 20–2 *First-Line Treatments of Acute Asthma*

Agent	Administration
Oxygen	High flow to maintain a $SaO_2 > 92$–95%; can be delivered by nasal prongs, a mask, or an endotracheal tube
β_2-Agonists	MDI: Initial dose is 4–8 puffs (salbutamol 100 µg/puff); it can be repeated every 15–20 min up to 3 times. In severe disease, the dose can be increased to 1 puff every 30–60 s, up to 20 puffs, as needed.
	Wet nebulizer: Initial dose is 5–10 mg of salbutamol (1–2 mL plus 3 mL of saline) every 15–20 min. For patients with severe attacks, wet nebulization can run continuously.
Corticosteroids	Prednisone 50 mg orally or methylprednisolone 125 mg IV stat then 40 mg IV daily if PO not possible, or hydrocortisone 500 mg IV; repeat every 8 hours for 24 hours

MDI = metered-dose inhaler; IV = intravenously; PO = per os (by mouth).

Corticosteroids

Corticosteroids should be started simultaneously with bronchodilators in the treatment of acute exacerbations of asthma—a recognition of the pivotal role of inflammation in the pathogenesis of this disease. There continues to be controversy regarding the optimum dose, route, and frequency of administration and the type of preparation used. Corticosteroids are now recommended for all but the mildest attacks of asthma. Unquestionably, the administration of corticosteroids favorably influences the outcome of both admitted and discharged patients. A recent meta-analysis by Rowe and colleagues (Level IA)[29] supports this view and showed that corticosteroids, if administered early, can prevent hospital admissions. Admission rates were significantly reduced: pooled OR 0.37, 95% CI 0.19 to 0.70; and for those with more severe asthma, OR 0.35, 95% CI 0.21 to 0.59. The effect was more marked in patients not previously receiving corticosteroids. The onset of action of corticosteroids was historically thought to be slow, but a number of recent studies assessing the role of inhaled corticosteroids in acute asthma suggest they may have an ability to modify the outcome when compared to oral corticosteroids alone. Rodrigo and Rodrigo[30] showed that in patients presenting to the ED, the addition of high-dose inhaled flunisolide (1 mg every 10 minutes for 3 hours) to inhaled salbutamol (400 µg every 10 minutes) led to greater bronchodilatation at 120, 150, and 180 minutes ($p = .041$) compared to inhaled salbutamol alone (Level IB).

Oral administration of corticosteroids is cheaper and has been found to be equally effective as other routes, even in severe asthma exacerbations (Level IA).[31] The parenteral preparations should probably be reserved for patients unable to take oral medications (see Table 20–2). Historically, the use of oral prednisone in patients discharged from the emergency department has been shown to reduce relapse.[29] More recently, we have shown that in patients given a loading dose of systemic corticosteroids and who have achieved an FEV_1 greater than 50%, an equivalent reduction in relapse can be achieved in patients who have been prescribed budesonide 2.4 mg by Turbuhaler in four divided doses when compared to prednisone 40 mg taken by mouth over a 10-day period (Level IB).[32] A number of other studies have also shown the benefit of inhaled corticosteroids in acute asthma.[33–37] In the most notable of these studies, Rowe et al[33] showed that the addition of inhaled budesonide (800 µg bid) to oral prednisone led to a reduced relapse in patients discharged from the ED, as compared to oral prednisone alone. After 21 days, 12 patients (12.8%) in the budesonide group experienced relapse compared with 23 patients (24.5%) in the placebo arm—a 48% reduction ($p = .49$).

Adjunct Therapy

Most patients will respond to first-line therapy with significant relief of bronchoconstriction; however, for those who do not improve, there are other pharmacologic agents worth consideration. These include anticholinergics, magnesium, adrenaline, intravenous salbutamol, and methylxanthines.

Anticholinergics

Ipratropium bromide, the anticholinergic agent most commonly used, has been shown to have a slower onset of action and produce less bronchodilatation than β_2-agonists. In recent years, a number of large studies have examined the additive effect of the two agents (Level IA).[38–40] Although the New Zealand study showed a greater improvement in FEV_1 equivalent to 150 mL in the combination therapy group, this effect is unlikely to be clinically significant and was lost when all three studies were combined.[41] Surprisingly, the benefit was less likely to be seen in the more severely obstructed patients. The doses recommended are empiric (Table 20–3). Of greater interest than the impact on spirometry has been the recent data suggesting that the combination leads to a significant reduction in hospitalization. This effect has been shown in a published pediatric meta-analysis[42] and, more recently, in a meta-analysis of adult studies (Level IA).[43] In their overview, Rodrigo et al showed an overall effect size of 0.13 (95% CI 0.03 to 0.23) with the addition of ipratropium bromide. Pooled results in the four studies that addressed the issue of hospitalization showed the addition of ipratropium bromide to a β_2-agonist reduced hospitalization significantly (OR 0.64, 95% CI 0.45 to 0.92) (Level IA). A potential limitation to these findings is the lack of standardization of admission criteria across studies. These data suggest that, in the more severe patients who do not respond promptly to β-agonists, ipratropium should be used as an additional bronchodilator.

Magnesium

The role of magnesium in acute asthma has, until relatively recently, been controversial. Rowe et al in a Cochrane review have clarified this therapy's role (Level IA).[44] In this overview, among seven studies there was a hospitalization rate of 23% in the magnesium sulfate group compared to 45% in the placebo group (relative risk reduction [RRR] 95% CI 2 to 49). In

Table 20–3 *Adjunct Therapy in Acute Asthma*

Agent	Administration
Anticholinergics	Ipratropium bromide should be given to patients with severe and near-fatal asthma (it may be helpful in addition to β_2-agonists for patients with moderate asthma). Frequency should be decreased in the recovery phase.
	MDI: Initial dose is 4–8 puffs (20 μg/puff) every 15–20 min, to be repeated 3 times. The dose can be increased to 1 puff every 30–60 s, to a maximum of 20 puffs, as needed.
	Wet nebulizer: initial dose is 0.25–0.5 mg (1–2 mL in 2–3 mL of saline) every 15–20 min, or continuous if necessary. It may be mixed with the β_2-agonists.
Magnesium sulfate	Intravenous infusion 25 mg/kg/h
Adrenaline	Adrenaline 0.3–0.5 mL (1:1,000) subcutaneously every 15–20 min, as required
	Adrenaline infusion: 4–8 μg/min (1 mL of 1:1,000 adrenaline in 250 mL of D5W gives 4 μg/mL solution); the infusion is started at 1–2 mL/min)
Intravenous β_2-agonists	Salbutamol 4 μg/kg, over 2–5 min; salbutamol can subsequently be given as an infusion at 0.1–0.2 μg/kg/min
Aminophylline	Aminophylline loading dose: 3–6 mg/kg intravenously over 1/2 h; the dose should be halved if the patient is already on theophylline; followed by an infusion at 0.2–1 mg/kg/h; blood level monitoring is recommended

MDI = metered-dose inhaler.

patients with more severe asthma, the results were more impressive with the magnesium sulfate patients, who had an admission rate of 51% compared to 91% among control patients (RRR 44% CI 29 to 56). Patients with an FEV_1 <30% at presentation and those who do not respond to initial treatment or improve beyond 60% of predicted FEV_1 at 1 hour should be considered eligible.[45] Rodrigo and colleagues' more recent overview confirms that there was no benefit in patients with less severe asthma.[46] In a further exciting study, the addition of magnesium sulfate as a vehicle for nebulized salbutamol in acute asthma led to an increase in FEV_1 to 61% in the combination arm versus salbutamol alone (31%; 95% CI 3 to 56; p = .03).[47] These results at 20 minutes need to be reassessed in larger and longer studies.

Adrenaline

Adrenaline has been used in the treatment of acute asthma since 1951. With the current availability of specific β_2-agonists, adrenaline is seldom needed. In certain circumstances, such as anaphylaxis with prominent bronchoconstriction, adrenaline is the drug of choice. Additionally, in circumstances in which inhaled bronchodilators are not available, subcutaneous adrenaline can be life saving (see Table 20–3).[48]

Intravenous Salbutamol

Aggressive treatment with inhaled salbutamol will eliminate the need to use intravenous salbutamol. However, in severely ill patients prior to endotracheal intubation and ventilation, or in patients responding poorly to inhaled salbutamol, the intravenous preparation can be tried (Level IC).[49]

Methylxanthines

Aminophylline has been used for many years in the treatment of acute asthma. It has been shown, however, that aminophylline confers no additional benefit to the use of β_2-agonists alone (Level ID). A meta-analysis by Littenberg of 13 adequately designed studies in patients with acute, severe asthma showed that the evidence for supporting its use was inconclusive.[50] Aminophylline has a narrow therapeutic margin and can cause significant toxicity, especially in hypoxic patients. The metabolism of theophylline is affected by multiple factors, making close monitoring of its levels during therapy imperative. The combination of the above factors has led to recent recommendations that methylxanthines should not be used during the first 4 hours of treatment of the patient in the ED. If one chooses to use aminophylline, recommended doses are shown in Table 20–3.

Intubation and Mechanical Ventilation

Most patients will respond promptly to bronchodilator and corticosteroid treatment. Attention should be paid to patients who do not respond, and timely preparations for intubation and mechanical ventilation should be made for the few patients who require them. The decision to intubate an asthma patient is ultimately made on clinical grounds (Level III). For patients in respiratory arrest, or for patients with decreased sensorium or coma who cannot protect their airways, endotracheal intubation is mandatory.[51] Otherwise, the decision usually evolves over minutes or hours, based on the ongoing clinical observations of the patient's response to treatment. Patients who deteriorate in spite of aggressive bronchodilator therapy and who become exhausted or confused, whose respiratory effort is decreasing, who are diaphoretic or cyanotic, or whose vital signs are unstable are not likely to improve without a period of respiratory support. These patients need endotracheal intubation and mechanical ventilation. Correctable conditions such as deterioration due to a pneumothorax should be sought and rapidly corrected. The arterial blood gases can be obtained to strengthen the clinical decision and may show hypoxia, increasing hypercapnia, and acidosis. However, the decision to intubate the patient should not be delayed while waiting to obtain arterial blood gases. A physician experienced with airway management should proceed with the intubation; an anesthetist should be contacted early if the attending physician is not comfortable intubating the patient.

It is important to decide which patients are likely to deteriorate and to proceed expeditiously with a rapid-sequence intubation, thereby avoiding "crash intubations." Patients who require intubation usually do so for a short period only (in general, less than 48 hours). Males, in particular, appear to deteriorate more quickly and are more likely to be extubated in the first 24 hours.

Patients must be preoxygenated with 100% oxygen. Ketamine is the induction agent of choice in asthma.[52] It is a phencyclidine analog that induces a state of dissociative anesthesia, putting the patient in a trance-like, cataleptic state. The patient maintains muscle tone, pharyngeal and laryngeal reflexes, and respiratory drive. In addition, ketamine is a bronchodilator, acting both directly and indirectly through catecholamine release. It is as effective as halothane or enflurane in preventing bronchoconstriction. One-quarter to one-third of adult patients receiving ketamine experience a postanesthesia emergence reaction, during which the patient experiences vividly dysphoric dreams and unpleasant experiences. The emergence reaction can be controlled with the use of benzodiazepines, particularly midazolam. The recommended dose is ketamine 1.5 mg/kg intravenously over 1 minute. The ketamine bolus can be repeated, as the bronchodilating effect wears off in 20 to 30 minutes. An infusion can also be started.

Succinylcholine, a depolarizing paralytic agent, is the agent of choice for paralyzing to facilitate endotracheal intubation. It is the fastest-acting agent, and it is effective and safe to be used in conjunction with ketamine for intubation of asthmatic patients. The recommended dose is succinylcholine 1.5 mg/kg intravenously as a bolus. Vecuronium, a nondepolarizing paralytic agent, should only be used for maintenance of paralysis.

Although the rate of complications for intubated asthmatic patients is high, the mortality rate should effectively be zero.[51] Strict attention should be paid to maintaining adequate paralysis and low flow rates or tidal volumes to reduce peak airway pressures and associated barotrauma. There should be caution to minimize the dose of corticosteroids used. The optimal dose of systemic corticosteroids appears to be, at most, 120 mg of methylprednisolone in divided doses.[53] In a recent case-control study, we found significantly more patients had muscle weakness following the use of continuous infusion of muscle relaxants combined with methylprednisolone 125 mg or greater daily (Level IID).[53]

Uncontrolled studies have shown that a number of other interventions may be used. These have included the suggestion that the use of inhalational anesthetics may reduce the duration of intubation.[54] Extracorporeal oxygenation[55] or bronchial lavage[56] have also been reported to be of benefit in patients who are being ventilated. The combination of helium and oxygen appears to reduce airway pressure and may be considered as adjunct therapy (Level IB).[57]

CRITERIA FOR ADMISSION OR DISCHARGE FOLLOWING THERAPY

Most patients presenting with exacerbations of asthma respond well to treatment and are discharged home safely (Level II). Hospital admission rates for adults vary between 10 and 25% and, depending on a variety of factors, between 5 and 25% of discharged patients suffer a relapse (Level II). Attempts have been made to predict the need for hospital admission from the initial patient evaluation.[58] Some broad guidelines for discharge are emerging; however, in no situation is the discharge of patients with treated asthma entirely free of risk. Spirometric measurements have limitations and should not be relied upon in isolation for decision making regarding the admission or discharge of asthmatic patients. However, data from several studies indicate that patients fall within discernible groups[59,60] (Table 20–4). The majority of patients who die from an acute asthma attack do so prior to reaching the hospital. The best way to identify asthma patients at risk of death is to identify those who have had a recent hospital admission and, in particular, those who have had one or more life-threatening attacks requiring mechanical ventilation, as outlined above (Level II). Patients with underlying severe disease, judged by chronic severe symptoms; systemic steroid requirement; and frequent, especially increasing, use of bronchodilators, are also at risk. Patients in this

Table 20–4 *Spirometric Admission and Discharge Criteria for Acute Asthma Patients*

Prebronchodilator treatment	FEV_1 < 1.0 L or PEF < 100 L/min or < 25% predicted or best will usually require admission
Postbronchodilator treatment	FEV_1 < 1.6 L or PEF < 200 L/min or < 40% predicted or best; admission is recommended
	FEV_1 between 1.6 and 2.1 L or PEF between 200 and 300 L/min or between 40 and 60% predicted or best; discharge may be possible after consideration of risk factors and follow-up care
	$FEV_1 \geq 2.1$ L or PEF $\geq$ 300 L/min or > 60% predicted or best; discharge is likely after consideration of risk factors and follow-up care

PEF = peak expiratory flow.

group also may have one or more of the following problems: recent discharge from the hospital for severe asthma, poor self-care or noncompliance with medications, depression or severe emotional disturbance, other significant psychologic factors, or shortcomings in education or supervision. Patients with these characteristics will clearly require careful consideration and close follow-up if discharged.

DISCHARGE PLANNING AND FOLLOW-UP

The goal of asthma therapy is the return of the patient to full function. With rare exceptions, disability is not acceptable. Patients should function with minimal or no symptoms, and their asthma should not affect their school, work, or exercise. Each patient, with a physician's help, should have a plan on discharge from the ED and instructions on how to deal with future exacerbations. A recent study has shown that the provision of a peak-flow meter in addition to asthma education can significantly reduce the risk of relapse.[60] In this study of 150 asthma patients discharged from the ED with either no action plan, a symptom action plan, or a peak-flow action plan, there was a striking reduction in the risk of relapse in the peak-flow action plan group (55 patients versus 45 versus only 5 [$p = .006$], respectively) (Level IB).

Regular use of β_2-agonists is often required for at least 48 hours after discharge, and patients should be advised how to modify treatment according to symptoms. If the patient is unable to control symptoms, he should return to the ED. Patients should know the results of their pulmonary function tests, thus facilitating treatment decisions at the time of their next presentation to the ED. Prior to discharging a patient, the physician should verify that the patient knows how to use the MDI and understands the role of bronchodilators and anti-inflammatory agents.

Corticosteroids are indicated upon discharge from the ED for all patients with severe asthma attacks. The treatment should be individualized, based on responses to past treatment and recent symptoms. Previously, the dose recommended was prednisone 30 to 60 mg/d for 7 to 14 days. More recently we have shown that inhaled budesonide at a dose of 2.4 mg in four divided doses can be used and provides at least the equivalent effect of oral prednisone.[32] If oral corticosteroids are used, they can usually be stopped rather than tapered in patients who are not steroid dependent (Level IA).[61] Given the most recent data from Rowe et al, patients being discharged from the ED should also have inhaled corticosteroids initiated.[33] Patients discharged from the ED should be re-evaluated within a week by their family physicians, and decisions regarding maintenance anti-inflammatory therapy should be made at this time (Level IIIA). There is also evidence that patients, especially those whose disease is poorly controlled, benefit from facilitated referrals to specialists (Level IA).[5] The provision of asthma education also can significantly reduce the risk of health care use, including unscheduled physician visits, ED visits, and hospitalizations for acute asthma (Level IA).[62]

FUTURE RESEARCH

Future studies should address the issue of the optimal interventions to prevent asthma exacerbations. Although long-acting β-agonists have been shown to reduce asthma exacerbations,[63] methodologic issues have been raised with regard to the design of this study.[64] Studies are needed to define the optimal strategy to prevent asthma exacerbations. There is a need to confirm, in prospective studies, the impact of ipratropium bromide and magnesium sulfate on hospitalization rates. Although guidelines have suggested that doubling the dose of inhaled corticosteroids is the optimal approach (Level III),[65] preliminary data from a randomized controlled trial showed that doubling the dose of inhaled corticosteroids did not alter the exacerbation when compared to the continued use of maintenance inhaled corticosteriods.[66] Intervention studies are also required to optimize the educational component of treatment for high-risk asthma patients (Level III).[67]

Conclusion

The following are evidence-based statements and recommendations regarding acute life-threatening asthma.

- Prevention of severe life-threatening attacks of asthma can be achieved with regular use of inhaled corticosteroids (Level II).
- Patients should have an objective assessment of airflow obstruction (Level III).
- Optimal therapy consists of short-acting β_2-agonists (Level I), oxygen (Level III), and corticosteroids (Level I). Ipratropium bromide does not have a significant effect on airflow but appears to reduce the need for hospitalization (Level I). More severe asthma patients appear to benefit from the addition of intravenous magnesium (Level I).
- Patients discharged from the emergency department should be treated with systemic corticosteroids (Level I) in combination with inhaled corticosteroids (Level I). Facilitated referral to a specialist after discharge from the emergency department has been shown to improve outcome (Level I).
- Education has an important role in reducing subsequent morbidity (Level I).

References

1. FitzGerald JM, Hargreave FE. The assessment and management of acute life threatening asthma. Chest 1989;95:888–94.
2. FitzGerald JM, Hargreave FE. Acute asthma: emergency department management and prospective evaluation of outcome. Can Med Assoc J 1990;142:591–5.
3. Grunfeld A, Beveridge RC, Bekowitz J, FitzGerald JM. Management of acute asthma in Canada: an assessment of physician behaviour. J Emerg Med 1997;15:547–56.
4. FitzGerald JM, Macklem PT. Proceedings of a workshop on near fatal asthma. Can Respir J 1995;2:113–26.
5. Zeiger RS, Heller S, Mellon MH, et al. Facilitated referral to asthma specialists reduces relapses in emergency department visits. J Allergy Clin Immunol 1991;87:1160–8.
6. Beveridge RC, Grunfeld AF, Hodder RV, Verbeek PR for the CAEP/CTS Asthma Advisory Committee. Guidelines for the emergency management of asthma in adults. Can Med Assoc J 1996;155:25–37.
7. Turner MT, Noertjojo K, Vedal S, et al. Risk factors for near fatal asthma: a case control study in hospitalised patients with asthma. Am J Respir Crit Care Med 1998;157:1804–9.
8. Fischl M, Pitchenik A, Gardner L. An index predicting relapse and need for hospitalisation in patients with acute bronchial asthma. N Engl J Med 1981;305:783–9.
9. Rose CC, Murphy JG, Schwartz JS. Performance of an index predicting the response of patients with bronchial asthma to intensive emergency department treatment. N Engl J Med 1984;310:573–7.
10. Centor RM, Yarborough B, Wood JP. Inability to predict relapse in acute asthma. N Engl J Med 1984;310:573–80.
11. Rodrigo G, Rodrigo C. Early prediction of poor response in acute asthma patients in the emergency department. Chest 1998;114:1016–21.
12. Shim CS, Williams MH. Evaluation of the severity of asthma: patients versus physicians. Am J Med 1980;93:11–3.
13. Awadh N, Shu S, Grunfeld A, et al. Comparisons of males and females presenting with acute asthma to the emergency department. Respir Med 1996;90:485–9.
14. Nowak RM, Tomlanovich S, Sarker DD, et al. Arterial blood gases and pulmonary function testing in acute bronchial asthma: predicting patient outcomes. JAMA 1983;249:2043–6.
15. Findley LJ, Sahn S. The value of chest roentgenograms in acute asthma in adults. Chest 1981;80:535–6.
16. Gershel JC, Goldman HS, Stein RE, et al. The usefulness of chest radiographs in first asthma attacks. N Engl J Med 1983;309:336–9.
17. Rebuck AS, Read J. Assessment and management of severe asthma. Am J Med 1971;51:788–98.
18. Rakes GP, Arruda E, Ingram JM, et al. Rhinovirus and respiratory syncytial virus in wheezing children requiring emergency care. Am J Respir Crit Care Med 1999;159:785–90.

19. Pizzichini MM, Pizzichini E, Cleeland L, et al. Sputum in severe exacerbations of asthma: kinetics of inflammatory indices after prednisone treatment. Am J Respir Crit Care Med 1997;155:1501–8.

20. Nowak RM, Gordon KR, Wroblewski DA. Spirometric evaluation of acute bronchial asthma. JACEP 1979;8:9–12.

21. Nowak RM, Pensler MI, Sarkar DD, et al. Comparison of peak expiratory and FEV1 admission criteria for acute bronchial asthma. Ann Emerg Med 1982;11:64–9.

22. FitzGerald JM, Grunfeld A. Status asthmaticus. In: Lichtenstein LM, Fauci AS, editors. Current therapy in allergy, immunology, and rheumatology. 5th ed. St. Louis (MO): Mosby; 1996. p. 63–7.

23. Spieri MA, Millar AB, Pavia D, Clark SW. Subcutaneous adrenaline versus terbutaline in the treatment of acute severe asthma. Thorax 1988;43:19–23.

24. Williams SJ, Winner SJ, Clark TJH. Comparison of inhaled and intravenous terbutaline in acute severe asthma. Thorax 1981;36:629–31.

25. Cheong B, Reynolds SR, Rajan G, et al. Intravenous beta-agonists in acute severe asthma. BMJ 1988;297:448–50.

26. Rossing TH, Fanta CH, McFadden ER Jr. The effect of outpatient treatment of asthma with beta-agonists on the response to sympathomimetics in the emergency department. Am J Med 1983;75:781–4.

27. Turner M, Patel A, Ginsberg S, FitzGerald JM. Bronchodilator therapy in acute airflow obstruction: a meta-analysis. Arch Intern Med 1997;158:1736–44.

28. Turner MO, Gafni A, Swan D, FitzGerald JM. A review and economic evaluation of bronchodilator delivery methods in hospitalised patients. Arch Intern Med 1996;156:2113–8.

29. Rowe BH, Spooner CH, Ducharme FM, et al. Early emergency department treatment of acute asthma with systemic corticosteroids. Cochrane Database of Systematic Reviews 2000; 2:CD002178.

30. Rodrigo G, Rodrigo C. Inhaled flunisolide for acute severe asthma. Am J Respir Crit Care Med 1998;157:698–703.

31. Harrison BD, Stokes TC, Hart GJ, et al. Need for intravenous hydrocortisone in addition to oral prednisolone in patients admitted to hospital with severe asthma without ventilatory failure. Lancet 1986;8474:181–4.

32. FitzGerald JM, Shragge DL, Haddon J, et al. A randomized controlled trial of high dose inhaled budesonide versus oral prednisone in patients discharged from the emergency department following an acute asthma exacerbation. Can Respir J 2000;7:61–7.

33. Rowe BH, Bota GW, Fabris L, et al. Inhaled budesonide in addition to oral corticosteroids to prevent asthma relapse following discharge from the emergency department: a randomised controlled trial. JAMA 1999;281:2119–26.

34. Sung L, Osmond M, Klassen T. Randomised, controlled trial of inhaled budesonide as adjunct to oral prednisone in acute asthma. Acad Emerg Med 1998;5:209–13.

35. Garrett J, Williams S, Wong C, Holdaway D. Treatment of acute asthmatic exacerbations with an increased dose of inhaled steroid. Arch Dis Child 1998;79:12–7.

36. Gussman A, Afilalo M, Colacone A, et al and the Asthma ED Study Group. The effects of combined intravenous and inhaled corticosteroids (beclomethasone dipropionate) for the emergency treatment of acute asthma. Acad Emerg Med 1997;4:100–6.

37. Levy ML, Stevenson C, Maslen T. Comparison of short courses of oral prednisolone and fluticasone propionate in the treatment of adults with acute exacerbations of asthma in primary care. Thorax 1996;51:1087–92.

38. FitzGerald JM, Grunfeld A, Pare PD, et al. The clinical efficacy of combination nebulized anticholinergic and adrenergic bronchodilators versus nebulized adrenergic bronchodilators alone in acute asthma. Chest 1997;111:311–5.

39. Garrett JE, Town GI, Rodwell P, et al. Nebulized salbutamol with and without ipratropium bromide in the treatment of acute asthma. J Allergy Clin Immunol 1997;100:165–70.

40. Karpel JP, Schacter EN, Fanta C, et al. A comparison of ipratropium and salbutamol versus salbutamol alone in the treatment of acute asthma. Chest 1996;110:611–6.

41. Lanes S, Garrett JE, Wentworth CE, et al. The effect of adding ipratropium bromide to salbutamol in the treatment of acute asthma: a pooled analysis of three trials. Chest 1998;114:365–72.

42. Plotnick LH, Ducharme FM. Should inhaled anticholinergics be added to β_2 agonists for treating acute childhood and adolescent asthma? A systematic review. BMJ 1998;317:971–7.

43. Rodrigo G, Rodrigo C, Burschtin O. Ipratropium in acute adult severe asthma: a meta-analysis of randomised controlled trials. Am J Med 1999;107:363–70.

44. Rowe BH, Bretzlaff JA, Bourdon C, et al. Magnesium sulphate for treating exacerbations of acute asthma in the emergency department. Cochrane Database of Systematic Reviews 2000;2:CD001490.

45. FitzGerald JM. Magnesium sulphate is effective for severe acute asthma treated in the emergency department. West J Med 2000;172:96.

46. Rodrigo G, Rodrigo C, Burschtin O. Efficacy of magnesium sulphate in acute adult asthma: a meta-analysis of randomized trials. Am J Emerg Med 2000;18:216–21.

47. Nannini LJ Jr, Pewdinao JC, Corna RA, et al. Magnesium sulphate as a vehicle for nebulized salbutamol in acute asthma. Am J Med 2000;108:193–7.

48. Spiteri MA, Millar AB, Pavia D, Clarke SW. Subcutaneous adrenaline versus terbutaline in the treatment of acute severe asthma. Thorax 1988;43:19–23.

49. Cheong B, Reynolds S, Rajan KG, Ward MJ. A comparison of intravenous with nebulised salbutamol in the treatment of acute, severe asthma. Br Med J 1988;297:448–50.

50. Littenberg B. Aminophylline treatment in severe, acute asthma. JAMA 1988;259:1670–84.

51. Darioli E, Perret C. Mechanical controlled hypoventilation in status asthmaticus. Am Rev Respir Dis 1984;129:385–7.

52. Sarama VJ. Use of ketamine in acute severe asthma. Acta Anaesthesiol Scand 1992;36:106–7.

53. Awadh N, Al-Mane F, Pare PD, FitzGerald JM. Acute myopathy after mechanical ventilation for acute asthma. Chest 1999;115:1627–31.

54. Schwartz SH. Treatment of status asthmaticus with halothane. JAMA 1984;257:2688–9.

55. MacDonnell KS. Extracorporeal membrane oxygenator support in a case of severe status asthmaticus. Ann Thorac Surg 1981;31:171–5.

56. Ramirez RJ, Obenour WH Jr. Bronchopulmonary lavage in asthma and chronic bronchitis: clinical and physiologic observations. Chest 1971;59:146–52.

57. Manthous CA, Hall JB, Caputo MA, et al. Heliox improves pulsus paradoxus and peak expiratory flow in non-intubated patients with severe asthma. Am J Respir Crit Care Med 1995;151:310–4.

58. Corre KA, Rothstein RJ. Assessing severity of adult asthma and need for hospitalisation. Ann Emerg Med 1985;14:45–52.

59. Grunfeld A, FitzGerald JM. Discharge considerations in acute asthma. Can Respir J 1996;3:322–4.

60. Cowie RL, Revitt S, Underwood MF, Field S. The effect of a peak flow–based action plan in the prevention of exacerbations of asthma. Chest 1997;112:1534–8.

61. O'Driscoll BR, Karla S, Wilson M, et al. Double blind trial of steroid tapering in acute asthma. Lancet 1993; 341:324–7.

62. Gibson PG, Coughlan J, Abramson M, et al. The effects of self-management and regular review in adults with asthma [update software]. Cochrane Review. Oxford: The Cochrane Library; February 1998.

63. Pauwels RA, Lofdahl C-G, Postma DS, et al. Effect of inhaled formoterol and budesonide on exacerbations of asthma. N Engl J Med 1997;337:1405–11.

64. FitzGerald JM. Effect of inhaled formoterol and budesonide on exacerbations of asthma [correspondence]. N Engl J Med 1998;338:1071–2.

65. Boulet LP, Becker A, Berube D, et al. Summary of recommendations from the Canadian Asthma Consensus Report 1999. Can Med Assoc J 1999;161:S1–12.

66. FitzGerald JM, Becker A, Chung K, Lee J, and the Canadian Asthma Exacerbation Study Group. A randomized controlled, multi-center study to compare double dose versus maintenance dose of inhaled corticosteroids · (ICS) during asthma exacerbations [abstract]. Am J Respir Crit Care Med 2000;161 Suppl:A187.

67. FitzGerald JM, Turner MO. Delivering asthma education to high risk groups. Patient Educ Counselling 1997;32:S77–86.

CHAPTER 21

Management of Asthma in the Intensive Care Unit

Avi Nahum, MD, PhD

David V. Tuxen, MBBS, FRACP, DipDHM, MD

The prevalence of asthma has in many countries increased from an estimated 4% prior to 1960 to estimates ranging from 8% in adults to 15 to 20% in children in the 1990s (Level II).[1–7] This was associated with an increase, in the 1980s, in emergency presentations, hospital admissions (Level II),[2,8,9] and deaths attributed to asthma (Level II).[10] Much attention was directed toward this problem and, by the 1990s, decreasing hospitalization and mortality rates were reported (Level II)[11–14] as well as decreasing intensive care admissions (Level IIIB). This has been attributed to increasing recognition of asthma and improvements in asthma treatment.

Acute severe asthma remains a medical emergency with a risk of respiratory arrest and death, and requires prompt clinical assessment with aggressive medical management. Life-threatening asthma events have been described in the setting of two distinct clinical backgrounds (Level III)[1,15–21]—acute severe airway obstruction superimposed on a poorly controlled asthma, and hyperacute asthma with a background of minimal airflow obstruction.

Acute severe asthma is the most common presentation of life-threatening asthma (and amount to approximately 70% of patients who require mechanical ventilation); it has a female preponderance and is associated with a poorly controlled moderate to severe asthma (Level III).[16,22,23] Nevertheless, asthma symptoms could have been minimal[24–26] before the episode because of underperception of breathlessness,[26] denial, and behavior modification. As a result, asthma severity may be underestimated by both patient and doctor, leading to delayed presentation and undertreatment (Level III).[22,27,28] Severe attacks may develop over hours to days, and presentation follows either a prolonged exacerbation refractory to therapy, or recurrent episodes.[16] In this setting, airway pathology is dominated by chronic inflammatory changes including edema, hypertrophy, and mucus plugging. Commonly there is a history of use of large doses of inhaled β_2-agonists. Since bronchospasm may be a minor component of the airway obstruction, the response to inhaled β_2-agonists may be limited. Improvement in airflow obstruction usually requires steroids and may be slow. Respiratory fatigue and the need for ventilatory support may arise before clinical improvement occurs.

Hyperacute fulminating asthma is less common and is usually seen in younger males who have normal or near normal lung function but with a high level of bronchial reactivity (Level III).[15–17,20,29–31] These patients may have had previous episodes of severe asthma or other evidence of high bronchial reactivity[32] such as marked diurnal variation of symptoms or exercise-induced asthma. However, there may be no history of asthma immediately prior to a life-threatening event. The attack is usually rapid and may lead to severe respiratory insufficiency within hours of onset and occasionally within minutes of a triggering event (Level III).[21,29] This group may suffer respiratory arrest before or soon after arrival at hospital[33] or may present with severe hypercapnia. The response to treatment is often prompt and aggressive treatment may avert the need for respiratory support.

There is a spectrum of illness between the two groups, and not all patients can be clearly categorized. However, both clinical patterns have been associated with the requirement for mechanical ventilation and asthma mortality.[22,23] Clinical triggers include upper respiratory tract infections, allergens, and irritants,[34] but no clear precipitant can be identified in over 30% of patients.[35]

CLINICAL PRESENTATION

Although expiratory wheeze is the clinical hallmark of asthma, the loudness of wheezing is not a good guide to the severity of airway obstruction (Level III).[36,37] Very soft breath sounds on auscultation or especially a "silent chest" may indicate grossly inadequate airflow ("locked lung syndrome"). Airflow obstruction results in pulmonary hyperinflation that may become clinically apparent as asthma becomes more severe.

Hypoxemia[36,38] and the requirement for increased minute ventilation[39–41] are invariably present due to increased ventilation-perfusion (V/Q) imbalance. The degree of these disturbances is roughly proportional to the severity of airflow obstruction.[36,38] Since hypoxemia is usually secondary to V/Q mismatch,[36,38,42] it is readily corrected with supplemental oxygen.[36] Refractory hypoxemia and central cyanosis may occur with severe asthma. Cyanosis may be clinically detected with as little as 1.5 g/100 mL deoxyhemoglobin (PaO$_2$ of approximately 60 mm Hg),[43] but it is a late sign, and hypoxemia must be sought using pulse oximetry or arterial blood gases and averted with high-flow oxygen therapy before it becomes clinically detectable. Persistent hypoxemia in the setting of high supplemental oxygen therapy should alert the physician to the possibility of shunt physiology such as pneumonia. Tachycardia and arrhythmias may be present and are often associated with stress, increased work of breathing, sympathomimetic drugs, electrolyte disturbances, and/or hypoxemia.

Increased work of breathing, due both to airflow obstruction and the mechanical disadvantage of hyperinflation, results in an increased requirement for respiratory muscle force generation and the use of accessory respiratory muscles.[24,44] This, in turn, results in the appearance and sensation of dyspnea[25,26] and, as airflow obstruction worsens, respiratory distress. The assessment of the degree of respiratory distress by both the patient and by an experienced treating doctor[45] can be valuable indicators of the severity of asthma and the need for ventilatory assistance in some patients with asthma. However, some patients may have minimal symptoms in the presence of severe airflow obstruction, (Level III)[24–26] and the patient's assessment of the response to treatment may also be inaccurate (Level III).[24,46] Small improvements in airflow obstruction have been shown to give symptom relief and can lead to underestimation of the severity of asthma and consequent undertreatment.[24] Increased work of breathing is also accompanied by assumption of an upright posture, sweating, and inability to speak, all of which are valuable indicators of severity of asthma.[47] Since severe airway obstruction limits the patient's capacity to increase tidal volume, increased minute ventilation requirement causes tachypnea.[39] As the severity of asthma worsens, ventilation requirement increases and tidal volume falls causing further increases in tachypnea. A reduction in tachypnea without improvement in asthma indicates fatigue and impending respiratory collapse.

The increased negative intrathoracic pressure generated during inspiration is also responsible for pulsus paradoxus, which is frequently present[24,48] and may be a useful clinical indicator of airways obstruction (Level IIIA). Pulsus paradoxus is an exaggeration of the normal slight fall in blood pressure and pulse volume on inspiration. A difference in systolic blood pressure between inspiration and expiration greater than 10 mm Hg (1.3 kPa) indicates severe asthma (Level III).[24,49,50] However, the degree of pulsus paradoxus does not necessarily correlate with the severity of the asthma, as it is also dependent on the capacity of the inspiratory muscles to generate negative intrathoracic pressure. If the inspiratory muscles are weak or impaired by hyperinflation and fatigue, then pulsus paradoxus may be small or may diminish as airflow obstruction becomes more severe.

When the patient with severe asthma is unable to achieve the ventilation required for normocapnia, ventilatory failure ensues and is manifested by a rising PaCO$_2$. This is usually accompanied by marked distress, restlessness, and anxiety. As higher levels of PaCO$_2$ are reached, flushing, further sweating, and bounding pulse occur and may be accompanied by exhaustion, obtundation, and a depressed level of consciousness. Once the patient with asthma has reached this level of severity, ventilatory assistance is almost invariably required and should be instigated urgently.

Usually two clinical patterns lead to hypercapnia in acute asthma. Early, severe hypercapnia may occur with hyperacute asthma due to the mechanical limitations imposed on ventilation by dynamic hyperinflation (see below). As this phenomenon is relatively independent of muscle fatigue, severe hypercapnia may be present in a patient who may not have impending respiratory collapse and who may respond rapidly to aggressive treatment. Although fatigue may occur, and provisions for rapid intubation should be made, such patients may avoid intubation if a rapid response to treatment occurs.

Conversely, patients with less fulminating but severe airflow obstruction, which is responding inadequately to treatment, may undergo fatigue at lower levels of PaCO₂. Such patients may be transiently capable of a higher level of minute ventilation (V_E) but not capable of sustaining it and may require ventilatory assistance.

AVOIDANCE OF MECHANICAL VENTILATIOIN

The wish to avoid the risk of cardiorespiratory arrest in patients with severe asthma must be balanced against the desire to avoid mechanical ventilation. In one series,[33] cardiorespiratory arrest was the initiator of mechanical ventilation for asthma in 10% of patients, and in a literature review,[51] cerebral hypoxia as a result of cardiorespiratory arrest was the most common cause of death. Whenever possible, patients who are in extremis should have mechanical ventilation instigated before the risk of cardiorespiratory arrest becomes high.

However, in the majority of patients with severe asthma who are not in extremis, every attempt should be made to avoid mechanical ventilation, provided it is safe to do so. Mechanical ventilation of patients with asthma can be difficult and is associated with significant risk of complications.[33,51] Its avoidance requires careful bedside assessment of the patient's ability to maintain ventilation. Patients with hypercapnia and respiratory distress may benefit from additional measures to reduce the need for mechanical ventilation. Full standard therapy should be undertaken and additional drug therapy that is not established should be considered. The use of heliox[52,53] and noninvasive mechanical ventilation[54] have both been shown to reduce the work of breathing and improve gas exchange (Level IIIA). Both have been suggested to reduce the requirement for mechanical ventilation (Level IIIB), but neither has been established in randomized clinical studies.

Drug Therapy

Drug therapy has been discussed in great detail in other sections of the text.

Full aggressive drug therapy should include continuous or 1 to 2 hourly nebulized salbutamol (albuterol),[55] ipratropium bromide nebulized 4 hourly,[56,57] early commencement of intravenous steroids, and nebulized budesonide.[58]

Intravenous aminophylline is no longer recommended as a first-line agent in the treatment of severe asthma. Although aminophylline is established as a bronchodilator, a recent review[59] found no evidence of benefit, in the majority of studies, in the presence of inhaled β-agonists and parenteral steroids. However, occasional studies have shown benefit,[60] and it continues to be recommended[51,61] for patients with severe asthma in whom the response to first-line agents has been suboptimal.

Intravenous salbutamol (albuterol) has been shown to be inferior to nebulized salbutamol (Level I),[62–64] but whether it confers additional benefit when added to nebulized salbutamol has not been adequately assessed. Intravenous salbutamol has the theoretic benefit of reaching airways that are not accessible to nebulized salbutamol because of sputum plugging. It is infrequently used in some countries (eg, United States, Canada) and commonly used in other countries (eg, Australia, New Zealand), which have a higher incidence of life-threatening asthma.

Epinephrine has the theoretic benefit of inducing mucosal shrinkage in addition to its bronchodilator properties, and there have been anecdotal reports suggesting its superiority to β-agonists.[65] Systematic studies comparing the two agents have failed to demonstrate this advantage,[66–68] but there have been no studies (to our knowledge) to assess whether adrenaline provides additional benefit in the presence of full β-agonist therapy. Although additional benefit from adrenaline has not been established, it has been increasingly used and recommended[59,61] for patients not responding to standard bronchodilator therapy.

Nonrandomized studies have suggested benefit from intravenous magnesium sulphate, (Level III),[69,70] but a larger randomized study has not confirmed this benefit (Level I).[71] A meta-analysis[72] of seven trials concluded that there was no evidence for routine use of magnesium sulphate in asthma but that there was evidence of benefit for presentations with acute severe asthma.

Bronchodilator sedatives and inhalational anesthetic agents have reported benefit in nonrandomized studies (Level IIIB)[72–75] but are contraindicated in nonintubated patients.

Antileukotriene agents have shown promising results in the management of chronic asthma,[76–78] but their role in acute severe asthma has not been established.

Heliox

Helium is not a bronchodilator but when a helium-oxygen mixture (Heliox, 80:20 or 60:40) is inhaled, overall gas density is lessened, reducing gas turbulence and, therefore, airflow resistance. This decreases the work of breathing (Level III)[52] and may allow improved penetration of inhaled bronchodilators to peripheral airways. These factors may avert respiratory fatigue in situations of life-threatening asthma and allow more time for bronchodilator and anti-inflammatory therapies to work. Manthous et al[52] found reductions in pulsus paradoxus and increases in peak flow in spontaneously breathing asthmatic patients given Heliox, and Gluck et al[53] found reductions in $PaCO_2$ and peak airway pressure when 60:40 Heliox was administered to patients requiring mechanical ventilation for severe asthma. Heliox can also be used in spontaneously breathing patients via a modified face mask, to avoid the need for intubation. The role of Heliox in acute asthma is far from established, but it is safe provided adequate oxygenation is maintained. It may be tried in critical asthma cases to avert intubation or during difficult mechanical ventilation (Level IIIB).

Application of Heliox through a mechanical ventilator requires a thorough understanding of the operation of the ventilator in the presence of Heliox. Due to the change in gas density, some ventilators' spirographs and O_2-blenders can no longer provide accurate information, necessitating adjustments in FIO_2, tidal volume (V_T), and inspiratory flow rate (V_1) and necessitating use of a calibrated volume spirometer to measure V_T periodically. Moreover, as the density of helium-oxygen gas mixture rises with increasing FIO_2, it is advisable to use the lowest possible FIO_2 that yields an adequate PaO_2. This also means that whenever FIO_2 is changed, V_T and V_1 need to be re-adjusted.

Noninvasive Ventilatory Assistance

Continuous positive airways pressure (CPAP), either by occlusive face or nasal mask or via the endotracheal tube, has been advocated to reduce the work of breathing, thus improving dyspnea in patients with acute asthma (Level IIIA).[79–81] It is believed that CPAP reduces the work of breathing by counterbalancing the positive pressure remaining in the alveoli at the end of expiration (PEEPi, intrinsic or auto-PEEP) as a result of gas trapping.[82,83] It may be used in patients with incipient respiratory failure to try and avert the need for mechanical ventilation, or during or after difficult weaning from the same. Continuous positive airways pressure is generally well tolerated, but pressure necrosis of the nose, ears, and cheeks; claustrophobia; and intolerance have been reported. In most cases, the beneficial clinical response to application of CPAP is usually evident within 30 minutes of its initiation. Patients who do not respond to CPAP quickly should be monitored carefully to detect any clinical deterioration;

its effect on dyspnea, respiratory rate, and blood gases should be carefully assessed before CPAP is continued.

Noninvasive mechanical ventilation (NIMV) may be delivered by occlusive nasal or face mask and has been used with a variety of ventilatory modes including volume control, pressure control, pressure support, and biphasic positive airways pressure (BiPAP). It has been used in acute respiratory failure from a variety of causes including exacerbations of chronic airflow limitation, where its benefit has now been established in randomized studies (Level I).[84–86] There is little data relating to its use in acute asthma.[54] Its increased level of ventilatory assistance may be of greater value than CPAP, but that same increased assistance may lead to increased risk from excessive pulmonary hyperinflation.

To date there is only one randomized controlled clinical study that has examined the effect of NIVM in patients with asthma.[87] Patients with moderate asthma that presented to the emergency department were randomized to receive two doses of aerosolized albuterol either by a small-volume nebulizer or via NIMV. Unfortunately, NIMV was not applied at any other time, and none of the patients required mechanical ventilation. Even though patients' response as judged by a peak expiratory flow rate measurement were better in the NIMV group,[87] it is impossible to gauge the clinical significance of this study with respect to NIMV as part of a clinical strategy to avoid intubation in asthmatic patients. In four case series (Level III)[54,88–90] that reported application of NIMV on 35 patients, five patients required intubation (14%). Even though most authors conclude that NIMV diminishes the need for intubation, it is difficult to put the current available data from case series into the proper clinical perspective. Note that in one group of asthmatic patients with hypercarbia, the required intubation rate was reported as only around 8%.[91] These observations underline the need for randomized controlled clinical trials of NIMV in moderate to severe asthma to assess its potential as a clinical tool to circumvent intubation.

MECHANICAL VENTILATION OF SEVERE ASTHMA

Decision to Intubate

Because of the different mechanisms of hypercapnia and the variable rate of response to treatment, the decision to intubate cannot be based solely on any numeric value of $PaCO_2$, respiratory rate, peak flow, or pulsus paradoxus. It must be based on bedside assessment by an experienced clinician, of the degree and evolution of respiratory distress and associated clinical symptoms. Patients who are drowsy or comatose (or who have experienced a respiratory arrest) require immediate intubation. Conscious patients with the clinical appearance of severe fatigue and inadequate or deteriorating respiratory patterns also need intubation. However, patients who are working hard but are not severely distressed may not need intubation despite the presence of marked hypercapnia (eg, $PaCO_2$ > 80 mm Hg). A useful adjunct to this decision is the patient's assessment of the degree of respiratory fatigue. Patients may underestimate their dyspnea but seldom overestimate it, and a complaint of severe fatigue or impending respiratory collapse should be taken seriously. Usually, patients with prior intubation episodes can inform the physician when to intubate quite accurately.

Dynamic Hyperinflation

Mechanical ventilation of patients with severe asthma continues to be associated with a high level of morbidity (hypotension 23%, barotrauma 12%) and mortality (overall 12% from 1261 episodes in 37 papers).[51] Hypotension and barotrauma are almost exclusively confined to patients with severe asthma who have been mechanically ventilated.[33] It now appears that this morbidity and up to one-third of the mortality may be due to unrecognized or undertreated dynamic hyperinflation (DHI) during mechanical ventilation.

In the setting of airflow obstruction, the tidal volume, either spontaneous or delivered by the ventilator during inspiration, cannot be fully exhaled during expiration, and gas is trapped within the thorax following each breath.[92] Initially, this leads to a progressive increased in lung volume, but after 6 to 20 breaths, a new equilibrium point is reached due to increased elastic recoil of the respiratory system and increases in small airway caliber as lung volume increases. At this equilibrium point, all the inspired tidal volume can be exhaled in the available expiratory time. If airflow obstruction is mild, this process is adaptive. It allows a higher V_E, and normocapnia that could not be achieved at functional residual capacity (FRC), to be achieved at a higher lung volume.

When airflow obstruction becomes more severe, DHI increases and the end-inspiratory lung volume required to achieve normocapnia approaches total lung capacity (TLC). During spontaneous ventilation, this dramatically decreases inspiratory muscle efficiency and increases respiratory effort. Inspiratory muscles operating at this lung volume are close to their minimum length and are at their minimum mechanical advantage for inspiration. This, combined with the increased load to breathing due to high airflow resistance and increased dead space, can easily lead to inspiratory muscles exceeding their maximum sustainable capacity and undergoing eventual fatigue with increasing hypercapnia.

When airflow obstruction rapidly becomes very severe, the end-inspiratory lung volume required to achieve the V_E for normocapnia significantly exceeds TLC. During spontaneous ventilation, the maximum end-inspiratory lung volume that can be achieved only minimally exceeds TLC and, hence, the V_E required cannot be achieved. Initial V_E required for normocapnia in mechanical ventilation for asthma is high.[33,39–41] It has been reported in one study[41] as 19 ± 2 L/min, whereas the V_E that achieved ventilation below the predicted normal TLC was 10 ± 1 L/min. Because of airflow obstruction, higher levels of ventilation would have required lung volumes above TLC, which cannot be achieved during spontaneous ventilation. Thus, a patient who requires a V_E of 19 L/min but who can only generate 10 L/min must be hypercapnic.

When the patient with very severe airflow obstruction receives mechanical ventilation, DHI is not limited by the inability of the inspiratory muscles to exceed TLC. Only moderate levels of V_E from a mechanical ventilator may drive DHI well above normal TLC (Figure 21–1) and lead to circulatory tamponade and pneumothorax.[33,40,41]

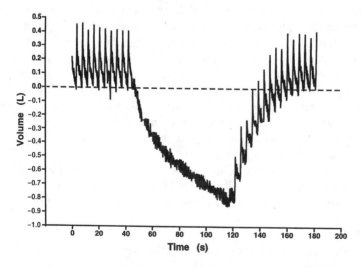

Figure 21–1 The effects of apnea and resumption of ventilation on lung volume measured by inductive plethysmography (Respitrace) in a patient requiring mechanical ventilation for severe asthma.

The extent of DHI during mechanical ventilation primarily depends on three interacting factors—the magnitude of inspired V_T, the expiratory time (T_E), and the severity of airflow obstruction. In practice, DHI is minimized best by using a low V_E achieved by a low V_T and a low rate of ventilation[41,93] and a high V_I.

In a paralyzed patient, DHI can be measured during mechanical ventilation by the volume of gas exhaled during a period of apnea long enough for expiratory flow to cease.[40] This has been termed the end-inspiratory lung volume above FRC (V_{EI}). When mechanical venti- lation resumes at the end of the period of apnea, DHI returns lung volume to its steady state within 8 to 12 breaths (see Figure 21–1). The evaluation of V_{EI} requires a volumetric mea- suring device, as flow transducing devices normally found on ventilators consistently under- estimate this volume. In a group of mechanically ventilated asthma patients, V_{EI} of 1.4 L (20 mL/kg) has been shown to be the most discriminating variable for prediction of risk of hypotension and barotrauma (Level II).[33] This level of V_{EI} was associated with an end-inspi- ratory lung volume that exceeded the normal TLC.[41] Thus, ventilatory patterns that maintain V_{EI} less than 1.4 L are probably safe, because they maintain lung volume below its normal maximum capacity (TLC). During initial mechanical ventilation of a group of severe asthma patients, normalizing $PaCO_2$ required a V_E of 16 L/min (range 10 to 25 L/min) and resulted in a V_{EI} of 2.1 ± 0.2 L, leading to hypotension in most patients.[40] A safe level of DHI ($V_{EI} <$ 1.4 L, < 20 mL/kg) required an initial V_E of < 8 L/min (115 mL/kg/min) and resulted in a $PaCO_2$ of 65 ± 15 mm Hg, indicating the necessity for hypoventilation to avoid excessive DHI (Level II). Use of a relatively low V_E during mechanical ventilation of asthma patients has also been suggested to improve outcome (Level II).[33,40,41,94–101]

Despite the fact that V_{EI} quantifies the extent of DHI during mechanical ventilation and can predict the risk of complications, it has not gained widespread clinical use because its measurement is technically complex and requires therapeutic paralysis. At the bedside, plateau airway pressure (Pplat, airway opening pressure after an end-inspiratory pause of 0.5 to 1.0 seconds) and auto-PEEP (airway opening pressure above the set PEEP after an end- expiratory pause 0.5 to 1.0 seconds) can be measured easily as indices of DHI. Moreover, other clinical indicators of DHI include changes in hemodynamics during a period of apnea or reduction in the ventilator rate. Plateau airway pressure should only be measured after a single breath, as application of an end-inspiratory pause in some ventilators automatically decreases T_E, and its presence during several breaths can increase DHI to dangerous levels. Under these conditions, the value of Pplat increases with each delivered V_T, leading to over- estimation of Pplat during baseline conditions.

Mechanical Ventilator Settings

Current recommendations (supported by these authors) for initial mechanical ventilation include sedation, with or without transient muscle relaxation, hypoventilation using an ini- tial V_E of 115 mL/min/kg, a V_T of ≤ 8 mL/kg, a rate of 10 to 12 breaths/min, and a peak flow rate of 80 to 100 L/min during constant-flow volume-controlled ventilation. Dynamic hyperinflation should be controlled by maintaining V_{EI} (if measured) < 1.4 L (20 mL/kg), Pplat < 25 cm H_2O, auto-PEEP < 10 to 12 cm H_2O, and no extrinsic PEEP. The Pplat of < 25 cm H_2O is recommended, because this is the pressure that corresponds most closely to the safe level of V_{EI}, to the avoidance of complications and to TLC.[33,40,41] This is lower than the Pplat limit commonly recommended for acute respiratory distress syndrome (ARDS) (Pplat < 30 to 35 cm H_2O), presumably because of higher respiratory system compliance in asthma.

There are, at present, no randomized controlled studies and only one study with historic controls to support any of these recommendations. Given these limitations, the evidence for each of the following recommendations needs careful assessment.

1. Initial V_E of 115 mL/min/kg:[41] the principle of a low V_E has good evidence and is widely accepted (Level IIIA) [33,40,41,95–101] with most authors recommending a V_E close to this level. Seventeen case series published in 16 papers after 1980 reported patients who received mechanical ventilation for asthma. Ten case series [17,33,102–109] that did not specify the use of a hypoventilation strategy reported 39 deaths in 352 patients (11% mortality). Seven case series[33,41,95–97,99] that specifically reported the

use of a hypoventilation strategy reported 11 deaths in 183 patients (6% mortality, $p < .05$). There were no significant differences in the incidence of pneumothorax (12% versus 10%) and hypotension (22% versus 23%) between these two groups; however, the latter may not be a valid comparison as it is likely that the threshold for reporting these complications was lower in series using hypoventilation (Level III).

2. $V_T \leq 8$ mL/kg:[41] the principle of a low V_T has moderately good evidence[40,98] and is widely accepted (Level IIIA).[40,41,98,99,106,110,111] Low V_T patterns have been shown to produce less DHI and lower V_{EI}s than high V_T patterns for the same V_E.[40]

3. Rate 10 to 12 breaths/min: low respiratory rate is closely allied to low V_E and is the most obvious way of ensuring an adequate T_E. Thus, the evidence for a low rate is that of low V_E (Level IIIA). Low rate is specifically recommended by a number of authors.[33,41,94,96,97,99,106,109–114]

4. Inspiratory flow rate of 80 to 100 L/min: a high inspiratory flow rate, although controversial, has also been recommended by a number of authors (Level IIIB),[41,93,100,101,115–117] because it incurs a shorter inspiratory time and, hence, a longer T_E for a given respiratory rate. The controversy[95–97,106,111] arises from the high peak inspiratory pressures caused by high inspiratory flow rates and the theoretic concerns that this may lead to increased distribution of ventilation to low-resistance lung units causing barotrauma.[118,119] These concerns are based on lung models[118,119] that do not contain important fundamental features present in severe asthma and have been refuted in clinical studies.[120] Although the evidence supporting high inspiratory flow is limited (Level IIIB),[41,93,116,120] there is no clinical evidence to support low inspiratory flow (Level IIIC).

5. $V_{EI} < 1.4$ L (20 mL/kg) (Level IIIA): V_{EI} has been shown to be a reliable measure of DHi[140] that correlated with complications,[33] that could be used to regulate mechanical ventilation,[41] and that has been shown to reduce the incidence of hypotension and barotrauma in a study with a historic control group.[98] Unfortunately, the technical complexity of this measurement and the desire to avoid neuromuscular blockade (see previous discussion), preclude this measurement from routine use in all patients.

6. Pplat < 25 cm H_2O (Level IIIB):[33] there have been no studies directly evaluating the use of Pplat to regulate mechanical ventilation or to avoid complications in asthma. In one study,[33] Pplat did not correlate with complications as well as V_{EI}. Although Pplat correlated with V_{EI} in individual patients, it did not correlate as well between patients due to wide variation of compliance.[33,41] This is not surprising considering that lung volume is close to or above TLC.[41] To maintain $V_{EI} < 20$ mL/kg (and, by implication, lung volume below TLC), the mean value of Pplat required is < 25 cm H_2O.[33,40,41] This value is less than the value of 30 to 35 cm H_2O usually recommended for ARDS to maintain lung units below their TLC.[121] One factor contributing to this may be that a number of lung units at a higher volume and pressure may not be communicating with the central airways due to airway closure[122]; hence, Pplat may be underestimating average alveolar pressure.

7. Auto-PEEP < 10 to 12 cm H_2O: auto-PEEP is a measure of the average alveolar pressure of lung units that remain in communication with the central airways at the end of expiration. As progressive airway closure occurs during expiration, a large number of lung units with alveolar pressures higher than measured auto-PEEP do not communicate that pressure to the central airways during the auto-PEEP maneuver (Figure 21–2). The consequence of this is that auto-PEEP underestimates the mean end-expiratory alveolar pressure and is insensitive to changes in the level of DHI.[122] Although a low level of auto-PEEP does not ensure a safe level of DHI, a high level of auto-PEEP still represents excessive DHI and indicates the need for its reduction.

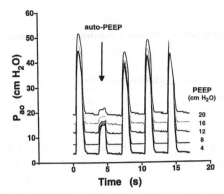

Figure 21–2 The effect of increasing PEEP on auto-PEEP in a mechanically ventilated patient with severe airflow obstruction. Notice that the level of auto-PEEP remains almost constant as PEEP increases from x to y; then there is an appearance of new auto-PEEP when PEEP is further increased, suggesting communication with higher pressure regions that did not previously contribute to measured auto-PEEP because of airway closure.

If DHI is excessive, as indicated by any of these variables exceeding their safe limit, the ventilator rate should be reduced, irrespective of $PaCO_2$. The ventilator should not be adjusted in response to $PaCO_2$, and, during controlled mechanical ventilation, PEEP should not be used to avoid further increases in lung volume.[93] Only if DHI is within safe limits can ventilation be liberalized by increasing the ventilator rate, thereby reducing hypercapnia. Plateau airway pressure and auto-PEEP can be used to regulate the level of hypoventilation during mechanical ventilation, and are the most practical measurements to avoid the complications associated with DHI.

Initial mechanical ventilation usually requires heavy sedation and transient muscle relaxation to achieve tolerance of hypercapnic acidosis and assessment of DHI. It is desirable to minimize or avoid the use of muscle relaxants because of the high risk of myopathy when they are used in association with parenteral corticosteroids (Level IIIE).[123–126] Approximately 20% of patients have rapidly resolving asthma[33,41] and should require only a brief or no period of muscle relaxation. Remaining patients should have one or two initial bolus doses of muscle relaxants to achieve initial stabilization and heavy sedation should be continued as required until airflow obstruction improves and DHI decreases. Continuous infusions of muscle relaxants should be avoided except in the most refractory patients who require prolonged profound hypoventilation that cannot be adequately achieved with heavy sedation and repeated bolus doses of muscle relaxants. If continuous infusions are required, they should be run at a low dose that maintains an initial response on train-of-4 nerve stimulation, and the infusion should be ceased every 24 hours to reassess ongoing need.

Initially, SIMV may be an appropriate ventilatory mode as it allows spontaneous breaths when paralysis has been ceased, but spontaneous breaths should not be supported (eg, by pressure support), as this may lead to unsafe increases in V_E and DHI.

Once airway obstruction begins to improve (as judged by decreasing Pplat and auto-PEEP or V_{EI}), the magnitude of DHI for a given V_E decreases. At this point, respiratory rate may be transiently increased and sedation reduced to allow commencement of weaning. Continuous positive airways pressure is believed to reduce the work of breathing. Studies have demonstrated that the use of low to medium levels of CPAP in acute asthma reduces respiratory rates, inspiratory work, and subjective sensations of dyspnea (Level IIIB).[79–81,127,128] Most of these studies are of nonintubated patients. There are no studies providing evidence of benefit during the weaning phase of mechanical ventilation.

Low levels of CPAP (equivalent to 80% of measured auto-PEEP) may be used in addition to pressure support in patients who are experiencing difficulty weaning. Auto-PEEP and Pplat should be assessed throughout this process to ensure that they remain within safe limits.

Hemodynamic Derangements during Mechanical Ventilation

Despite the improved outcomes from hypoventilation strategies, infrequent individual patients with very severe airflow obstruction may still develop excessive pulmonary hyperinflation during these strategies. The most severe cases may develop life-threatening levels of hypotension or apparent circulatory arrest, without the cause being immediately obvious.[129,130] Any unexplained hypotension or electromechanical dissociation occurring during mechanical ventilation of a patient with airflow obstruction should first be given an apnea test[129] or a period of profound hypoventilation (two to three breaths/min)[101] before any other delaying or potentially harmful diagnostic or therapeutic procedures are attempted.

An apnea test consists of complete disconnection from the ventilator to allow unimpeded expiration for a minimum of 1 minute and observation of the effects on blood pressure and (if possible) central venous pressure. If, during the apnea period, the blood pressure improves significantly (and CVP falls), ventilation should be recommenced at a lower V_E—using V_T and V_I recommendations (above) and a substantially reduced ventilator rate, as low as three to six breaths/min. As the mechanism of hypotension is primarily decreased venous return secondary to excessive intrathoracic pressure and increased pulmonary vascular resistance, the resolution of hypotension may be aided by fluid loading. With the application of hypoventilation, varying degrees of hypercapnic acidosis may occur and occasionally $PaCO_2$ may exceed 100 mm Hg with pH < 7.00, raising the question of whether to use bicarbonate therapy. In patients with moderately severe hypercapnic acidosis, bicarbonate has been shown to have no circulatory or respiratory benefits[131]; however, whether this is also true in very severe respiratory acidosis is unknown. Theoretically, bicarbonate may reduce respiratory drive and distress by reducing the level of acidosis, thereby diminishing sedative needs, but this has not been shown.

Rare patients with exceptionally severe airflow obstruction may remain excessively hyperinflated with high airway pressures, hypotension, and risk of pneumothorax despite profound hypoventilation. Such patients require maximal conventional bronchodilator therapy including continuous nebulized and intravenous salbutamol, full-dose corticosteroids, and intravenous aminophylline.

In patients who are refractory to full medical therapy, less established drug therapies may be tried. These include adrenaline (Level IIIC),[65,132] magnesium (Level IIID),[69–71,133] ketamine (Level IIIC),[72,73] and inhalational anesthetic agents (Level IIIC),[134,135] all of which have reported benefit in observational studies on patients with asthma in less extreme circumstances but lack randomized controlled studies (except magnesium) in a large group of ventilated asthma patients. Whether there is a component of airflow obstruction (bronchospasm, or in the case of adrenaline, edema) that is capable of improvement despite full conventional therapy is uncertain.

The two therapies that do not require an improvement in airway caliber for an effect are cardiopulmonary bypass and Heliox. Cardiopulmonary bypass (two case reports, Level IIIC)[136,137] has been used to maintain gas exchange while awaiting bronchodilator response for this very severe subset of patients. Cardiopulmonary bypass is limited by availability, invasiveness and technical complexity, and delays before commencement. Uncontrolled reports exist of success of Heliox in nonintubated patients,[52,53] and Heliox has been used with success in a patient in this extreme circumstance (Dr. Nerina Harley, November 1998; personal communication) (Level IIIC). Heliox has the advantage of being less invasive and more readily available; however, it remains technically complex. Heliox connections do not fit the standard air and oxygen inlets of mechanical ventilators. The very different flow characteristics of the gas alter the V_T and rate delivered by the ventilator. Not all ventilators function adequately with this gas, and those that do require careful calibration and monitoring of V_T and rate delivery.

Management of Pneumothorax during Mechanical Ventilation

Pneumothorax was reported in 10% of episodes of mechanical ventilation for asthma and was estimated to be the cause of 6% of deaths in 1,261 of episodes of mechanical ventilation reported in 37 studies.[51] Excessive DHI was thought to be the likely mechanism for the majority of these complications (Level III).[33,40,51] A pneumothorax in a mechanically ventilated asthma patient remains a potentially life-threatening problem. This is probably due to the high propensity of pneumothoraces in asthma to be under tension and to become bilateral during mechanical ventilation.

Despite the presence of a pneumothorax, the presence of severe airflow obstruction with delayed emptying and airway closure prevents lung collapse. Consequently, a lung unit that develops an air leak does not have collapse as a mechanism to stop continued air leak. Such lung units continue to be filled by the ventilator but more readily empty down the lower resistance air leak pathway than via the expiratory airways. This functional one-way valve mechanism may quickly lead to the development of considerable tension. Once tension develops in one hemithorax, V_E delivered to that lung decreases due to the decreased compliance of that lung. In this setting, a larger fraction of the V_E is subsequently delivered by the ventilator to the contralateral lung. As the primary reason for the pneumothorax was most likely excessive DHI (occurring bilaterally), a further increase in V_E to the contralateral lung increases the already excessive level of DHI in that lung, leading to a high risk of a second tension pneumothorax.

The possibility of a pneumothorax should be promptly excluded in patients who develop a sudden deterioration in status—tachypnea, respiratory distress, desaturation, high airway pressures, high pressure alarms, tachycardia, or hypotension. This will often occur following a ventilator setting change or a procedure (suctioning, physiotherapy, or central venous catheter insertion), which may themselves cause some of these changes in the patient's status, thereby disguising the presence of a pneumothorax. Inequality of air entry and tracheal shift are not always reliable signs of a pneumothorax during mechanical ventilation. Because the lung in severe airflow obstruction resists deflation, blind intercostal catheter insertion in the absence of a pneumothorax carries a high risk of lung injury. Hence, a chest radiography should always be urgently performed in preference to blind intercostal catheter insertion, unless the patient is severely hypotensive (systolic blood pressure < 70 mm Hg) and does not respond properly to an apnea test. Nevertheless, when the presence of a pneumothorax is suspected clinically, the first course of action should be to protect the contralateral lung from developing a pneumothorax. This can be achieved by immediately reducing the ventilator rate, increasing sedation and/or paralyzing the patient to prevent excessive spontaneous ventilation, and fluid loading as required to assist any hypotension.

Complications of Specific Therapies

Parenteral side effects of β-agonists include tremor, tachycardia, tachyarrhythmias, hypokalemia and lactic acidosis; patients should be monitored for all of these problems. Lactic acidosis may occur in patients receiving parenteral salbutamol and occasionally continuous nebulized salbutamol with lactate levels as high as 12 mmol/L.[51] Intravenous salbutamol infusions should not exceed 10 μg/min, and patients should be monitored for the presence of lactic acidosis by regular assessment of the blood gas bicarbonate level and measurement of the serum lactate level if the former is low or falling. If lactic acidosis is detected, intravenous salbutamol should be reduced or ceased altogether.

Patients who receive high doses of intravenous corticosteroids with neuromuscular blocking agents (NMBAs) are at risk of acute necrotizing myopathy (Level III).[123–126] Effects may range from mild motor weakness to functional quadriparesis. Weakness may delay weaning from the ventilator, prolong hospital stay, and require prolonged rehabilitation, all of which represent substantial detriment to patient care and hospital cost.[138] The etiology appears to be functional muscle denervation from the use of any NMBA.[139] Muscle denervation has been shown to increase the expression of steroid receptors on muscle fibers, thereby sensitizing them to the potential effect of corticosteroids.[140]

All patients who receive intravenous corticosteroids should have their creatinine kinase (CK) levels monitored daily, and corticosteroids should be commenced at the minimum effective dose (eg, hydrocortisone 200 mg IV 6 hourly) and have dose reductions commenced after 24 to 48 hours, unless asthma is exceptionally refractory.[58] Neuromuscular blocking agents use should be minimized. Careful neurologic assessments should be undertaken following cessation of paralysis. If any weakness is detected, the presence of myopathy should be confirmed by electromyography.

LONG-TERM OUTCOMES

Even though severe asthma is recognized as a life-threatening event, recurrent life-threatening episodes and mortality following such events remains substantial. Nine percent of patients who undergo mechanical ventilation for asthma have had a previous episode of mechanical ventilation for the same indication. Long-term follow-up studies of survivors of mechanical ventilation for asthma have reported posthospital mortalities ranging from 7.5 to 24% over a follow-up period of 1 to 7 years.[141-144] This highlights the need for careful follow-up and aggressive medical management after an episode of mechanical ventilation.

In conclusion, the physician faces a number of unique problems associated with significant morbidity and mortality during and after management of patients with life-threatening asthma. The best and simplest solution to these problems remains patient management that prevents the need for mechanical ventilation altogether. Improvements in community and medical information, education of all patients with acute asthma, and detailed management strategies following a severe episode are needed. Hopefully these measures will make life-threatening asthma increasingly rare.   .

REFERENCES

1. Pingleton S. Asthma mortality has increased not only in the United States but also across the world. JAMA 1997;273:1717–8.
2. National Institutes of Health, National Heart, Lung and Blood Institute. National Heart, Lung, and Blood Institute Data Fact Sheet; Asthma Statistics. Bethesda (MD): US Dept of Health and Human Services, Public Health Service; 1989.
3. Bauman A, Young L, Peat J, et al. Asthma under-recognition and under-treatment in an Australian community. Aust N Z J Med 1992;22:36–40.
4. Musk A, Ryan G, Perera D, et al. Mortality from asthma in Western Australia. Med J Aust 1987;147:423–7.
5. Fleming D, Crombie D. Prevalence of asthma and hay fever in England and Wales. Br Med J 1987;294:279–83.
6. Anderson H, Butland B, Strachan D. Trends in prevalence and severity of childhood asthma. BMJ 1994;308:1600–4.
7. Peat J, van den Berg R, Green W, et al. Changing prevalence of asthma in Australian children. BMJ 1994;308:1591–6.
8. Mitchell E. International trends in hospital admission rates for asthma. Arch Dis Child 1985;60:376–8.
9. Anderson H. Increase in hospital admissions for childhood asthma: trends in referral, severity and readmissions from 1970 to 1985 in a health region of the United Kingdom. Thorax 1989;44:614–9.
10. Sly M. Changing asthma mortality. Ann Allergy 1994;73:259–68.
11. Wilson J, Jenkins C. Asthma mortality: where is it going? Med J Aust 1996;164:391–2.
12. Kemp T, Pearce N. The decline in asthma hospitalisations in persons aged 30–40 years in New Zealand. Aust N Z J Med 1997;27:578–81.

13. Australian Bureau of Statistics. Causes of death—Australia. 1989–94. Catalogue No.: 3303.0.

14. Comino E, Bauman A. Trends in asthma-mortality in Australia, 1960–1996. Med J Aust 1998;168:525–7.

15. Johnson A, Nunn A, Somner A, et al. Circumstances of death from asthma. Br Med J 1984;288:1870–2.

16. Wasserfallen J, Schaller M, Feihl F, Perret C. Sudden asphyxic asthma: a distinct entity? Am Rev Respir Dis 1990;142:108–11.

17. Kallenbach J, Frankel A, Lapinski S, et al. Determinants of near fatality in acute severe asthma. Am J Med 1993;95:265–72.

18. Molfino N, Nannini L, Martelli A, Slutsky A. Respiratory arrest in near-fatal asthma. N Engl J Med 1991;324:285–8.

19. Sur S, Crotty T, Kephart G. Sudden-onset fatal asthma: a distinct entity with few eosinophils and relatively more neutrophils in the airway submucosa. Am Rev Respir Dis 1993;148:713–9.

20. Hetzel M, Clark T, Branthwaite M. Asthma: analysis of sudden deaths and ventilatory arrests in hospital. Br Med J 1977;1:808–11.

21. Robin E, Lewiston N. Unexpected, unexplained sudden death in young asthmatic subjects. Chest 1989;96:790–3.

22. Benatar S. Fatal asthma. N Engl J Med 1986;314:423–9.

23. Sears M, Rea H, Fenwick J, et al. Deaths from asthma in New Zealand. Arch Dis Child 1986;61:6–10.

24. McFadden EJ, Kiser R, DeGroot W. Acute bronchial asthma. Relations between clinical and physiologic manifestations. N Engl J Med 1973;228:221–5.

25. Burdon J, Juniper E, Hargreave F, Campbell E. The perception of breathlessness in asthma. Am Rev Respir Dis 1982;126:825–8.

26. Rubinfeld A, Pain M. Perception of asthma. Lancet 1976;1:882–4.

27. Westerman D, Benatar S, Potgieter P, Ferguson A. Identification of the high-risk asthmatic patient. Experience with 39 patients undergoing ventilation for status asthmaticus. Am J Med 1979;66:565–72.

28. Karetzky M. Asthma mortality associated with pneumothorax and intermittent positive pressure breathing. Lancet 1975;1:828–9.

29. McDonald J, Seaton A, Williams D. Asthma deaths in Cardiff 1963–1974: 90 deaths outside hospital. Br Med J 1976;1:1493–5.

30. Ferrer A, Torres A, Roca J, et al. Characteristics of patients with soybean dust–induced acute severe asthma requiring mechanical ventilation. Eur Respir J 1990;3:429–33.

31. Strunk R. Death due to asthma: new insights into sudden unexpected deaths but the focus remains on prevention. Am Rev Respir Dis 1993;148:550–2.

32. Pouw E, Koeter G, deMonchy J, et al. Clinical assessment after a life-threatening attack of asthma; the role of bronchial reactivity. Eur Respir J 1990;3:861–6.

33. Williams T, Tuxen D, Scheinkestel C, et al. Risk factors for morbidity in mechanically ventilated patients with acute severe asthma. Am Rev Respir Dis 1992;146:607–15.

34. Stevenson D, Mathison D, Tan E, Vaughan J. Provoking factors in bronchial asthma. Arch Intern Med 1975;135:777–83.

35. Bellamy D, Collins J. Acute asthma in adults. Thorax 1979;34:36–9.

36. Rees H, Millar J, Donald J. A study of the clinical course and arterial blood gas tensions of patients in status asthmaticus. Q J Med 1968;37:234–43.

37. Shim C, Williams MJ. Relationship of wheezing to the severity of obstruction in asthma. Arch Intern Med 1983;143:890–2.

38. McFadden E, Lyons H. Arterial blood gas tension in asthma. N Engl J Med 1968;278:1027–32.

39. Hedstrand V. Physiological derangements in acute bronchial asthma with special reference to the intensity of the attacks as classified from clinical signs. Ups Dissertations Fac Med Abstracts 1970;84:1–19.

40. Tuxen D, Lane S. The effects of ventilatory pattern on hyperinflation, airway pressures, and circulation in mechanical ventilation of patients with severe airflow obstruction. Am Rev Respir Dis 1987;136:872–9.

41. Tuxen D, Williams T, Scheinkestel C, et al. Use of a measurement of pulmonary hyperinflation to control the level of mechanical ventilation in patients with severe asthma. Am Rev Respir Dis 1992;146:1136–42.

42. Nowak R, Tomlanovich M, Sarker D, et al. Arterial blood gases and pulmonary function testing in acute bronchial asthma. Predicting patient outcomes. JAMA 1983;249:2043–6.

43. Goss G, Hayes J, Burdon J. Deoxyhaemoglobin concentrations in the detection of central cyanosis. Thorax 1988;43:212–3.

44. Rebuck A, Read J. Assessment and management of severe asthma. Am J Med 1971;51:788–98.

45. Shim C, Williams MJ. Evaluation of the severity of asthma: patients versus physicians. Am J Med 1980;68:11–3.

46. Kelsen S, Kelsen D, Fleegler B, et al. Emergency department assessment and treatment of patients with acute asthma. Adequacy of the conventional approach. Am J Med 1978;64:622–8.

47. Brenner B, Abraham E, Simon R. Position and diaphoresis in acute asthma. Am J Med 1983;74:1005–9.

48. Martin J, Jardim J, Sampson M, Engel L. Factors influencing pulsus paradoxus in asthma. Chest 1981;80:543–9.

49. Knowles G, Clark T. Pulsus paradoxus as a valuable sign indicating severity of asthma. Lancet 1973;2:1356–9.

50. Fitzgerald J, Hargreave F. The assessment and management of life-threatening asthma. Chest 1989;95:888–94.

51. Tuxen D. Mechanical ventilation in asthma. In: Recent advances in critical care medicine. No. 4. Evans T, Hinds C, editors. London: Churchill Livingstone; 1996. p. 165–89.

52. Manthous C, Hall J, Caputo M, et al. Heliox improves pulsus paradoxus and peak expiratory flow in nonintubated patients with severe asthma. Am J Respir Crit Care Med 1995;151:310–4.

53. Gluck E, Onorato D, Castriotta R. Helium-oxygen mixtures in intubated patients with status asthmaticus and respiratory acidosis. Chest 1990;98:693–8.

54. Meduri G, Cook T, Turner R, et al. Noninvasive positive pressure ventilation in status asthma. Chest 1996;110:767–74.

55. Mandelberg A, Chen E, Noviski N, Priel I. Nebulized wet aerosol treatment in emergency department—is it essential? Chest 1997;112:1501–5.

56. Schuh S, Johnson D, Callahan S, et al. Efficacy of frequent nebulized ipratropium bromide added to frequent high-dose albuterol therapy in severe childhood asthma. J Pediatr 1995;126:639–45.

57. Karpel J, Schacter E, Fanta C, et al. A comparison of ipratropium and albuterol vs albuterol alone for the treatment of acute asthma. Chest 1996;110:611–6.

58. Rodrigo G, Rodrigo C. Inhaled flunisolide for acute severe asthma. Am J Respir Crit Care Med 1998;157:698–703.

59. Beveridge R, Grunfeld A, Hodder R, Verbeek P. Guidelines for the emergency management of asthma in adults. Can Med Assoc J 1996;155:25–37.

60. Huang D, O'Brien RG, Harmen E, et al. Does aminophylline benefit adults admitted to the hospital for an acute exacerbation of asthma? Ann Intern Med 1993;119:1155–60.

61. Levy B, Kitch B, Fanta C. Medical and ventilatory management of status asthmaticus. Intensive Care Med 1998;24(2):105–17.

62. Lawford P, Jones B, Milledge J. Comparison of intravenous and nebulized salbutamol in initial treatment of severe asthma. BMJ 1978;1:84.

63. Williams S, Winner S, Clark T. Comparison of inhaled and intravenous terbutaline in acute severe asthma. Thorax 1981;36:629–31.

64. Salmeron S, Brochard L, Mal H, et al. Nebulized versus intravenous albuterol in hypercapnic acute asthma: a multicenter, double-blind, randomized study. Am J Respir Crit Care Med 1994;149:1466–70.

65. Appel D, Karpel J, Sherman M. Epinephrine improves expiratory flow rates in patients with asthma who do not respond to inhaled metaproterenol sulfate. J Allergy Clin Immunol 1989;84:90–8.

66. Baughman R, Ploysongsang Y, James W. A comparative study of aerosolized terbutaline and subcutaneously administered epinephrine in the treatment of acute bronchial asthma. Ann Allergy 1984;53:131–4.

67. Tinkelman D, Webb C, Vanderpool G, et al. The use of ketotifen in the prophylaxis of seasonal allergic asthma. Ann Allergy 1986;56:213–7.

68. Spiteri M, Millar A, Pavia D, Clarke S. Subcutaneous adrenaline vs terbutaline in the treatment of acute severe asthma. Thorax 1988;43:19–23.

69. Okayama H, Aikawa T, Okayama M, et al. Bronchodilator effect of intravenous magnesium sulfate in bronchial asthma. JAMA 1987;257:1076–8.

70. Noppen M, Luc Vanmaele L, Impens N, Schandevyl W. Bronchodilating effect of intravenous magnesium sulfate in acute severe bronchial asthma. Chest 1990;97:373–6.

71. Green S, Rothrock S. Intravenous magnesium for acute asthma: failure to decrease emergency treatment duration or need for hospitalization. Ann Emerg Med 1992;21:260–5.

72. Rowe BH, Bretzlaff JA, Bourdon D, et al. Magnesium sulphate for treating exacerbations of acute asthma in the emergency department. Cochrane Database Syst Rev 2000;(2):CD001490.

73. Fisher M. Ketamine hydrochloride in severe bronchospasm. Anaesthesia 1977;32:771–2.

74. Grunberg G, Cohen J, Keslin J, Gassner S. Facilitation of mechanical ventilation in status asthmaticus with continuous intravenous thiopental. Chest 1991;99:1216–9.

75. Prezant D, Aldrich T. Intravenous droperidol for the treatment of status asthmaticus. Crit Care Med 1988;16:96–7.

76. Drazen J. Effects of leukotrienes on airway function. In: The lung: scientific foundations. Crystal R, editor. Philadelphia: Lippincott-Raven; 1997. p. 1287–96.

77. Holgate S, Bradding P, Sampson A. Leukotriene antagonists and synthesis inhibitors: new directions in asthma therapy. J Allergy Clin Immunol 1996;98:1–13.

78. Horwitz R, McGill K, Busse W. The role of leukotriene modifiers in the treatment of asthma. Am J Respir Crit Care Med 1998;157:1363–71.

79. Tenaillon A, Salmona J, Burdin M, Lissac J. Continuous positive airway pressure in asthma. Am Rev Respir Dis 1983;127:658.

80. Weng J, Smith D, Graybar G, Kirby R. Hypotension secondary to air trapping treated with expiratory flow retard. Anesthesiology 1984;60:350–3.

81. Mathieu M, Tonneau M, Zarka D, Sartene R. Effects of positive end-expiratory pressure in severe acute asthma. Crit Care Med 1987;15:1164.

82. Martin J, Shore S, Engel L. Effect of continuous positive airway pressure on respiratory mechanics and pattern of breathing in induced asthma. Am Rev Respir Dis 1982;126:812–7.

83. Gottfried S, Rossi A, Milic-Emili J. Dynamic hyperinflation, intrinsic PEEP and the mechanically ventilated patient. Intensive Crit Care Digest 1986;5:30–3.

84. Brochard L, Mancebo J, Wysocki M, et al. Noninvasive ventilation for acute exacerbations of chronic obstructive pulmonary disease. N Engl J Med 1995;333:817–22.

85. Kramer N, Meyer T, Meharg J, et al. Randomised prospective trial of noninvasive positive pressure ventilation in acute respiratory failure. Am J Respir Crit Care Med 1995;151:1799–806.

86. Bott J, Carroll MP, Conway J, et al. Randomised controlled trial of nasal ventilation in acute ventilatory failure due to chronic obstructive airways disease. Lancet 1993;341:1555–7.

87. Pollack C, Fleisch K, Dowsey K. Treatment of acute bronchospasm with beta-adrenergic agonist aerosols delivered by a nasal bilevel positive airway pressure circuit. Ann Emerg Med 1995;26:552–7.

88. Meduri G, Abou-Shala N, Fox R. Noninvasive face mask mechanical ventilation in patients with acute hypercapnic respiratory failure. Chest 1991;100:445–54.

89. Meduri G, Turner R, Abou-Shala N, et al. Non-invasive mechanical ventilation via a face mask: first line intervention in patients with acute hypercapnic and hypoxemic respiratory failure. Chest 1996;109:179–92.

90. Patrick W, Webster K, Ludwig L, et al. Noninvasive positive pressure ventilation in acute respiratory distress without prior chronic respiratory failure. Am J Respir Crit Care Med 1996;153:1005–11.

91. Mountain R, Sahn S. Clinical features and outcome in patients with acute asthma presenting with hypercapnia. Am Rev Respir Dis 1988;138:535–9.

92. Oh T, editor. Intensive care manual. 2nd ed. Boston: Butterworths; 1985.

93. Tuxen D. Detrimental effects of positive end-expiratory pressure during controlled mechanical ventilation of patients with severe airflow obstruction. Am Rev Respir Dis 1989;140:5–9.

94. Webb A, Bilton A, Hanson G. Severe bronchial asthma requiring ventilation. A review of 20 cases and advice on management. Postgrad Med J 1979;55:161–70.

95. Darioli R, Perret C. Mechanical controlled hypoventilation in status asthmaticus. Am Rev Respir Dis 1984;129:385–7.

96. Lissac J, Labrousse J, Tenaillon A, et al. Traitment des asthmes aigus graves de l'adulte. Ann Med Interne (Paris) 1986;137(1):34–7.

97. Limthongkul S, Udompanich V, Wongthim S, et al. Status asthmaticus: an analysis of 560 episodes and comparison between mechanical and non-mechanical ventilation groups. J Med Assoc Thai 1990;73:321–7.

98. Tuxen D, Williams T, Scheinkestel C, et al. Limiting dynamic hyperinflation in mechanically ventilated patients

with severe asthma reduces complications [abstract]. Anaesth Intensive Care 1993;21:718.

99. Bellomo R, McLaughlan P, Tai E, Parkin G. Asthma requiring mechanical ventilation. A low morbidity approach. Chest 1994;105:891–6.

100. Hall J, Wood L. Management of the critically ill asthmatic patient. Med Clin North Am 1990;74:779–96.

101. Corbridge T, Hall J. The assessment and management of adults with status asthmaticus. Respir Crit Care Med 1995;151:1296–316.

102. Santiago S, Klaustermeyer W. Mortality in status asthmaticus: 9 year experience in a respiratory intensive care. J Asthma Res 1980;17:75–9.

103. Halttunen P, Luomanmaki K, Takkunen O, Viljanen A. Management of severe asthma in an intensive care unit. Ann Clin Res 1980;12:109–11.

104. Petheram I, Branthwaite M. Mechanical ventilation for pulmonary disease. Anaesthesia 1980;35:467–73.

105. Picado C, Montserrat J, Roca J, et al. Mechanical ventilation in severe exacerbation of asthma. Eur J Respir Dis 1983;84:102–7.

106. Lukska A, Smith P, Coakley J, et al. Acute severe asthma treated by mechanical ventilation: 10 years experience from a district general hospital. Thorax 1986;41:459–63.

107. Higgins B, Greening A, Crompton G. Assisted ventilation in severe acute asthma. Thorax 1986;41:464–7.

108. Moss S, Rudolf M, Owen R, Ind P. Mechanical ventilation for acute severe asthma in a district general hospital (DGH) in the United Kingdom in the 1980's [abstract]. Am Rev Respir Dis 1990;141:A398.

109. Mansel J, Stogner S, Petrini M, Norman J. Mechanical ventilation in patients with acute severe asthma. Am J Med 1990;89:42–8.

110. Riding W, Ambiavagar M. Resuscitation of the moribund asthmatic. Postgrad Med J 1967;43:234–43.

111. Williams N, Crook J. The practical management of severe status asthmaticus. Lancet 1968;i:1081–3.

112. Marchand P, Van Hesselt H. Last-resort treatment of status asthmaticus. Lancet 1966;1:227–30.

113. Misuraca L. Mechanical ventilation in status asthmaticus. N Engl J Med 1966;257:318–20.

114. Scoggin C, Sahn S, Petty T. Status asthmaticus. A nine year experience. JAMA 1977;238:1158–62.

115. Petty T. Oxygen and mechanical ventilation in status asthmaticus. In: Weiss EB, editor. Status asthmaticus. Baltimore: Univ Park Press; 1978. p. 285–92.

116. Connors A, McCaffree D, Gray B. Effect of inspiratory flow rate on gas exchange during mechanical ventilation. Am Rev Respir Dis 1981;124:537–43.

117. Bone R, Burch S. Management of status asthmaticus. Ann Allergy 1991;67:461–9.

118. Otis A, McKerrow C, Bartlett R, et al. Mechanical factors in distribution of pulmonary ventilation. J Appl Physiol 1956;8:427–43.

119. Bates J, Rossi A, Milic-Emili J. Analysis of the behavior of the respiratory system with constant inspiratory flow. J Appl Physiol 1985;58:1840–8.

120. Leatherman J, Ravenscraft S, Iber C, et al. High peak inflation pressures do not predict barotrauma during mechanical ventilation of status asthma [abstract]. Am Rev Respir Dis 1989;139:154A.

121. Artigas A, Bernard GR, Carlet J, et al. The American-European Consensus Conference on ARDS, part 2. Ventilatory pharmacologic, supportive therapy, study design strategies and issues related to recovery and remodeling. Acute respiratory distress syndrome. Am J Respir Crit Care Med 1998;157:1332–47.

122. Leatherman J, Ravenscraft S. Low measured auto-positive end-expiratory pressure during mechanical ventilation of patients with severe asthma: hidden auto-positive end-expiratory pressure. Crit Care Med 1996;24(3):541–6.

123. Williams T, O'Hehir R, Czarny D, et al. Acute myopathy in severe asthma treated with intravenously administered corticosteroids. Am Rev Respir Dis 1988;137:460–3.

124. Douglass J, Tuxen D, Horne M, et al. Myopathy in severe asthma. Am Rev Respir Dis 1992;146:517–9.

125. Hansen-Flaschen J, Cowen J, Raps E. Neuromuscular blockade in the Intensive Care Unit. More than we bargained for. Am Rev Respir Dis 1993;147:234–6.

126. Nates J, Cooper D, Tuxen D. Acute weakness syndromes in critically ill patients—a reappraisal. Anaesth Intensive Care 1997;25:502–13.

127. Shivaram U, Donath J, Khan F, Juliano J. Effects of continuous positive airway pressure in acute asthma. Respiration 1987;52:157–62.

128. Shivaram U, Miro A, Cast M, et al. Cardiopulmonary responses to continuous positive airway pressure in acute asthma. J Crit Care 1993;8(2):87–92.

129. Rosengarten P, Tuxen D, Dziukas L, et al. Circulatory arrest induced by intermittent positive pressure ventilation in a patient with severe asthma. Anaesth Intensive Care 1990;19:118–21.

130. Kollef MH. Lung hyperinflation caused by inappropriate ventilation resulting in electromechanical dissociation: a case report. Heart Lung 1992;21:74–7.

131. Cooper D, Cailes J, Scheinkestel C, Tuxen D. Acute severe asthma and acidosis—effect of bicarbonate on cardiac and respiratory function. Anaesth Intensive Care 1993;22:212–3.

132. Tirot P, Bouachour G, Varache N, et al. Use of intravenous adrenaline in severe acute asthma. Rev Mal Respir 1992;9:319–23.

133. Sydow M, Crozier T, Zielman S, et al. High-dose intravenous magnesium sulfate in the management of life threatening status asthmaticus. Intensive Care Med 1993;19:467–71.

134. Parnass S, Feld J, Chamberlin W, Segil L. Status asthmaticus treated with isoflurane and enflurane. Anesth Analg 1987;66:193–5.

135. Saulnier F, Durocher A, Deturck R, et al. Respiratory and hemodynamic effects of halothane in status asthmaticus. Intensive Care Med 1990;16:104–7.

136. King D, Smales C, Arnold A, Jones O. Extracorporeal membrane oxygenation as emergency treatment for life threatening acute severe asthma. Postgrad Med J 1986;62:555–7.

137. Shapiro M, Kleaveland A, Bartlett R. Extracorporeal life support for status asthmaticus. Chest 1993;103:1651–4.

138. Rudis M, Guslits B, Peterson E, et al. Economic impact of prolonged motor weakness complicating neuromuscular blockade in the intensive care unit. Crit Care Med 1996;24:1749–56.

139. Leatherman J. Life-threatening asthma. Clin Chest Med 1994;15:453–79.

140. DuBois D, Almon R. Disuse atrophy of skeletal muscle is associated with an increase in number of glucocorticoid receptors. Endocrinology 1980;107:1649–51.

141. Marquette C, Saulnier F, Leroy O, et al. Long-term prognosis of near-fatal asthma. Am Rev Respir Dis 1992;146:76–81.

142. Maynard R, Hillman K. Intensive care admission as a predictor of asthma mortality. Anaesth Intensive Care 1993;21:712.

143. Richards G, Kolbe J, Fenwick J, Rea H. Demographic characteristics of patients with severe life threatening asthma: comparison with asthma deaths. Thorax 1993;48:1105–9.

144. Seddon P, Heaf D. Long term outcome of ventilated asthmatic patients. Arch Dis Child 1990;65:1324–8.

CHAPTER 22

Severe Acute Asthma in Children

Gerard J. Canny, MD, FRCPC, FAAP, FCCP
Suzanne Schuh, MD, FRCPC, AB PEM

Acute asthma is a common, potentially life-threatening medical emergency that is often suboptimally managed (Level IIA).[1-3] Although deaths from pediatric asthma are relatively rare, it is the most common medical emergency and a major cause of hospitalization among children.[4] This chapter will focus on the assessment and treatment of severe asthma exacerbations, based on an extensive review of the pediatric literature relating to the topic.

RECOGNITION AND ASSESSMENT OF SEVERE ASTHMA

The intensity of treatment in acute asthma is based on an accurate assessment of the severity of the event, which should be based on history, physical examination, and simple physiologic measurements.

Clinical Evaluation

Historic features that indicate the potential for life-threatening asthma and the need for close monitoring and possible hospital admission are listed in Table 22–1 (Level IIA).[5-7] In particular, children who have needed mechanical ventilation or admission to the intensive care unit (ICU) for asthma in the past should be treated very cautiously.[8] Physical signs and physiologic features of severe acute asthma are outlined in Table 22–2 and should be serially documented throughout treatment. Of these signs, the degree of accessory muscle use has been shown to correlate most closely with the severity of airway obstruction and level of hypoxemia.[9] Although a large pulsus paradoxus usually indicates significant airway obstruction,[9,10] its absence is not necessarily a reassuring finding.[9] Since accurate measurement of pulsus paradoxus in young children is difficult, this sign is most useful in older children.

Table 22–1 *Risk Factors for Potentially Fatal Asthma in Children*

Previous life-threatening episodes, requiring ICU admission or mechanical ventilation
Recent hospitalization or multiple ED visits for asthma
Dependency on multiple medications (particularly oral corticosteroids)
Previous pneumothorax or pneumomediastinum associated with asthma
Psychosocial problems resulting in noncompliance or erratic medical care
Excessive use of short-acting β_2-agonists, especially in the absence of inhaled corticosteroids

ICU = intensive care unit; ED = emergency department.

Investigations

In older children (> 5 to 6 years old), the assessment of acute asthma is incomplete without an objective measurement of the degree of airflow obstruction with a portable spirometer or a simple peak-flow meter. Measurements should be made at baseline and serially to follow the response to treatment. The results should be expressed as a percent of the predicted normal values for height and sex,[11] or of the child's "personal best" value. A peak expiratory flow (PEF) or forced expiratory volume in 1 second (FEV_1) value of less than 50% predicted indicates severe asthma.

Table 22–2 *Physical and Physiologic Features of Severe Acute Asthma*

Recognition of severe acute asthma

      Respiratory rate > 2 SD for age*

      Too breathless to talk or feed

      Accessory muscle use (eg, sternomastoid muscles, nasal flaring)

      Pulsus paradoxus > 15 mm Hg (useful in older children)

Potentially life-threatening features

      A silent chest or feeble respiratory effort

      Cyanosis

      Reduced level of consciousness or excessive fatigue

      Pneumothorax or pneumomediastinum or subcutaneous air

Physiologic features

      $SaO_2 \leq 91\%$ (in room air, before treatment)

      PEF ≤ 50% predicted or "personal best" value

      $PaCO_2 > 40$ mm Hg (5.3 kPa) if measured

SD = standard deviation; PEF = peak expiratory flow.
*Normal respiratory rates are provided by Pasterkamp H. The history and physical examination. In: Chernick V, Boat TF, editors. Disorders of the respiratory tract in children. 6th ed. Philadelphia: W.B. Saunders Co.; 1988. p. 88.

Arterial blood gas determination is rarely necessary prior to or during treatment. However, this procedure is mandatory in the presence of cyanosis, confusion, fatigue, or severe persistent lung function impairment ($FEV_1 \leq 25\%$ predicted) and in children who are not responding to aggressive treatment. A normal, high, or rising $PaCO_2$ value and a low pH are markers of severe (potentially life-threatening) acute asthma.[12] Pulse oximetry is a noninvasive method of measuring systemic oxygenation, and it can be used to determine supplementary oxygen requirements. Some studies suggest that children with acute asthma who have SaO_2 values of ≤ 91% (in room air) before treatment should be hospitalized (Level IIB).[13,14]

Chest radiography is not routinely performed in acute asthma (Level IIA)[1] but should be performed in patients who are critically ill if a complication (eg, pneumothorax) is suspected, if there is a poor response to therapy, or if another diagnosis is strongly suspected.

TREATMENT

Children with severe acute asthma require expeditious treatment, close observation, and serial measurements of physical signs, oxygen saturation, and lung function. The goals of treatment are to relieve hypoxemia, to quickly reverse airway obstruction, and to prevent early relapse. First-line treatment, therefore, consists of supplementary oxygen, aggressive use of bronchodilators, and systemic corticosteroids (Figure 22–1).

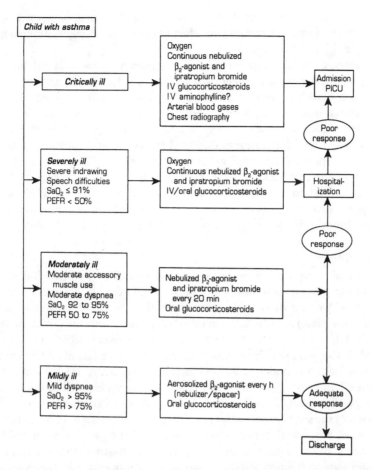

Figure 22–1 Algorithm for the management of asthma of different degrees of severity. PEFR = peak expiratory flow; IV = intravenous; PICU = pediatric intensive care unit. (Reproduced with kind permission from Canny GJ. Treatment of acute asthma. In: Reissman JJ, editor. Pediatric asthma: management strategies for primary care physicians. Canadian Medical Association disease management/patient counselling series. Toronto: Grosvenor House Press Inc.; 1997. p. 41–52.)

Oxygen

Children with severe exacerbations of asthma are usually hypoxemic as a result of ventilation-perfusion mismatch.[9,12] Supplementary oxygen should be administered by face mask or nasal cannulas to maintain $SaO_2 \geq 92$ to 95% (Level IIIB).[15,16] Nebulized medications should be delivered with oxygen, rather than air, as bronchodilators occasionally can cause transient oxygen desaturation.[17]

Bronchodilators

β₂-Agonists

A short-acting β_2-agonist, such as albuterol (salbutamol) or terbutaline, administered by the inhaled route is now considered the first-line treatment for acute asthma and has replaced the use of subcutaneous epinephrine (Level IA).[18] Several studies have demonstrated the efficacy and safety of frequent nebulizations of β_2-agonists in children with acute asthma.[19–21] Based on these studies, nebulized albuterol can be administered in a dose of 150 µg/kg (0.03 mL/kg) up to a maximum dose of 5 mg (1 mL) every 20 minutes (or continuously) to children with severe asthma, until a clinical response is achieved. In children who are less severely ill, hourly nebulizations of albuterol may suffice.[21,22] If the child responds to treatment, the frequency of administration can be decreased. Possible side effects of nebulized β_2-agonists include tremor, tachycardia, and mild hypokalemia.[20,21]

In recent years, there has been an increasing tendency to use metered-dose inhalers (MDIs) with spacer devices to administer β_2-agonists to children with acute asthma. Amirav and Newhouse[23] reviewed 10 pediatric studies that have compared the efficacy of bronchodilator therapy administered by MDI-spacer versus nebulizer; they concluded that nebulizers are no more efficacious in the treatment of acute asthma (Level IA). Further studies will be necessary to determine the optimum dose and frequency of β_2-agonist administration with a spacer device, particularly in infants and young children. The American Academy of Pediatrics guidelines[16] recommend 2 to 4 puffs of albuterol by MDI-spacer every 20 minutes in acute asthma. In children with mild to moderate asthma exacerbations (FEV$_1$ 50 to 79%), a recent emergency department (ED) study found that 2 puffs of albuterol by MDI-spacer achieved similar bronchodilation as 6 to 10 puffs, or 150 µg/kg albuterol by nebulizer.[24]

Anticholinergic Agents

Ipratropium bromide is the most widely used anticholinergic agent. Although it has a slower onset of action and provides less maximal bronchodilation than β_2-agonists, it has a longer duration of action. A recent meta-analysis concluded that the addition of ipratropium to a nebulized β_2-agonist has an additive effect in improving pulmonary function in children with acute asthma.[25] It appears to be most effective in severe asthma,[26] which may explain why Ducharme and Davis[22] were unable to demonstrate a beneficial effect of adding ipratropium in children with mild to moderate asthma exacerbations being treated with nebulized albuterol. Some,[26,27] but not all,[28] studies have reported reduced hospitalization rates in children with severe asthma being treated in the ED with a nebulized albuterol/ipratropium combination. In view of the safety profile of ipratropium,[26–28] it seems appropriate to recommend that both classes of bronchodilators be given in acute asthma, particularly in children with severe disease and in the early hours of treatment (Level IB). Based on the dose-response relationship for ipratropium,[29] a dose of 125 µg has been recommended in preschool children, and a dose of 250 µg in older children. In two studies, a beneficial effect with no significant side effects was reported when 250 µg ipratropium by nebulizer was administered with albuterol every 20 minutes for the first hour of treatment.[26,28] In a recent study, an even larger dose (500 µg) of ipratropium was administered with nebulized albuterol, even in preschool children.[27]

Theophylline

Relatively few studies have examined the role of aminophylline in children with acute asthma. In a double-blind controlled pediatric study, Pierson et al[30] found that intravenous aminophylline had a beneficial therapeutic effect when given in combination with nebulized sympathomimetics and systemic corticosteroids. Relatively weak, nonselective sympathomimetic agents were used in this study. In contrast, three more recent studies[31–33] of hospitalized children with acute asthma found no beneficial effects of theophylline over and above those provided by nebulized albuterol and systemic corticosteroids, and theophylline therapy was associated with an increased incidence of adverse side effects. Theophylline is, therefore, no longer considered a first-line treatment for acute asthma (Level ID). Based on the recent study of Yung and South,[34] theophylline may still have a role in children with severe asthma unresponsive to initial treatment with oxygen, bronchodilators, and systemic corticosteroids.

Corticosteroids

Systemic corticosteroids should be considered part of the initial treatment of all but the mildest asthma exacerbations (Level IA). Most trials of corticosteroids in acute asthma have

Table 22-3 *Drug Dosages for Severe Acute Asthma*

Medications	Dosages		Comments
Bronchodilators			
Albuterol—nebulizing solution (0.5%; 5 mg/mL)	150 µg/kg (maximum 5 mg/dose) every 20 min × 3 doses, then every 1–4 h or 0.5mg/kg/h by continuous nebulization		Dilute to 4 mL with normal saline O₂ flow at 6–10 L/min
Albuterol—MDI-spacer (100 µg/puff)	0.3 puffs/kg up to 6–10 puffs every 20 min × 3 doses, then every 1–4 h		Nebulization preferable in children with severe distress and in young children
Albuterol—intravenous infusion	Initial rate: 1 µg/kg/min Increase by 1 µg/kg/min every 15 min as required to a maximum of 10 µg/kg/min		ICU setting Check serum K+
Ipratropium bromide—nebulizing solution (0.025%; 250 µg/mL)	125–500 µg/dose every 20 min × 3 doses, then every 1–4 h		May mix with albuterol solution Titrate to response
Theophylline—aminophylline = (80% theophylline)	Loading dose: 6 mg/kg IV over 30 min Maintenance infusion rate:		Use 3 mg/kg in children on maintenance oral theophylline Monitor serum concentrations
	2–6 mo	0.4 mg/kg/h	
	6–11mo	0.7 mg/kg/h	
	1–9 yr	1.0 mg/kg/h	
	9–12 yr	0.8 mg/kg/h	
	>16 yr	0.6 mg/kg/h	
	cardiac or liver failure	0.2 mg/kg/h	
Corticosteroids			
Prednisone/prednisolone	1–2 mg/kg/d po (maximum 60 mg/d)		
Dexamethasone	0.3 mg/kg/d po		
Hydrocortisone	5 mg/kg every 6 h IV		
Methylprednisolone	1–2 mg/kg every 6 h IV		Convert to po corticosteroids when stabilized

MDI = metered dose inhaler; ICU = intensive care unit; po = per os (by mouth); IV = intravenously.

demonstrated beneficial effects in terms of the rate of improvement in symptoms, airway obstruction, and systemic oxygenation.[35–39] The administration of oral corticosteroids can decrease the need for hospitalization in children with acute asthma within 4 hours of therapy in the ED;[39] it can also shorten the duration of admission.[36–38] Since they take several hours to take effect, corticosteroids should be given as soon as possible after arrival to the ED.

The dose of systemic corticosteroids in asthma is somewhat arbitrary, and very high doses certainly are not necessary. Oral corticosteroids appear to be as effective as intravenous corticosteroids, provided children are not vomiting and are able to swallow the steroid tablets or syrup. There is no agreement as to the optimal duration of corticosteroid therapy; 5- to 7-day courses generally are used. In some children, a single dose of corticosteroids may suffice.[38,39] If a longer course of oral corticosteroids is used, tapering of dosage is not necessary, even after 10 days of therapy.[40]

Although it is commonly recommended that inhaled corticosteroids (ICSs) be introduced or increased in acute asthma exacerbations, the data to support this in children are scant[41–43] and, in one study, nonsupportive.[44] In a recent ED study, Rodrigo and Rodrigo[45] reported improved lung function in adults with moderately severe acute asthma ($FEV_1 = 40$ to 70%) treated with high-dose flunisolide (1 mg every 10 minutes for 3 hours). The authors postulated that this improvement may reflect a vasoconstrictor effect of ICS in the airways rather than an anti-inflammatory effect per se. In contrast, Schuh et al[46] in an ED study found that children with severe acute asthma ($FEV_1 < 60\%$) derived a greater bronchodilator response and a hospitalization benefit from treatment with oral prednisone (2 mg/kg) than from inhaled fluticasone proprionate (2 mg). Thus, although ICS may have a role in the treatment of children with mild asthma exacerbations at home (Level IB),[41–43] pending further studies, systemic corticosteroids should be used in severe acute asthma.

PRACTICAL ASPECTS OF MANAGEMENT

Children can present with all levels of asthma severity to the ED, and the intensity and duration of therapy will vary accordingly. Figure 22–1 outlines a practical treatment plan, and drug doses are provided in Table 22–3.

After appropriate treatment in the ED, up to 75% of children with acute asthma can be discharged;[1] the need for hospitalization can be further reduced if an observation unit is available in which children can be observed and treated for a longer time.[47] The decision to hospitalize a child with acute asthma should be based on the initial assessment and subsequent response to treatment. It should be emphasized that there is no single pretreatment objective measure that reliably can predict the need for hospitalization in the pediatric population.[14,48] In a recent study, Schuh et al[48] found that an $FEV_1 \leq 30\%$ after 2 hours of treatment in the ED was associated with a high likelihood of hospitalization, whereas an $FEV_1 \geq 60\%$ was associated with successful discharge. Table 22–4 outlines admission guidelines that have been suggested for children (Level IIB/C).

Table 22–4 *Guidelines for Hospital Admission of Children with Acute Asthma*

Critical illness

Poor response to ED treatment or, eg, persistent accessory muscle use or PEFR < 60% predicted

High-risk patients, eg, those with past admission to ICU

$SaO_2 \leq 91\%$ (in room air) with evidence of severe respiratory distress before treatment

Pneumothorax or pneumomediastinum

Nonmedical or social factors, eg, suspected noncompliance, child living a long distance from hospital

ED = emergency department; PEFR = peak expiratory flow; ICU = intensive care unit.

IN-HOSPITAL MANAGEMENT

Virtually all hospitalized children with acute asthma will have moderate to severe airway obstruction with an inadequate response to ED therapy, mandating careful ongoing assessment. Pulmonary function measurements, before and after bronchodilators, should be repeated several times each day, and SaO_2 monitored by oximetry. Particular attention should be given to children with $FEV_1 < 25\%$ predicted or $PaO_2 \geq 40$ mm Hg (5.3 kPa). In-hospital treatment consists of oxygenation, regular inhalations of β_2-agonists with ipratropium, systemic corticosteroids, and possibly aminophylline. Recent studies have indicated that β_2-agonists can be administered as effectively by MDI-spacer as by nebulizer in hospitalized children with asthma (Level IA).[23,49] Potassium supplementation may be necessary in children requiring aggressive therapy with β_2-agonists.[20]

TREATMENT OF RESPIRATORY FAILURE

Despite optimal therapy, a small number of children with severe acute asthma develop respiratory failure with progressive hypoxemia, hypercapnia, and fatigue, and require transfer to an intensive care facility.[50] Ideally, these children should be managed by an experienced critical care team skilled in intubation and ventilation techniques. The usual cause of death in asthma is severe asphyxia and acidosis, and correction of these abnormalities is of prime importance. On admission to the intensive care unit, children who do not require immediate intubation are placed in 100% oxygen until arterial blood gas results are available. Nebulized albuterol can be administered continuously,[51] a strategy that may avert the need for ventilation in some children with impending or actual respiratory failure (Level IIB).[18] Nebulized ipratropium can be added every 20 minutes.[26,28] Intravenous corticosteroids (and possibly aminophylline) are given concurrently. Arterial blood gas tensions (obtained from an indwelling arterial catheter) are measured at 15- to 30-minute intervals, as demanded by the child's course. In the presence of severe acidosis (pH < 7.2), the judicious use of sodium bicarbonate may be helpful (Level IIB).[52] In children who fail to respond to these measures, a continuous intravenous infusion of albuterol is warranted (Level IIB), although efficacy data on intravenous β_2-agonists in pediatric asthma are limited.[53,54] Finally, magnesium sulfate,[55] ketamine,[56] and the use of a helium-oxygen (Heliox) gas mixture[57] should as yet be considered experimental therapeutic modalities in the management of acute asthma in children.

If intubation becomes necessary, it should be done on an elective basis prior to development of cardiorespiratory arrest.[58] The decision to intervene is based on an assessment of the child's clinical condition and response to therapy. Increasing fatigue and somnolence are particularly ominous signs (Level IIIA). There is no absolute $PaCO_2$ value above which intubation is mandatory, as some children with very high $PaCO_2$ values can rapidly respond to therapy. Intubation should be effected with the least systemic disturbance to the child by experienced physicians. The achieve this, the use of ketamine combined with a short-acting muscle relaxant (succinylcholine) is recommended (Level IIIA). The ventilatory strategies used in children with severe asthma are described elsewhere by one of the authors (GJC).[58] Throughout the period of ventilation, bronchodilator and steroid therapy should be continued. β_2-Agonists can be administered by intravenous infusion or aerosolized into the inspiratory circuit of the ventilator—a topic that recently has been reviewed.[59,60]

DISCHARGE PLANNING AND FOLLOW-UP

During the recovery phase of acute asthma, the frequency of inhalation therapy gradually should be reduced, and children should be switched to the inhalation device most appropriate for age, with proper attention to inhalation technique. Oral drugs should be substituted for intravenous medications. Children can be discharged home once symptoms have cleared and pulmonary function has stabilized (eg, PEFR > 75% predicted). Over the subsequent few days, β_2-agonists should be used regularly and then tapered. A course of oral corticosteroids can be completed over 3 to 7 days. A prophylactic anti-inflammatory agent (usually an inhaled corticosteroid) should be introduced. High-dose inhaled steroid therapy may be an alternative to oral corticosteroids in the postdischarge period,[46] but requires further evaluation.

Re-education of the child and family with respect to the long-term management of asthma and the home treatment of exacerbations is essential. In this regard, a recent study highlighted the value of a nurse-led home management training program for children admitted to hospital with acute asthma.[61] For older children with more severe asthma, consideration should be given to providing for PEF monitoring at home.

The child's primary care physician should be informed of the acute illness and treatment given on discharge. Early follow-up by the child's physician is mandatory to allow for reassessment and an opportunity for the physician to provide further education, proper long-term prophylactic treatment, and ongoing supervision (Level IIIA). In selected cases, referral to an asthma specialist may be advisable.

ACUTE ASTHMA IN INFANTS AND YOUNG CHILDREN

A variety of anatomic and physiologic factors account for the increased vulnerability of infants and young children to develop airway obstruction and respiratory failure.[62] It is not surprising, therefore, that hospitalization rates[1] and the need for mechanical ventilation in acute asthma are disproportionately high in this age group. Lung function measurements at the bedside are difficult in young children,[22] which underscores the importance of clinical parameters, oximetry (and possibly arterial blood gases) in assessing asthma severity, and the response to treatment. The management of acute asthma in young children essentially is similar to that already outlined. While the efficacy of β_2-agonists in children less than 18 months has been questioned,[63] a beneficial clinical response to nebulized albuterol in young children (< 2 years old) with acute asthma has been reported by the authors.[64,65] A trial of β_2-agonists is, therefore, warranted in infants and young children with acute asthma (Level IB). A favorable response to β_2-agonists delivered by MDI-spacer with a face mask also has been reported in preschool children with acute asthma.[23] In addition, systemic corticosteroids in conjunction with β_2-agonists have successfully been used in acute asthma in this age group.[66,67] Nebulized ipratropium appears to be effective in about 40% of wheezy infants.[68] If theophylline is used, the dose will need to be modified (see Table 22–3) in view of the reduced rate of theophylline metabolism during the first year of life.

SUMMARY

The following are concluding statements and recommendations regarding management of severe acute asthma in children.

- Acute asthma is a common pediatric emergency that requires careful initial and ongoing assessment.
- Supplemental oxygen should be the initial treatment for hypoxemic patients (Level IIIB).
- An aerosolized β_2-agonist is the bronchodilator of first choice (Level IA).
- Inhalation of ipratropium may add to the bronchodilation induced by β_2-agonists (Level IB).
- Early use of systemic corticosteroids is essential in all but the mildest exacerbations (Level IA).
- Aminophylline is rarely necessary in acute asthma and may increase adverse effects (Level ID).
- Intravenous β_2-agonists may have a role in life-threatening exacerbations (Level IIB).
- Patient fatigue is an absolute indication for mechanical ventilation (Level IIIA).
- Adequate supervision, education, and prophylactic treatment are indicated to prevent further severe asthma episodes (Level IIIA).

The authors thank Miriam McCleane for secretarial assistance.

REFERENCES

1. Canny GJ, Reisman J, Healy R, et al. Acute asthma: observations regarding the management of a pediatric emergency department. Pediatrics 1989;83:507–12.

2. Crain EF, Weiss KB, Fagan MJ. Pediatric asthma care in US emergency departments. Arch Pediatr Adolesc Med 1995;149:893–901.

3. Neville RG, Hoskins G, Smith B, Clarke RA. How general practitioners manage acute asthma attacks. Thorax 1997;52:153–6.

4. Wilkins K, Mao Y. Trends in rates of admission to hospital and death from asthma among children and young adults in Canada during the 1980s. Can Med Assoc J 1993;148:185–90.

5. Strunk RC. Workshop on the identification of the fatality-prone patient with asthma: summary of workshop discussion. J Allergy Clin Immunol 1987;80 Suppl:455–7.

6. Lieu TA, Quesenberry CP, Sorel ME, et al. Computer-based models to identify high-risk children with asthma. Am J Respir Crit Care Med 1998;157:1173–80.

7. Ernst P, Spitzer WO, Suissa S, et al. Risk of fatal and near-fatal asthma in relation to inhaled corticosteroid use. JAMA 1992;268:3462–4.

8. Turner MO, Noertjojo K, Vedal S, et al. Risk factors for near fatal asthma: a case control study in hospitalized patients with asthma. Am J Respir Crit Care Med 1998;157:1804–9.

9. Kerem E, Canny G, Tibshirani R, et al. Clinical-physiological correlations in acute asthma in childhood. Pediatrics 1991;87:481–6.

10. Wright RO, Steele DW, Santucci KA, et al. Continuous, noninvasive measurement of pulsus paradoxus in patients with acute asthma. Arch Pediatr Adolesc Med 1996;150:914–8.

11. Weng TR, Levison H. Standards of pulmonary function tests in children. Am Rev Respir Dis 1969;99:879–94.

12. Weng TR, Langer HM, Featherby EA, Levison H. Arterial blood gas tensions and acid-base balance in symptomatic and asymptomatic asthma. Am Rev Respir Dis 1970;101:274–82.

13. Geelhoed GC, Landau LI, LeSouef PN. Predictive value of oxygen saturation in emergency evaluation of asthmatic children. Br Med J 1988;297:395–6.

14. Kerem E, Tibshirani R, Canny G, et al. Predicting the need for hospitalization in children with acute asthma. Chest 1990;98:1355–66.

15. The British Thoracic Society. The British guidelines on asthma management. Thorax 1997:52:S1–21.

16. American Academy of Pediatrics. Practice parameter: the office management of acute exacerbations of asthma in children. Pediatrics 1994;93:119–26.

17. Seidenberg J, Mir Y, van der Hardt H. Hypoxaemia after nebulized salbutamol in wheezy infants: the importance of aerosol acidity. Arch Dis Child 1991;66:672–5.

18. Canny GJ, Bohn D, Levison H. Sympathomimetics in acute asthma: inhaled or parenteral? Am J Asthma Allergy Pediatr 1989;2:165–70.

19. Robertson CF, Smith F, Beck R, Levison H. Response to frequent low doses of nebulized salbutamol in acute asthma. J Pediatr 1985;106:672–4.

20. Schuh S, Parkin P, Rajan A, et al. High- versus low-dose, frequently administered, nebulized albuterol in children with severe, acute asthma. Pediatrics 1989;83:513–8.

21. Schuh S, Reider MJ, Canny G, et al. Nebulized albuterol in acute childhood asthma: comparison of two doses. Pediatrics 1990;86:509–13.

22. Ducharme FM, Davis GM. Randomised controlled trial of ipratropium bromide and frequent low doses of salbutamol in the management of mild and moderate acute pediatric asthma. J Pediatr 1998;133:479–85.

23. Amirav I, Newhouse MT. Metered-dose inhaler accessory devices in acute asthma: efficacy and comparison with nebulizers: a literature review. Arch Pediatr Adolesc Med 1997;151:876–82.

24. Schuh S, Johnson DW, Stephens D, et al. Comparison of albuterol delivered by metered dose inhaler with spacer versus a nebulizer in children with mild acute asthma. J Pediatr 1999;135:22–7.

25. Osmond MH, Klassen TP. Efficacy of ipratropium bromide in acute childhood asthma: a meta-analysis. Acad Emerg Med 1995;2:651–6.

26. Schuh S, Johnson DW, Callahan S, et al. Efficacy of frequent nebulized ipratropium bromide added to frequent high-dose albuterol therapy in severe childhood asthma. J Pediatr 1995;126:639–45.

27. Qureshi F, Pestian J, Davis P, Zaritsky A. Effect of nebulized ipratropium on the hospitalization rates of children with asthma. N Engl J Med 1998;339:1030–5.

28. Zorc JJ, Pusic MV, Ogborn J, et al. Ipratropium bromide added to asthma treatment in the pediatric emergency department. Pediatrics 1999;103:748–52.

29. Davis A, Vickerson F, Worsley G, et al. Determination of dose-response relationship for nebulized ipratropium in asthmatic children. J Pediatr 1984;105:1002–5.

30. Pierson WE, Bierman CW, Stamm SJ, Van Arsdel PP. Double blind trial of aminophylline in status asthmaticus. Pediatrics 1971;48:642–6.

31. DiGiulio GA, Kercsmar CM, Krug SE, et al. Hospital treatment of asthma: lack of benefit from theophylline given in addition to nebulized albuterol and intravenously administered corticosteroid. J Pediatr 1993;122:464–9.

32. Carter E, Cruz M, Chesrowan S, et al. Efficacy of intravenously administered theophylline in children hospitalized with severe asthma. J Pediatr 1993;122:470–6.

33. Strauss RE, Wertheim DL, Bonagura VR, Valacer DJ. Aminophylline therapy does not improve outcome and increases adverse effects in children hospitalized with acute asthmatic exacerbations. Pediatrics 1994;93:205–10.

34. Yung M, South M. Randomised controlled trial of aminophylline for severe acute asthma. Arch Dis Child 1998;79:405–10.

35. Shapiro GG, Furukawa CT, Pierson WE, et al. Double-blind evaluation of methylprednisolone versus placebo for acute asthma episodes. Pediatrics 1983;71:510–4.

36. Connett GJ, Warde C, Wooler E, Lenney W. Prednisolone and salbutamol in the hospital treatment of acute asthma. Arch Dis Child 1994;70:170–3.

37. Younger RE, Gerber PS, Harrod HG, et al. Intravenous methylprednisolone efficacy in status asthmaticus of childhood. Pediatrics 1987;80:225–30.

38. Storr J, Barrell E, Barry W, Lenney W. Effect of a single oral dose of prednisolone in acute childhood asthma. Lancet 1987;1:879–82.

39. Scarfone RJ, Fuchs SM, Nager AL, Shane SA. Controlled trial of oral prednisone in the emergency department treatment of children with acute asthma. Pediatrics 1993;92:513–8.

40. O'Driscoll BR, Kalra S, Wilson M, et al. Double-blind trial of steroid tapering in acute asthma. Lancet 1993;341:324–7.

41. Wilson NM, Silverman M. Treatment of acute, episodic asthma in preschool children using intermittent high dose inhaled corticosteroids at home. Arch Dis Child 1990;65:407–10.

42. Connett G, Lenney W. Prevention of viral induced asthma attacks using inhaled budesonide. Arch Dis Child 1993;68:85–7.

43. Scarfone RJ, Loiselle JM, Wiley JF, et al. Nebulized dexamethasone versus oral prednisone in the emergency treatment of asthmatic children. Ann Emerg Med 1995;26:480–6.

44. Garrett J, Williams S, Wong C, Holdaway D. Treatment of acute asthma exacerbations with an increased dose of inhaled steroid. Arch Dis Child 1998;79:12–7.

45. Rodrigo G, Rodrigo C. Inhaled flunisolide for acute severe asthma. Am J Respir Crit Care Med 1998;157:698–703.

46. Schuh S, Reisman J, Al-Shehri M, et al. A comparison of inhaled fluticasone and oral prednisone for children with severe acute asthma. N Engl J Med. 2000;343:684–94.

47. Willert C, Davis AT, Herman JJ, et al. Short-term holding room treatment of asthmatic children. J Pediatr 1985;106:707–11.

48. Schuh S, Johnson D, Stephens D, et al. Hospitalization patterns in severe acute asthma in children. Pediatr Pulmonol 1997;23:184–92.

49. Dewar AL, Stewart A, Cogswell JJ, Connett GJ. A randomised controlled trial to assess the relative benefits of large volume spacers and nebulizer to treat acute asthma in hospital. Arch Dis Child 1999;80:421–3.

50. Stein R, Canny GJ, Bohn D, et al. Severe acute asthma in a pediatric intensive care unit: six years' experience. Pediatrics 1989;83:1023–8.

51. Papo MC, Frank J, Thompson AE. A prospective randomized study of continuous versus intermittent nebulized albuterol for severe status asthmaticus in children. Crit Care Med 1993;21:1479–86.

52. Menitobe SM, Goldring RM. Combined ventilator and bicarbonate strategy in the management of status asthmaticus. Am J Med 1983;74:898–901.

53. Bohn DJ, Kalloghlian A, Jenkins J, et al. Intravenous salbutamol in the treatment of status asthmaticus in children. Crit Care Med 1984;12:892–6.

54. Browne GJ, Penna AS, Phung X, Soo M. Randomized trial of intravenous salbutamol in early management of acute severe asthma in children. Lancet 1997;349:301–5.

55. Ciarallo L, Sauer AH, Shannon MW. Intravenous magnesium therapy for moderate to severe pediatric asthma: results of a randomized, placebo-controlled trial. J Pediatr 1996;129:809–14.

56. Rock MJ, Reyes de la Rocha S, LiHommedieu S, Truemper E. Use of ketamine in asthmatic children to treat respiratory failure refractory to conventional therapy. Crit Care Med 1986;14:514–6.

57. Manthous CA, Hall JB, Melmed A, et al. Heliox improves pulsus paradoxus and peak expiratory flow in non-intubated patients with severe asthma. Am J Respir Crit Care Med 1995;151:310–4.

58. Canny GJ, Bohn DJ, Reisman JJ, Levison H. Childhood asthma. In: Weiss EB, Stein M, editors. Bronchial asthma: mechanisms and therapeutics. 3rd ed. Boston: Little, Brown and Co.; 1993. p. 1062–84.

59. Dhand R, Tobin MJ. Inhaled bronchodilator therapy in mechanically ventilated patients. Am J Respir Crit Care Med 1997;156:3–10.

60. Smalldone GC. Aerosolized bronchodilators in the intensive care unit: much ado about nothing? Am J Respir Crit Care Med 1999;159:1029–30.

61. Madge P, McColl J, Paton J. Impact of a nurse-led home management training programme in children admitted to hospital with acute asthma: a randomised controlled trial. Thorax 1997;52:223–8.

62. Reisman JJ, Canny GJ, Levison H. The wheezing infant. In: Tinkelman DG, Napitz CK, editors. Childhood asthma: pathophysiology and treatment. 2nd ed. New York: Marcel Dekker Inc; 1993. p. 255–82.

63. Silverman M. Bronchodilators for wheezy infants? Arch Dis Child 1984;59:84–7.

64. Bentur L, Canny GJ, Shields MD, et al. A controlled trial of nebulized albuterol in children under the age of 2 years with acute asthma. Pediatrics 1992;89:133–7.

65. Bentur L, Kerem E, Canny GJ, et al. Response of acute asthma to a β_2 agonist in children less than two years of age. Ann Allergy 1990;65:122–6.

66. Tal A, Bavilski C, Yohai D. Dexamethasone and salbutamol in the treatment of acute wheezing in infants. Pediatrics 1983;71:13–8.

67. Tal A, Levy N, Bearman JE. Methylprednisolone therapy for acute asthma in infants and toddlers: a controlled clinical trial. Pediatrics 1990;86:350–6.

68. Reisman JJ, Canny GJ, Levison H. The role of anticholinergic drugs in pediatric airways disease. In: Gross N, editor. Anticholinergic therapy. 1st ed. London: Franklin Scientific Projects; 1993. p. 169–80.

CHAPTER 23

Role of Asthma Education

Peter G. Gibson, MBBS(Hons), FRACP
Louis-Philippe Boulet, MD, FRCPC

There are global problems with asthma management, which include undertreatment with corticosteroids, limited knowledge, and poor asthma management skills among patients with severe asthma.[1] Morbidity and mortality from asthma are high; however, much of this is believed to be preventable and associated with factors such as delay, denial by the patient, and suboptimal management.[2] There is an evident need to educate both patients and health care providers to optimize asthma management and ensure the successful application of pharmacotherapy.

Patient education has been defined as "a planned learning experience using a combination of methods such as teaching, counseling, and behavior modification techniques which influence patients' knowledge and health behavior and involving an interactive process which assists patients to participate actively in their health care."[3] Asthma patient education is recommended as a key component of many asthma management guidelines.[4-6] Some guidelines advise that verbal information alone does not alter behavior, and they propose the use of written self-management plans in combination with written and audiovisual reinforcement of spoken messages.[7] This chapter describes the psychoeducational models that have been applied to asthma education and identifies the evidence supporting the effects of asthma education in adults. We have gathered evidence from high-quality studies that examine the effects of patient asthma education programs on morbidity from asthma.

THEORETIC MODELS FOR EDUCATIONAL INTERVENTIONS

For asthma education to be effective in modifying patient behavior, a series of complex strategies may be required, based on the principles of social learning theories.[8] The theories of education and their application to asthma are reviewed by Green and Frankish[9] and include the health belief model, the locus of control theory, and the social learning theory.[10-12] Basic principles from these theories have been used in asthma education including feedback, reinforcement, individualization of the interventions, facilitation, and relevance.[13]

Different models have been developed to plan teaching interventions for individuals and groups. The PRECEDE model is one of the most commonly used models.[9,14,15] PRECEDE is the acronym for "Predisposing, Reinforcing and Enabling Causes in Educational Diagnosis and Evaluation." In the PRECEDE model (Table 23–1), the first steps include establishing educational diagnoses in regard to (1) patient's quality of life; (2) definition of health problems (physical, psychological, or social) affecting asthma patient's quality of life; (3) recognized behaviors associated with the specific health problems; (4) identification of factors associated with behaviors linked to health problems (predisposing factors, enabling factors or barriers, and reinforcement factors); and finally, (5) a determination of the administrative aspects of the educational program.

Preparation for Educational Intervention

The types of behavior that people with asthma must adopt to adequately control their asthma in regard to medication, environment, lifestyle habits, and other aspects are initially deter-

Table 23–1 *The PRECEDE Model of Educational Intervention*

Asthma education
    Care provider as unit of analysis
    Definition of provider's tasks
    Integral to medical care
    Individually administered
    Phased administration
    Focus on medical self care
    Feedback incorporated
    Active role of parents

Educational diagnosis
    Predisposing factors
        Sufficient knowledge about asthma
            Detailed information
            Interconnected information
            Purposeful information
        Positive attitude about asthma care
        Realistic outcome expectations
            About self-management
            About medical care
        Moderate level of anxiety

    Enabling factors
        Continuity of education
        Appropriate referral
        Objective criteria estimation of severity of episode
        Skills needed for self-management behaviors

    Reinforcing factors
        Communication with care provider
        Feedback on management attempts
        Patient-oriented problem solving
        Clinical management of asthma
        Clinical diagnosis

Behavioral diagnosis
    Behavioral factors
        Prevention of asthma attacks
            Predicting asthma attacks
            Complying with medication
            Administering prescribed medication correctly
            Managing side effects
            Avoiding or reducing known triggers
        Attack management
            Symptom discrimination
            Administering prescribed medication correctly
            Managing side effects
            Remaining calm and avoiding panic
            Monitoring progress of attack

    Other behaviors
        Normalizing patient's physical and social activities
        Effective communication with health care providers

Social and epidemiologic diagnosis
    Quality of life—reduction of
        Social isolation
        Restriction of activities

    Patient's health status—reduction of
        Emergency department visits
        Visits to general practitioners
        Hospital admissions

mined. The educator then chooses which behaviors should be modified in priority and identifies the factors affecting the adoption or maintenance of these behaviors. The PRECEDE model identifies three sets of variables to consider when planning an educational intervention: predisposing factors, enabling factors, and reinforcing factors.

Predisposing factors are the knowledge, attitudes, beliefs, and perceptions that set up a motivation to undertake an action. The attitude and beliefs of the patient and the health care providers in regard to the need for asthma education are important when beginning this type of intervention. The degree of self-confidence and perception of benefits of the intervention by the health professional will play a role in his/her motivation to change the patient's behavior.

Enabling factors include resources available both at the individual level (eg, knowledge on asthma and treatment, intellectual capacities, current skills in the practice of asthma management, financial status) and in the community (eg, access to human resources and health services).

Reinforcing factors are the rewards that help the behavior to be repeated or sustained over time. The support of peers and health care providers as well as the perception of an improvement following proper self management are among reinforcing factors.

These three factors have a hierarchical order. Factors predisposing the adoption of the targeted behavior should be considered first, then the enabling and, finally, the reinforcing factors.

Application of Educational Interventions

This second stage concerns choosing and applying the educational methods to facilitate the acquisition of knowledge, attitudes, and skills needed to manage asthma. There are general principles to be respected to promote learning.[14]

Motivation is influenced by the patient's adaptation mechanisms. Success in learning is a source of motivation, as is personal satisfaction. The degree to which a person develops a feeling of personal efficacy will determine how motivated he or she will be to adopt the behavior targeted by the teaching intervention. This feeling is considered one of the main factors in social and health learning.

Motivation to learn is also influenced by the stage of adaptation to the disease. Patients with a recent diagnosis of asthma will behave differently from those with long-standing asthma, and this should influence the type of intervention chosen. Adaptation mechanisms to chronic disease often depend on disease severity, patient and family perception of the problem, and options for lifestyle changes.[16]

Types of Asthma Educational Interventions

The specific components of the asthma educational interventions that are described in the literature can be divided into provision of information about asthma, self monitoring, regular medical review, and the use of a written action plan (Figure 23–1, Table 23–2).

To define the level of evidence supporting these interventions, we conducted a search for Level I evidence (systematic reviews, randomized controlled trials [RCTs], and controlled clinical trials) on asthma education. The Cochrane Airways Review Group database and Cochrane Controlled Trials Register (CENTRAL) were searched, bibliographies were reviewed, and advice was sought from experts. This approach identified two systematic reviews[17,18] that examined 36 RCTs published between 1979 and 1998. Those asthma education programs that offered only education about asthma were termed "limited education" or "information only." They were distinguished from those that taught self-management skills such as self monitoring or use of a written action plan (self-management education) and those that optimized asthma therapy by including a regular medical review (optimal education).

Limited Asthma Education

Limited asthma education consists of the provision of knowledge about asthma by way of written pamphlets, videos, or lectures. Limited asthma education (information only) is appealing in several ways. It generally is easy to implement and can be adapted readily to suit

Figure 23–1 Components of asthma education.

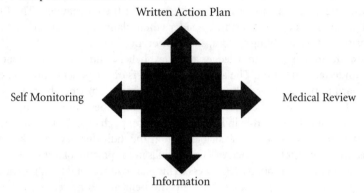

Written Action Plan

Self Monitoring

Medical Review

Information

Table 23–2 *Components of Asthma Education*

Information about asthma	
Mode	Interactive or noninteractive
Content	Knowledge about asthma prevention and self management
Setting and duration	Hospital, emergency department, community
Self monitoring	Recording of PEF or symptoms or both in diary
Medical review	Regular review of asthma severity and medications
Action plan	Individualized
	Written
	Details of what do to in an exacerbation and how to access medical help

PEF = peak expiratory flow.

a busy medical practice. In addition, it is cheaper than more intensive forms of intervention and superficially appears to satisfy the stated desires of patients for more information about their condition (Level II).[19] The effects of limited asthma education on asthma outcomes in adults have been reported in 11 RCTs, which have been compiled in a systematic review.[17]

Figure 23–2 Effects of limited education on visits to the doctor for asthma. WMD = weighted mean difference for individual trials; χ^2 = test for heterogeneity across different trials; Z = test statistic for WMD; area of square (■) is proportional to amount of information contributed for WMD for individual trials; diamond (◆) = WMD and 95% CI for all trials combined; SD = standard deviation.

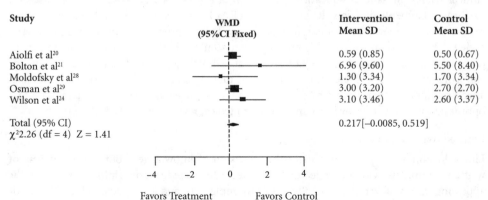

Study	WMD (95%CI Fixed)	Intervention Mean SD	Control Mean SD
Aiolfi et al[20]		0.59 (0.85)	0.50 (0.67)
Bolton et al[21]		6.96 (9.60)	5.50 (8.40)
Moldofsky et al[28]		1.30 (3.34)	1.70 (3.34)
Osman et al[29]		3.00 (3.20)	2.70 (2.70)
Wilson et al[24]		3.10 (3.46)	2.60 (3.37)
Total (95% CI)		0.217[–0.0085, 0.519]	
$\chi^2$2.26 (df = 4) Z = 1.41			

−4   −2   0   2   4

Favors Treatment   Favors Control

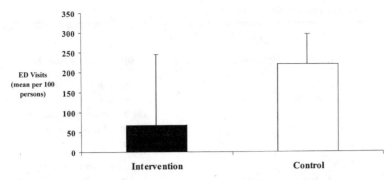

Figure 23–3 Emergency department (ED) visits are reduced by limited asthma education in patients recruited from the emergency department (mean + SD; $p < .05$). (Reprinted with permission from Bolton MB, Tilley BC, Kuder J, et al. The cost and effectiveness of an education program for adults who have asthma. J Gen Intern Med 1991;6:401–7.)

There are six RCTs that used interactive asthma education programs (Table 23–3).[20–25] Most of the interactive programs used group educational modalities. Most of these studies showed significant improvements in asthma symptoms. There was little difference in results between group or individual educational interventions.

There are five noninteractive programs that describe a combination of written, audio, and video modalities used to provide information about asthma.[24,26–29] These were administered without direct contact with an educator (noninteractive). While most of these studies showed significant improvement in asthma knowledge, there were no significant effects shown on asthma morbidity (Table 23–4).[24,26–29]

Limited asthma education programs that offer only the opportunity to increase knowledge and that make no attempt to influence self-management skills, behaviors, or attitudes for adult asthmatic patients do not reduce hospitalization rates or visits to the doctor for asthma attacks (Level I) (Figure 23–2). These results are consistent with the theoretic proposition

Table 23–3 *Interactive Asthma Education Trials*

		Number of Subjects		
Study	*Intervention*	*Intervention*	*Control*	*Significant Outcomes*
Aiolfi et al[20]	Group sessions	22	22	Nil
Bolton et al[21]	Group sessions	119	122	Fewer ED visits, fewer days of limited activity*
Huss et al[22]	Computer	26	26	Higher adherence, less allergen in bedrooms, reduction in β_2-agonist use, fewer symptoms*
Maiman et al[23]	Individual sessions with nurse-educator	245	249	Fewer ED visits*
Wilson et al[24]	Group sessions Individual sessions	83 81	71	Fewer symptom days, better symptom control, better asthma status, better physical control*
Ringsberg et al[25]	Group sessions	20	18	Decrease in number of hospital days*

ED = emergency department.
*For intervention group.

Table 23–4 *Noninteractive Asthma Education Trials*

		Number of Subjects		
Study	Intervention	Intervention	Control	Significant Outcomes
Hilton et al[26]	1. Booklet and audiocassette 2. Booklet alone	88 86	100	For both intervention groups, time missed from work was decreased and satisfaction of asthma understanding was increased.
Jenkinson et al[27]	1. Book 2. Audiocassette 3. Book and audiocassette	44 41 41	40	All intervention groups had an increase in knowledge of asthma and related drugs.
Moldofsky et al[28]	Video	31	31	Immediately after video there was improvement in asthma knowledge, but this was lost 16 months later.
Osman et al[29]	Booklets	397	404	There were no significant differences for all outcomes.
Wilson et al[24]	Workbook	75	71	Intervention group experienced fewer symptomatic days and better asthma status.

that limited educational interventions, as they have been practiced, have little influence on health-related behaviors and skills.[30] There are two positive findings that deserve further consideration: reductions in reported symptoms and emergency department (ED) attendances (Figure 23–3).

Limited Education and Asthma Symptoms

For more severe degrees of disruption, such as days off work or school, there was no clear beneficial effect of limited educational interventions (Level I). However, patients reported that they perceived a reduction of symptoms following limited asthma education (information only) (Level I). It is not clear whether this was a true effect of the intervention or the result of anticipation bias, as the interventions were administered in an unblinded fashion.

Limited Education and Emergency Department Visits

Patients attending the ED for asthma exacerbations have a high risk for future ED visits and tend to have more severe asthma and poor asthma management skills (Level II).[31] As such, they represent an appropriate group to target for asthma education. Two studies reported positive effects of asthma education in patients recruited from the emergency department.[21,23]

Bolton randomized adults either to usual care or an educational intervention, consisting of three 1-hour educational group sessions with a nurse-educator. The sessions gave a basic introduction to asthma, prevention and control of asthma attacks, asthma medication, devices and how to use them, and avoidance of asthma triggers. Subjects were also provided with a handout at each session to use at home. There were significantly fewer asthma-related visits to an ED and limited-activity days for the intervention group in the initial 4 months after the intervention (Level I). These effects, however, were not sustained at the 12-month follow-up. Emergency department visits were initially reduced by a mean of 2.4 per persons per year (95% CI 1.18 to 4.34) (see Figure 23–2). Although the effect size was small, the low cost of limited asthma education makes this an appealing adjunct to therapy in this setting.[21]

Table 23–5 *Characteristics of Randomized Trials of Optimal Asthma Self-Management Education**

Study	Intervention Type*	Setting	Number of Patients† Intervention	Control	Outcomes‡
Ayres et al[32]	I, SM, RR, AP	Outpatient	21	29	FEV_1, PEF
Côté et al[33]	I, SM, RR, AP	Doctor-led education in tertiary care setting	95	54	Hospitalizations, ED visits, days off school/work
Cowie et al[34]	I, SM, RR, AP	Nurse-led education in hospital clinic	91	48	Hospitalizations, ED visits
GRASSIC[35]	I, SM, RR, AP	Doctor-led instruction in hospital clinic and GP	230	228	Hospitalizations, unscheduled doctor visits, FEV_1, PEF
Ignacio-Garcia and Gonzalez-Santos[36]	I, SM, RR, AP	Outpatient	35	35	Hospitalizations, unscheduled doctor visits, days off school/work, FEV_1, PEF
Jones et al[37]	I, SM, RR, AP	GP	33	39	FEV_1, PEF
Lahdensuo et al[38]	I, SM, RR, AP	Outpatient	56	59	Hospitalizations, unscheduled doctor visits, days off school/work, FEV_1
Sommaruga et al[39]	I, SM, RR, AP	Inpatient	20	16	ED visits, days off school/work
Yoon et al[40]	I, SM, RR, AP	Hospital-based asthma education center	28	28	Hospitalizations, ED visits, days off school/work, FEV_1, PEF
Zeiger et al[41]	I, SM, RR, AP	HMO investigation of ED users	110	139	Hospitalizations, ED visits, days off school/work, nocturnal asthma, FEV_1, PEF

I = information; SM = self monitoring; RR = regular review of medications; AP = action plan; ED = emergency department; PEF = peak expiratory flow; FEV_1 = forced expiratory volume in 1 second; GP = general practice; HMO = health maintenance organization.

*Versus usual care.
†At study completion.
‡Used in meta-analysis.

Table 23–6 *Characteristics of Randomized Trials of Symptom- versus PEF-Based Asthma Self Management*

Study	Setting	Number of Participants*		Additional Interventions	Outcomes†
		Symptom-Based SM	PEF-Based SM		
Charlton et al[42]	Nurse-led asthma clinic; primary care	33	27	Information and regular medical review	OCS courses, doctor visits
Côté et al[33]	Doctor-led education; tertiary care	45	50	Information and regular medical review	Hospitalizations, ED visits, days off work/school
Cowie et al[34]	Nurse-led education; tertiary care	45	46	Information and regular medical review	Hospitalizations, ED visits
Turner et al[43]	Primary care	48	44	Information and regular medical review	Hospitalizations, ED visits, OCS courses, days off work/school

PEF = peak expiratory flow; SM = self management; OCS = oral corticosteroids; ED = emergency department.
*At study completion.
†Used in meta-analysis.

Asthma Self-Management Education

Asthma self-management programs have been developed to teach people with asthma how to monitor the severity of their condition, identify deterioration in asthma control, act appropriately in this situation, and adhere to recommended therapy and follow-up. A systematic review that reports the results of 28 papers describing 23 RCTs that examined asthma self-management education has been published on the Cochrane Database of Systematic Reviews.[18] Self-management interventions involved self monitoring of symptoms and/or peak expiratory flow (PEF) (n = 25), review of treatment and asthma severity by a medical practitioner (n = 22), and provision of a written action plan (n = 14). In three RCTs, two active treatments were compared without a control group, whereas each of the other studies had a control group (Table 23–5).[32–41] Four studies (Table 23–6) compared symptom- versus PEF-based self management.[34,35,42,43] One study compared self management with regular medical review (see below).[32]

Optimal Asthma Self-Management Education

Self-management education providing all four of the asthma educational components (see Figure 23–1 and Table 23–5) was described as "optimal asthma self-management education."[18] These programs included

1. Patient asthma education, which is a program that delivers information about asthma and its management
2. Self monitoring, which is the regular measurement and recording by the patient of either PEF or asthma symptoms using diary cards
3. Medical review, which includes assessment of asthma control, asthma severity, and medications by a medical practitioner (in some programs this assessment was a formal part of the intervention, whereas, in others, the patients were advised to consult their own doctor)

4. A written action plan, which is an individualized plan produced for the purpose of patient self management of deteriorating asthma (action plans were written to accommodate individual patients' asthma severity and treatment, and contained information on when and how to access the medical system in response to worsening asthma—an example of a written action plan is provided in Figure 23–4)[2,4]

Optimal self-management education including regular review, self monitoring, and provision of a written action plan led to clinically important improvements in morbidity from asthma (Level I). This review[32] showed that with self-management education there was a reduction in the proportion of participants reporting hospitalizations (Figure 23–5), ED visits (Figure 23–6), unscheduled doctors visits, days lost from work due to asthma, and episodes of nocturnal asthma (Level I). The effects were large enough to be both clinically and statistically significant. Those interventions that included a written action plan and regular medical review consistently showed an effect; whereas, less intense interventions were not always of obvious benefit. These results support the use of self-management education as an important part of asthma management, although self-management education did not consistently improve clinical measures of lung function (FEV_1) (Figure 23–7)(Level IA).

Self Monitoring

The regular measurement and recording of either PEF or symptoms is a part of many asthma education programs. Self monitoring is promoted as an aid to both the patient and the physician in assessing asthma severity, determining how well the individual responds to treatment, and identifying deteriorating asthma.[44] The potential benefits of this are to improve asthma control, to improve medication compliance, and to reduce hospitalizations and emergency department visits by facilitating the early detection and treatment of exacerbations of asthma. For the purposes of this chapter and the systematic reviews, PEF monitoring was defined as the regular (usually daily) recording of morning and/or evening PEF (before and/or after use of bronchodilator). Symptom-based self monitoring was defined as the regular (usually daily) recording of asthma symptoms, including nocturnal waking, day and night use of β-agonists, breathlessness, wheezing, and chest tightness.

Symptom- versus peak flow–based self monitoring. Self management using a written action plan based on PEF-based self management was compared with symptom-based self management in four studies (see Table 23–6).[33,34,42,43] These studies reported similar reductions in hospitalizations, ED visits, unscheduled doctor visits, and days off work or school due to asthma in both groups ($p > .05$) (Table 23–7) (Level I). Action plans based on symptoms are therefore equally effective to those based on peak-flow levels (Level I). This suggests that regular PEF monitoring is not mandatory for all asthmatic patients. The focus should be on optimizing asthma control, regular review, and provision of a written action plan. There are, however, opportunities to identify whether specific groups, such as those with poor perception of symptoms,[45] would do better with peak flow–based action plans.

Self monitoring without a written action plan. Five studies examined the effects of asthma education and self monitoring of symptoms or PEF (Table 23–8).[46–50] These studies did not include provision of a written action plan or regular medical review. Berg et al reported a significant increase in compliance with use of inhaled medications in the intervention group but saw no difference between the intervention and control groups in asthma symptoms, PEF, or self management.[50] Brewin and Hughes[46] found a significantly higher level of asthma knowledge and management. In 1995, Kotses et al[47] saw a short-term (2-month) improvement in management skills and cognitive abilities, and a long-term decrease in frequency of asthma attacks and medication use. In 1996, Kotses et al[48] compared group and individual education

Figure 23–4 Example of a written action plan. (Reproduced with permission from Australian asthma management handbook 1998. Australia: National Asthma Campaign; 1998.)

WHEN WELL

———————————————— Dosage ————————————————
———————————————— Dosage ————————————————
———————————————— Dosage ————————————————

Take_____10 minutes before exercise

WHEN NOT WELL

If your peak flow reading does not reach _____following your medication for a 24-h period

If you are getting a cold
If you are waking at night due to your asthma or have symptoms when you wake in the morning
Or
If you require your bronchodilator (_____) frequently and are not getting the same effect

Then

Increase your _____
Have extra _____
Other _____

Continue this treatment for 2 weeks
See your doctor if _____

FOR A SEVERE ATTACK

If your peak flows do not reach _____
If you have severe shortness of breath and can only speak in short sentences
If you are having a severe attack of asthma and are frightened
Or
If you are needing your _____ more than 4-hourly and are not gaining an effect

Then

Take _____; **repeat if you do not improve**
Take _____ **of prednisone**
Seek medical attention immediately by calling an ambulance
Continue to use your _____**until help arrives**

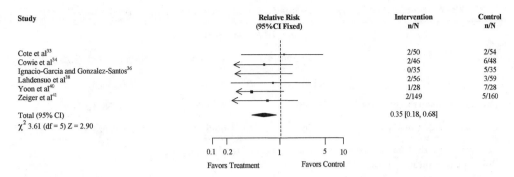

Figure 23–5 Effects of optimal asthma self-management education on hospitalization for asthma. χ^2 = test for heterogeneity across different trials; Z = test statistic for relative risk; area of square (■) is proportional to amount of information contributed for relative risk for individual trials; diamond (◆) = relative risk and 95% CI for all trials combined.

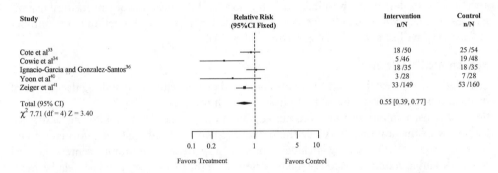

Figure 23–6 Effects of optimal asthma self-management education on emergency department visits for asthma. χ^2 = test for heterogeneity across different trials; Z = test statistic for relative risk; area of square (■) is proportional to amount of information contributed for relative risk for individual trials; diamond (◆) = relative risk and 95% CI for all trials combined.

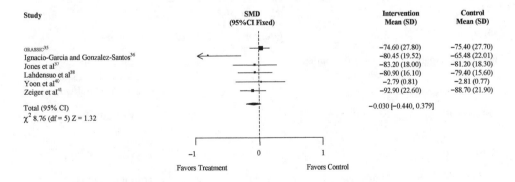

Figure 23–7 Effects of optimal asthma self-management education on FEV_1. The convention of favorable results being displayed to the left-hand side of null effect warrants negative signs being placed before results. Results are reported as % predicted, except for Yoon R et al[40] which is in liters. SMD = standardized mean difference for individual trials; χ^2 = test for heterogeneity across different trials; Z = test statistic for SMD; area of square (■) is proportional to amount of information contributed for SMD for individual trials; diamond (◆) = SMD and 95% CI for all trials combined; SD = standard deviation.

Table 23–7 *The Effect of Symptom- versus PEF-based Self Management on Asthma Outcomes*

| Outcome | Number of Participants* | | Relative Risk (95% CI) |
	Intervention*	Control	
Hospitalization	4/140	3/138	1.22 (0.33, 4.55)
Emergency department visits	30/140	32/138	0.90 (0.58, 1.39)
Unscheduled doctor visits	55/76	66/85	0.93 (0.78, 1.10)

*Experiencing the outcome of interest as a function of total sample size.
PEF = peak expiratory flow.

and found a reduction in asthma symptoms, and an increase in PEF in both groups; however, only the individual group reported a decrease in asthma attacks. Neri et al[49] compared two levels of intervention. Both intervention groups had significant reduction in days of admission to the hospital. The more comprehensive intervention saw significant differences in asthma attacks, days in the hospital, work days lost, and the need for urgent medical examinations. The less comprehensive intervention resulted in a trend for reduction in the number of working days lost and hospital admissions (Level I).

Regular Medical Review

Five studies with a total of 1,062 patients compared asthma education and regular review of medications and asthma control by a physician, with usual care (Table 23–9).[26,51–54] Three of the studies used an intervention combining patient information, self monitoring, and regular review of medications,[51–53] while the remaining two used only patient information and regular review.[26,54] The setting included hospital outpatients, community centers, general practices, and telephone calls to the subjects' homes. In the two studies in which regular medical review was not provided, participants were advised to visit their own doctor for regular review.[52,54] The outcomes examined included nocturnal asthma, visits to the ED, unscheduled doctor visits, days off normal activities, and hospitalizations.

Table 23–8 *Randomized Controlled Trials of Asthma Education and Self Monitoring*

| Study | Setting | Number of Patients* | | Outcomes† |
		Intervention	Control	
Brewin and Hughes[46]	Nurse-led inpatient education	33	45	Hospitalizations, unscheduled doctor visits, days off school/work, FEV$_1$
Kotses et al[47]	Not stated	36	40	ED visits, days off school/work
Kotses et al[48]	Not stated	22	12	ED visits, PEF
Neri et al[49]	Outpatient	33	32	Hospitalizations, unscheduled doctor visits, days off school/work, FEV$_1$
Berg et al[50]	Outpatient	31	24	PEF

FEV$_1$ = forced expiratory volume in 1 second; ED = emergency department; PEF = peak expiratory flow.
*At study completion.
†Used in meta-analysis.

Interventions that included regular review of medications led to a significant reduction in ED visits (Level I). Bailey et al[52] reported significantly better compliance and an increase in functional status in the intervention group. There was a significant decrease in hospital and ED visits in both the control and intervention groups (Level I). Hilton et al[26] reported significant improvements in asthma knowledge and satisfaction of understanding of asthma. Shields et al[54] found a nonsignificant trend in a decrease of visits to the ED ($p < .15$). Allen et al[51] reported significant improvements in asthma knowledge, compliance, and perceived morbidity. There was no difference in any clinical measure of morbidity. Garrett et al's intervention group used more preventative medication, had more peak-flow meters, better PEF-monitoring technique, more self-management plans, and better knowledge of how to manage an asthma attack than the control group.[53] The intervention group also had less nocturnal waking and better self-reported asthma control. There was no difference in compliance, hospital admissions, days lost from work, or emergency department visits between the groups (Level I).

Table 23–9 *Characteristics of Randomized Trials of Asthma Education and Regular Medical Review**

| Study | Intervention | Setting | Number of Patients[†] | | Outcomes[‡] |
			Intervention	Control	
Allen et al[51]	I, SM, RR	Hospital-based community service asthma education	56	57	Nocturnal asthma
Bailey et al[52]	I, SM, RR	Outpatient	124	101	ED visits
Garrett et al[53]	I, SM, RR	Nurse-run community education center	228	223	Hospitalizations, ED visits, unscheduled doctor visits, days off school/work, nocturnal asthma
Hilton et al[26]	I, RR	GP; doctor-led education	86	100	ED visits, days off school/work
Shields et al[54]	I, RR	HMO classes and/or nurse-led phone counseling	44	43	ED visits

I = information; SM = self monitoring; RR = regular review of medications; ED = emergency department; GP = general practice; HMO = health maintenance organization.
*Versus usual care.
[†]At study completion.
[‡]Used in meta-analysis.

CONCLUSION

The results of this review can be used to improve the precision of the recommendations in current asthma management guidelines. Most guidelines do not specify the nature of the educational intervention required in asthma management. Verbal information alone does not alter behavior or improve outcomes (Level IC). Effective asthma education requires the use of written self-management plans with written and audiovisual reinforcement of spoken messages (Level IA). Information needs to be combined with instruction on self management to reduce asthma morbidity (Level IA). Action plans based on symptoms are equally effective to those based on monitoring of PEF. Educating people with asthma who attend the ED can lead to important reductions in morbidity from asthma (Level IB).

The authors thank Amanda Wilson and Jennifer Coughlan for outstanding editorial support and NSW Health for their financial assistance.

REFERENCES

1. Bauman A, Mitchell CA, Henry RL et al. Asthma morbidity in Australia: an epidemiological study. Med J Aust 1992;156:827–31.
2. Gibson PG, Wilson AJ. The use of continuous quality improvement methods to implement practice guidelines in asthma. J Qual Clin Pract 1996;16:87–102.
3. Bauman A, Browne G. The role of education in adult asthma management. Patient Management 1987;June: 94–103.
4. Australian asthma management handbook 1998. Australia: National Asthma Campaign; 1998.
5. Boulet LP, Becker A, Berube D, et al. Summary of recommendations from the Canadian Asthma Consensus Report 1999. Can Med Assoc J 1999;161:S1–12.
6. National Institutes of Health, NHLBI. Guidelines for the diagnosis and management of asthma. Bethesda (MD): NIH; 1997 Publication No.:97-4051. Available at:http://www.nhlbi.nih.gov/nhlbi/lung/asthma /prof/asthgdln.pdf.
7. British Thoracic Society. The British guidelines on asthma management. Thorax 1997;52 Suppl:S2–21.
8. Boulet L, Chapman K, Green L, FitzGerald JM. Asthma education. Chest 1994;106 Suppl:184–196S.
9. Green LW, Frankish CJ. Theories and principles of health education applied to asthma. Chest 1994;106:219–30S.
10. Glanz KM, Lewis FK, Rimer B. Health behavior and health education: theory research and practice. Josey Bass; 1990. p. 460.
11. Bandura A. Self-efficacy: towards a unifying theory of behavioral change. Psychol Rev 1977;84:191–215.
12. Gonzalez V, Geoppinger J, Lorig K. Four psychosocial theories and their application to patient education and clinical practice. Arthritis Care Res 1990;3:132–43.
13. Mullen P, Green L. Educating and counselling for prevention from theory and research to principles. In: Goldbloom R, Lawrence T, editors. Preventing disease: beyond the rhetoric. New York: Springer-Verlag; 1990.
14. Hagan L. L'asthme: notions de base-éducation-intervention. Chapitre 14: Éduquer pour maîtriser l'asthme: principes et méthodes. Laval: Presses de l'Université Laval; 1997. p. 193–219.
15. Green LN, Marshall WK. Health promotion planning: an educational and environmental approach. Mayfield Publishers; 1991. p. 506.
16. Redman BK. The process of patient education. 7th ed. Toronto: Mosby; 1993. p. 337.
17. Gibson PG, Coughlan J, Wilson AJ, et al. The effects of limited (information-only) asthma education on health outcomes of adults with asthma [update software]. Cochrane Database of Systematic Reviews. Oxford: The Cochrane Collaboration; Issue 3, 1998.
18. Gibson PG, Coughlan J, Wilson AJ, et al. The effects of self-management asthma education and regular practitioner review in adults with asthma [update software]. Oxford: The Cochrane Collaboration; Issue 1, 1998.
19. Gibson PG, Talbot PI, Toneguzzi RC. Self-management autonomy and quality of life in asthma. Chest 1995;107:1003–8.
20. Aiolfi S, Confalomieri M, Scartabellati A, et al. International guidelines and educational experiences in an out-patient clinic for asthma. Monaldi Arch Chest Dis 1995:50;477–81.
21. Bolton MB, Tilley BC, Kuder J, et al. The cost and effectiveness of an education program for adults who have asthma. J Gen Intern Med 1991;6:401–7.
22. Huss K, Huss RW, Squire EN, et al. Computer education for asthmatic patients: what effects? J Nurs Care Qual 1992;6:57–66.

23. Maiman LA, Green LW, Gibson G, MacKenzie EJ. Education for self-treatment by adult asthmatic patients. JAMA 1979;241:1919–22.

24. Wilson SR, Scamagas P, German DF, et al. A controlled trial of two forms of self-management education for adults with asthma. Am J Med 1993;94:564–76.

25. Ringsberg KC, Wiklund I, Wihelmsen L. Education of adult patients at an "asthma school": effects on quality of life, knowledge and need for nursing. Eur Respir J 1990;3:33–7.

26. Hilton S, Sibbald B, Anderson HR, Freeling P. Controlled evaluation of the effects of patient education on asthma morbidity in general practice. Lancet 1986;1:26–9.

27. Jenkinson D, Davison J, Jones S, Hawtin P. Comparison of effects of a self management booklet and audiocassette for patients with asthma. BMJ 1988;297:267–70.

28. Moldofsky H, Broder I, Davies G, Leznoff A. Videotape education program for people with asthma. Can Med Assoc J 1979;120:669–72.

29. Osman LM, Abdalla MI, Beattie JAG, et al. Reducing hospital admission through computer supported education for asthma patients. BMJ 1994:308:568–71.

30. Bauman AE, Craig AR, Dunsmore J, et al. Removing barriers to effective self-management of asthma. Patient Educ Counseling 1989;14:217–26.

31. Gibson PG, Talbot PI, Hancock J, et al. A prospective audit of asthma management following emergency asthma treatment at a teaching hospital. Med J Aust 1993;158:775–8.

32. Ayres JG, Campbell LM, Follows RMA. A controlled assessment of an asthma self-management plan involving a budesonide dose regimen. Eur Respir J 1996;9:886–92.

33. Cote J, Cartier A, Robichaud P. Influence on asthma morbidity of asthma education programs based on self-management plans following treatment optimization. Am J Respir Crit Care Med 1997;155:1509–14.

34. Cowie RL, Revitt SG, Underwood MF, Field SK. The effect of a peak-flow based action plan in the prevention of exacerbations of asthma. Chest 1997;112:1134–8.

35. Grampian Asthma Study of Integrated Care (GRASSIC). Effectiveness of routine self-monitoring of peak flow in patients with asthma. BMJ 1994;308:564–7.

36. Ignacio-Garcia JM, Gonzalez-Santos P. Asthma self-management education program by home monitoring of peak expiratory flow. Am J Respir Crit Care Med 1995;151:353–9.

37. Jones KP, Mullee MA, Middleton M, et al. Peak flow based asthma self-management: a randomised controlled study in general practice. Thorax 1995;50:851–7.

38. Lahdensuo A, Haahtela T, Herrala J, et al. Randomised comparison of guided self-management. Br Med J 1990;312:748–52.

39. Sommaruga M, Spanevello A, Migliori GB, et al. The effects of a cognitive behavioural intervention in asthmatic patients. Monaldi Arch Chest Dis 1995;50:398–402.

40. Yoon R, McKenzie DK, Bauman A, Miles DA. Controlled trial evaluation of an asthma education program for adults. Thorax 1993;48:1110–6.

41. Zeiger RS, Heller S, Mellon MH, et al. Facilitated referral to asthma specialist reduces relapses in asthma emergency department visits. J Allergy Clin Immunol 1991;87:1160–8.

42. Charlton I, Charlton G, Broomfield, Mulle MA. Evaluation of peak flow and symptoms only self management plans for control of asthma in general practice. BMJ 1990;301:1355–9.

43. Turner MO, Taylor D, Bennett R, FitzGerald JM. A randomised trial comparing peak expiratory flow and symptom self-management plans for patients with asthma attending a primary care clinic. Am J Respir Crit Care Med 1998;157:540–6.

44. Thoracic Society of Australia and New Zealand. The Australian asthma management plan. Med J Aust 1996;164:727–30.

45. Rubinfield AR, Pain MCF. Perception of asthma. Lancet 1976;1:882–4.

46. Brewin AM, Hughes JA. Effect of patient education on asthma management. Br J Nurs 1995;4:81–101.

47. Kotses H, Berstein IL, Bernstein DI, et al. A self-management program for adult asthma. Part 1: development and evaluation. J Allergy Clin Immunol 1995;95:529–40.

48. Kotses H, Stout C, McConnaughty K, et al. Evaluation of individualized asthma self-management programs. J Asthma 1996;33:113–8.

49.   Neri M, Migliori GB, Spanevello A, et al. Economic analysis of two structured treatment and teaching programs on asthma. Allergy 1996;51:313–9.

50.   Berg J, Jacqueline DJ, Sereika S. An evaluation of a self-management program for adults with asthma. Clin Nurse Res 1997:6;225–38.

51.   Allen RM, Jones MP, Oldenburg B. Randomised trial of an asthma self-management programme for adults. Thorax 1995;50:731–8.

52.   Bailey WC, Richards JM, Brooks M, et al. A randomized trial to improve self-management practices of adults with asthma. Arch Intern Med 1990:150;1664–8.

53.   Garrett J, Fenwick JM, Taylor G, et al. Prospective controlled evaluation of the effect of a community based asthma education centre in a multi-racial working class neighbourhood. Thorax 1994;49:976–83.

54.   Shields MC, Vail MJ, Reinhard JD, et al. Counselling is better accepted than classes in patient education of adult inner city asthmatic patients. New Health Care Systems: HMOs & Beyond. Group Health Association 1986;June:289–98.

CHAPTER 24

Asthma Unresponsive to Usual Therapy

Kenneth R. Chapman, MD, MSc, FRCPC, FACP

———•———

This chapter addresses the problem of asthma that fails to respond to usual antiasthma therapy with adequate disease control. This topic presents special problems in a text that aims to be "evidence based," because there is no widely accepted definition of "asthma unresponsive to usual therapy." Thus, there is no body of research addressing the issue in a consistent fashion. This chapter reviews disparate bodies of research and attempts to weigh the value of various approaches suggested to deal with this common problem. The most defensible recommendation arising from this review is the need for comprehensive and consistent research in this area of study.

DEFINITION

We lack a definition of "unresponsive asthma," in part, because our treatment strategies are evolving rapidly and our goals for therapy have changed dramatically. During the past 10 to 15 years, our "usual therapy" has shifted from a crisis-oriented bronchodilator-driven approach to an anti-inflammatory approach that aims to control airway irritability.[1,2] A decade ago, many physicians regarded control of asthma as freedom from emergency department visits and hospitalizations. Now, most national and international guidelines have defined asthma control in much more rigorous terms, including complete or nearly complete freedom from the need to inhale short-acting bronchodilators while enjoying an unrestricted lifestyle.[3] More fundamentally, we lack a definition of unresponsive asthma because we lack a useful clinical definition of asthma itself. As will become clear in this chapter, our inability to diagnose and quantify asthma in the primary practice setting is a major reason that many patients with apparent asthma are unresponsive to usual forms of treatment. An additional barrier to our understanding of the problem is the lack of a comprehensive approach by researchers. Typical research addresses one area of particular interest to the investigator and leaves other potential causes of unresponsive asthma neglected. It is plausible, for example, that many patients whose asthma has appeared to improve following treatment of gastroesophageal reflux in an uncontrolled trial actually improved by means of incidental improvements in compliance or inhaler technique.

A review of this area of study reveals that many different terms are used to describe the problem of asthma that fails to respond to typical first- or second-line therapy. Published articles speak of refractory asthma, difficult asthma, brittle asthma, steroid-resistant asthma, and steroid-dependent asthma, and one can find relevant data in articles addressing simply severe asthma or near-fatal asthma. Throughout this chapter, the term unresponsive asthma will be used. As a working definition, asthma will be regarded as unresponsive if desired endpoints of symptom control and normal or nearly normal pulmonary function cannot be achieved or are achieved only with the administration of systemic corticosteroids on a regular maintenance basis.

CAUSES AND RECOMMENDATIONS

Many of the common causes of unresponsive asthma are listed in Table 24–1. These might be categorized into four main groups. In the first group, the diagnosis of asthma is incorrect either because the patient does not have asthma at all or because the patient has asthma but has complained of symptoms that are not caused by asthma. In the second group, the diagnosis of asthma is correct, but the desired response is not achieved because a fundamental element of management has been overlooked, has been prescribed incorrectly, or has not been adhered to by the patient. The third broad category of unresponsive asthma is that of asthma made worse by coexisting conditions. Finally, some patients appear to have correctly diagnosed asthma that is optimally managed in the absence of complicating factors, but they continue to suffer unrelenting asthma symptoms and require systemic corticosteroids or other intrusive therapy.

Table 24–1 *Common Causes of Unresponsive Asthma*

Wrong diagnosis
    Chronic obstructive pulmonary disease
    Left ventricular failure
    Deconditioning
    Angina
    Localized obstruction
    Cystic fibrosis
    Vocal cord dysfunction
    Factitious asthma
    Nonasthmatic cough (eg, postnasal drip)

Poor compliance

Suboptimal inhaler technique

Tobacco smoke (including secondhand smoke)

Significant environmental allergen

Significant occupational exposure

Drugs
    β-blockers
    Nonsteroidal anti-inflammatory drugs
    Angiotensin converting enzyme inhibitors

Concurrent disease
    Chronic obstructive pulmonary disease
    Gastroesophageal reflux
    Chronic Sinusitis
    Rhinitis
    Systemic diseases
    Thyrotoxicosis
    Vasculitides

Complicated asthma
    Allergic bronchopulmonary aspergillosis
    Brittle asthma—types I and II
    Steroid-resistant asthma
    Steroid-dependent asthma
    Asthmatic bronchitis
    Poor perceivers
    Heightened perceivers

Misdiagnosis

For many years, specialists in the field of asthma have contended that asthma is underdiagnosed. Typical reports include that of Speight who reviewed the referral notes that accompanied asthmatic children referred for specialist assessment.[4] He noted that only 1 in 5 was thought likely to have asthma while numerous other nonpulmonary diseases were considered to be likelier explanations for their chronic cough, wheezing, and breathlessness. Such underdiagnosis may no longer be the norm in affluent countries, however. As primary care physicians are reminded that asthma has become increasingly common and that effective therapy is available, they are more likely to consider antiasthma therapy for patients who report respiratory symptoms. There is growing evidence that overdiagnosis of asthma is now a substantial problem. The most likely explanation for this difficulty with diagnosis is the failure of primary care doctors to use objective measures of lung function to confirm their clinical impressions. Essentially all national and international guidelines for the management of asthma recommend the use of lung function measurements, in particular, spirometry, to confirm the presence of variable airflow obstruction.[3,5,6] Patients with symptoms consistent with asthma should exhibit either a bronchodilator response or bronchoconstriction after exposure to a triggering agent such as cold air or methacholine. Regrettably, surveys of primary care physicians suggest that only 5% are likely to request spirometry for a patient who has persistent cough accompanied by wheezes on physical examination.[7] A lack of familiarity with simple lung function measurements may result in substantial problems with diagnosis. In one survey of patients whose physicians suspected asthma and requested pulmonary function testing, a report of normal resting spirometry was usually treated as final and diagnostic; only 10% of patients were returned the laboratory for some form of challenge test.[8] Instead, most received diagnoses and treatment based on their clinical presentations and the family physicians' interpretation or misinterpretation of the normal spirometry. Follow-up of such patients showed little concordance between their actual methacholine challenge test results and the clinical diagnosis they had received; the odds of correct diagnosis were little better than chance alone. The false-positive diagnosis of asthma does not appear to be a transient problem with a provisional diagnosis that is soon rejected. In one survey of patients with negative methacholine challenge testing after referral to an asthma center, approximately two-thirds were receiving regular antiasthma therapy for the treatment of their presumed asthma.[9] These patients had been receiving a median of two medications for an average of more than 2 years at the time of their methacholine challenge tests. Most such patients had been referred for the assessment of refractory or unresponsive asthma, and most had either no respiratory disease or suffered from allergic rhinitis with postnasal drip or simple chronic bronchitis associated with chronic cigarette smoking. A minority of patients had other significant medical illnesses such as undetected congestive heart failure or coronary artery disease. Almost a decade ago, one newly created asthma center reported that approximately one in seven patients referred for assessment and management of troublesome asthma did not suffer from the disease.[10]

There is growing awareness of a problem usually termed "vocal cord dysfunction." Long recognized, the term vocal cord dysfunction describes the patient whose episodic wheezing and breathlessness is an upper airway phenomenon of voluntary or unconscious narrowing of the vocal cords.[11] Few systematic reviews of this problem are available, and its true prevalence is probably unknown. Most available literature is anecdotal in nature and describes one or a handful of patients with bizarre clinical courses. Patients recognized to have the disorder may have presented to the emergency department on multiple occasions and, in extreme instances, may have been intubated for apparent status asthmaticus.[12] Among cases reported in literature, women outnumber men, and frequently the sufferers of vocal cord dysfunction have worked in medical or medically related occupations. Such patients have significant underlying psychiatric disease, and some may suffer from Munchausen syndrome. For some patients, there may be an element of secondary gain. This motive may be at play in patients who are seeking compensation for occupational asthma. Milder forms of the disorder are thought to arise from inflammatory conditions of the upper airway and may be responsive to appropriate medication and speech therapy. Regrettably, the diagnosis of the disorder may be difficult, particularly if vocal cord dysfunction and true asthma coexist in the same patient. The "gold standard" for diagnosis is laryngoscopy during an acute episode of breathlessness, either spontaneous or induced, demonstrating inappropriate vocal cord motion with abduction of the vocal cords on inspiration with a small anterior chink remaining for airflow.

The problem of establishing diagnoses in infants and children represents a special problem given their inability to perform pulmonary function tests. As a practical consequence, most diagnoses are made clinically. Under such circumstances, physicians must be particularly alert to the possibility that unresponsive asthma may be the consequence of an incorrect provisional diagnosis.

Recommendation

Patients thought to have unresponsive asthma should have their diagnoses verified objectively by demonstration of variable airflow obstruction—a bronchodilator response, steroid response, or bronchoconstrictor response. In patients with atypical presentations (eg, late-onset disease) or symptoms unresponsive to therapy, other disease possibilities should be considered and investigated (Level IIIA).

Noncompliance

Compliance with therapy is a problem in the management of all chronic medical conditions and asthma is no exception. However, ensuring compliance with regular, preventive antiasthma therapy represents particular problems. First, asthma is a highly variable disease, and noncompliance does not always invoke inevitable consequences of disease worsening. The noncompliant patient may suffer few or no adverse effects for many months before the consequences of noncompliance are apparent. Second, our reliance on the inhaled medications may make monitoring of compliance difficult. Inhaled medications exert their effects topically, and it is not feasible in most clinical settings to measure blood or serum levels of the therapeutic agent to verify patient compliance. Third, inhaled corticosteroids are our most effective agents in the maintenance therapy of troublesome asthma, but many patients are fearful of using corticosteroids.[13]

It is axiomatic that physicians are poor judges of whether patients are compliant or noncompliant.[14] Many of the factors that physicians assume to be helpful in predicting compliance (education, income, gender, and disease severity) are not valuable predictive factors when studied objectively.[14] Most estimates of compliance with maintenance therapy in either clinical trials or clinical practice approximate 40% of prescribed doses. This estimate varies, of course, with the age of the patient population being studied, the type of medication being prescribed, and the frequency of drug administration. Most studies of compliance employ pharmacy records, pill counts, and weighing of canisters to provide these estimates. Of particular concern are the results of a small number of clinical trials that employ electronic dose counting to track metered-dose inhaler adherence.[15] These studies indicate that compliance with prescribed doses may be far less. Indeed, the extent of noncompliance with prescribed anti-inflammatory therapy leads one to marvel that any patient achieves disease control under usual practice circumstances. Our current treatment successes with twice-daily inhaled corticosteroid drugs are probably the consequence of the higher concentration formulations now in use, which provide a useful topical anti-inflammatory effect, even in the face of haphazard administration. The development of low-cost electronic dose counters will make it feasible for clinicians to monitor patient use of inhaled medications.[16] Similarly, the incorporation of dose counters in novel inhalation devices will make such monitoring a more routine part of usual clinical care.[17]

Recommendation

Patients thought to have unresponsive asthma should have their compliance with antiasthma therapy verified by whatever means is feasible (eg, a review of pharmacy records) (Level IIA).

Inhaler Misuse

Although the pressurized dry-suspension metered-dose inhaler has been available for almost 50 years and is now the most popular means of delivering treatment to patients with asthma, our patients' use of these devices remains suboptimal. Surveys of inhaler use estimate that between 14 and 89% of patients are not using their pressurized aerosols optimally.[18,19] On average, 40% of patients newly referred to a specialized center or pulmonary function laboratory are not using their inhalers adequately. This misuse should not be surprising; most caregivers are unfamiliar with the rudiments of proper inhalation technique.[20–23] Although dry-powder devices are considered simpler for patients to use, problems of inhaler misuse can still be identified. The clinical consequences of inhaler misuse are variable. Short-acting β_2-agonists such as salbutamol are typically administered in a dosage that is on the plateau of the dosage-response curve. Even in the face of suboptimal inhaler technique, enough of the drug may be deposited to provide useful bronchodilator response. Moreover, patients are invited to self administer bronchodilator at times of need; in the face of suboptimal inhaler technique, they can titrate the number of doses upward to achieve desired clinical effect. By contrast, the clinical effects of inhaled corticosteroids are much more dependent upon adequate inhaler technique. These well-known findings suggest that many patients with true asthma whose disease responds transiently to β_2-agonist but poorly to a maintenance drug are suffering the consequences of undetected inadequacy in their inhaler technique. Physicians unfamiliar with inhaler use themselves may be in a poor position to detect and remedy this cause of unresponsive asthma. Even for the expert, suboptimal inhaler technique might be difficult to detect by visual inspection alone. In one survey of elderly individuals using a conventional and breath-actuated pressurized aerosol, trained laboratory technicians overestimated the success of inhalation maneuvers; flaws in inhalation technique were better detected by an objective monitor of inspiratory flow rate and timing.[24] The fact that a patient has once used an inhaler with good technique should not dissuade physicians from re-examining this essential element of care; studies show that patients often acquire habits of poor inhaler technique over time, making reassessment and retraining essential.[25]

Recommendation

Patients thought to have unresponsive asthma should have their inhaler technique reviewed by a health care provider familiar with the optimal use of these devices. Ideally, an objective monitor of inhaler technique should be used (Level IIA).

Environmental and Other External Factors

There is substantial indirect evidence that poorly controlled asthma often is the consequence of significant environmental exposures. The evidence is strongest in the emergency department literature, which reports that patients with severe asthma requiring emergency department care are likely to be sensitized to common domestic allergens and have elevated allergen levels in their households. Studies of inner city children with poorly controlled asthma describe many factors that might account for a lack of disease control.[26,27] Among them is a significant and continuing exposure to domestic antigens including cockroach antigen.[28] Among adults with asthma, there is a correlation between antigen exposures at home and disease severity; of particular importance is the presence of a fur-bearing pet.[29] The most important nonallergic exposure appears to be tobacco smoke; children exposed their parents' secondhand cigarette smoke are more likely to require emergency department care than are children whose parents don't smoke. These associations between poorly controlled asthma and environmental exposures strongly suggest a causal relationship. Nonetheless, from the clinical perspective, the most important aspect of the association is the implication for treatment and disease control. A number of studies address attempts to control the environment and describe variable success.

The first studies to address environmental control are from the 1920s. Patients with severe asthma were moved to sanitaria high in the European Alps where allergen exposure is minimal.[30] In the anecdotal literature of the day, improvement in asthma symptoms described in some cases was apparently dramatic. Modern studies have confirmed the benefit of removing allergic asthmatic patients from their usual environments to spend time in a special environment made as allergen free as possible.[31] Among asthma patients sensitive to dust mite, removal to a dust mite–free environment can produce a gradual improvement in asthma symptom scores as well as a decrease in bronchial hyper-reactivity. Such studies are typically conducted in small numbers of carefully characterized patients. Of course, removing patients from their usual environments is an impractical intervention that cannot be translated into usual clinical practice.

A more feasible clinical intervention is controlling allergens in the patient's usual environment. A number of studies have described interventions to control dust mite exposure and cat dander exposure. Interventions typically require considerable patient effort and, for sustained benefit, a long-term lifestyle change. For example, a decrease in the dust mite antigen is not as simple as the purchase of mattress and pillow encasements but requires a change in the laundering of bedclothes, a reduction in the relative humidity of the household and bedroom, removal of dust-catching drapes and carpeting, and avoidance of stuffed animals. Under clinical trial conditions, it is possible to demonstrate modest improvements in asthma symptoms or the need for asthma medication, but group results reported are seldom dramatic.[32] However, it is difficult, if not impossible, to blind such studies adequately and produce a control intervention for comparison. Nevertheless, there is little question that clinicians should seek important environmental exposures when asthma is not responding well to usual therapy. In particular, the importance of household pets must be emphasized. Many clinicians are loathe to address this issue in their practices; many patients are reluctant to remove a valued pet from their homes. Those who do may be disappointed at the modest benefit they enjoy and the slowness with which the improvement takes place.

Recommendation

In patients whose asthma appears unresponsive to usual therapy, the environment must be examined for allergen and nonallergen exposures that may be making asthma worse. This assessment is accomplished first by an adequate history and subsequently by adjunctive skin testing. Environmental control measures may have modest benefit in improving symptoms and reducing need for medication (Level IIA).

Occupational Asthma

Occupational exposures are said to cause or contribute to 10% of asthma cases.[33,34] This figure is difficult to substantiate, and there may be real confusion between cases of pre-existing asthma that are aggravated by an irritant exposure and asthma that is newly induced by an occupational exposure. Detection of occupational asthma requires painstaking history taking supplemented by careful testing that may include prolonged periods of peak-flow monitoring, skin testing, and even challenge testing. Such an approach often is not discussed as part of the approach to refractory or unresponsive asthma, but it should not be overlooked by the clinician. The reader is referred to Chapter 9 for further discussion of this problem.

Chronic Obstructive Pulmonary Disease and Other Forms of Minimally Reversible Obstruction

Distinguishing asthma from chronic obstructive pulmonary disease (COPD) can sometimes be difficult. Some patients regarded as having unresponsive asthma because of persisting dyspnea and airflow obstruction actually may suffer from COPD as well as or instead of asthma. This diagnostic confusion is most likely to arise in smokers or ex-smokers who are middle-aged or older and who have some atopic background or family history of asthma. Clinicians may find it difficult to distinguish the two disease processes because our working definitions of COPD and asthma overlap and are sometimes hopelessly circular. Both asthma and COPD are characterized by airflow obstruction, and current definitions of both disorders mention airway inflammation.[3,35] Although the type of airway inflammation may differ between the two diseases, induced sputum measurements and other diagnostic studies that might distinguish between types of airway inflammation are not widely available in the clinical setting. Variability of airflow obstruction is regarded as a characteristic of asthma, but current descriptions of COPD also make mention of some responsiveness to therapy. Presumably, patients whose response to therapy is substantial enough to be consistent with asthma can be diagnosed confidently as having this disease. However, when such patients fail to achieve normal lung function with therapy, how can the clinician confidently exclude the possibility of coexisting COPD? One approach is to use the oral corticosteroid trial, an approach advocated in many guidelines for the management of COPD.[36] However, such a strategy may not be as effective in individual patients as it might appear to be from controlled trials. A meta-analysis reported by Callaghan and colleagues suggests that only 10% of patients with COPD will have potentially useful responses to oral steroid.[37] Unfortunately, this 10% response figure represents the difference between the percentage of patients responding to prednisone (30%) and the percentage of patients responding to placebo (20%). In clinical practice, the incautious trial of oral corticosteroids will lead practitioners to overestimate the corticosteroid responsiveness of individual COPD patients and, presumably, to overestimate the percentage of their patients who exhibit features of coexisting asthma. To further complicate the use of the oral steroid trial, some apparent nonresponders to corticosteroids are actually noncompliant.[38]

Although tobacco-related COPD might be the most common reason that patients have incomplete resolution of airflow obstruction with antiasthma treatment, other possibilities must be considered. Postviral, idiopathic, or collagen vascular–associated bronchiolitis may account for some unresponsive asthma. Long-standing and undertreated asthma can engender airway remodeling and the phenomenon once described as "asthmatic bronchitis."[39]

Recommendation

A period of aggressive therapy should be used at the outset of asthma management to determine the best symptom control and spirometric function that can be achieved. In patients with persistently abnormal spirometry, COPD and other causes of nonreversible airflow obstruction must be considered (Level IIIC).

Gastroesophageal Reflux

In 1962, Kennedy drew attention to the association between gastroesophageal reflux (GER) and troublesome asthma symptoms.[40] Many patients with asthma describe increased wheezing, dyspnea, or cough in association with episodes of symptomatic GER, and some such patients will report improvement in asthma symptoms when their GER is treated. The importance of this putative relationship is often overstated. For example, Irwin and colleagues describe GER as the most common factor making asthma difficult to control, and report that approximately two-thirds of their poorly controlled patients responded favorably to antireflux treatment.[41] They argue that all difficult-to-control asthma patients must be evaluated for GER, even in the absence of symptoms. Such an expensive approach seems to overlook the more prosaic explanations for poor asthma control, such as poor compliance or continued exposure to potent asthma-inducing allergens.

Physiologic studies suggest high rates of GER in patients with asthma. Sontag and colleagues, for example, have reported that 40% of the asthma patients they studied had erosive esophagitis, 58% had hiatus hernias, and more than 80% had abnormal 24-hour esophageal pH monitoring studies.[42,43] However, in the absence of a control population, the significance of these prevalence rates is uncertain. Moreover, some older reports of GER and asthma are confounded by the concurrent use of theophylline, an agent well known for decreasing lower esophageal sphincter tone and increasing gastric acid secretion.

Drug treatment of asthma is not the only cause of some instances of GER. Asthma itself can lead to increased GER. The resistive pressure load of airflow limitation results in increasingly negative intrathoracic inspiratory pressures, and, if expiratory airflow limitation is severe, it can increase positive intra-abdominal pressures, thereby raising the likelihood that gastric content will reflux.

Originally, GER was thought to worsen asthma by means of microaspiration of gastric acid and irritation of airway epithelium. However, it is difficult to demonstrate that actual aspiration of gastric content occurs. A more plausible mechanism is vagally mediated reflex bronchospasm. In animal models, acid perfusion of the distal esophagus is followed by increased airways resistance, an effect abolished by cervical vagotomy.

The clinical relevance of GER to asthma management is best evaluated by trials of antiacid and antireflux therapy in patients with asthma and suspected GER. A recent review of the literature revealed 242 papers on the subject; 12 were original peer-reviewed trials published in English.[44] Of these, only eight were placebo-controlled trials.[45–52] The typical trial involved small numbers of subjects, 20 to 30 patients, and monitored outcomes for a relatively short period of time, such as 4 to 6 weeks. The results of these studies show modest improvements in symptoms of asthma, slightly decreased medication use, and no change in spirometry or peak flow. Many explanations can be offered for such modest results. It is possible that the antireflux therapy given in the trial was insufficient to abolish physiologically important reflux; few studies documented abolition of reflux and reflux symptoms with therapy. It is also possible that spirometry and peak flows are insensitive measures of the phenomenon being studied and that a measure of airway hyper-reactivity would be more revealing. However, one must question the nature of the symptoms that improved. Is it possible that improved "asthma" symptoms were actually the symptoms of GER? Do some patients with unresponsive asthma have thoracic symptoms of GER that have been mistakenly attributed to the airway disease? The potentially deceptive nature of symptom-based therapeutic trials is highlighted by the magnitude of the placebo responses in studies of GER. Those studies incorporating a control population or a placebo treatment arm reported a 40% response rate to placebo "therapy."

Recommendation

Symptoms of GER in asthma patients warrant appropriate antiacid and antireflux therapy. There is no convincing evidence that searches for asymptomatic GER are essential to the investigation of unresponsive asthma or that trials of GER therapy are warranted (Level IIIC).

Allergic Rhinitis and Chronic Sinusitis

Rhinitis, chronic sinusitis, and allergic rhinitis are all described as factors that may make preexisting asthma worse. The coexistence of allergic rhinitis and unresponsive asthma is not surprising; most patients with asthma suffer from atopy, and allergic rhinitis may be the most common atopic manifestation. If severe and refractory allergic rhinitis is associated with severe and unresponsive asthma, the rhinitis does not necessarily cause the asthma, but the two conditions may be related by the severity of the underlying atopic diathesis or by the degree of environmental exposure. However, many clinicians and investigators have advocated aggressive treatment of allergic rhinitis and other nasal conditions as a means of improving unresponsive asthma. These recommendations are usually accompanied by speculation on a biologic pathway by which rhinitis could make coexisting asthma worse. The simplest explanation offered is that nasal congestion causes mouth breathing, thereby exposing the lower airway to air that has not been warmed, humidified, and filtered by the nose. Alternatively, irritation or stimulation of inflamed nasal mucosa could increase lower airway resistance by a reflex mechanism.[53] A somewhat different mechanical explanation is offered by investigators who have reported improvement in unresponsive asthma when patients use nasal continuous positive airway pressure (CPAP) therapy at night.[54] They speculate that nasal congestion can lead to snoring and that the vibration triggers reflex bronchospasm. A less mechanical explanation is that the inflamed nasal mucosa triggers the inflammatory cascade so pivotal in the development of airway inflammation and airway hyper-reactivity of asthma. Some argue that inflammatory mediators drip directly into the lower airway. Seldom considered is the possibility that troublesome and refractory "asthma symptoms" may, in truth, be symptoms more appropriately attributed to allergic rhinitis. For example, nocturnal cough and awakening may be caused by postnasal drip, but in a patient with asthma, it may be in misidentified as a sign of poor asthma control. If treatment of the allergic rhinitis and improvement in postnasal drip decrease the nocturnal awakenings, both patient and practitioner may regard asthma control as having been improved.

There are surprisingly few studies that address the role of treating allergic rhinitis in the management of asthma; few or none have reported the prevalence of uncontrolled allergic rhinitis or sinusitis in patients regarded as having unresponsive asthma. A handful of controlled trials have attempted to study the impact of allergic rhinitis treatment in controlling asthma symptoms. Such studies typically describe a crossover intervention in a small number of carefully selected patients with atopy, allergic rhinitis, and asthma. In general, the use of nasal corticosteroids to treat allergic rhinitis, can produce statistically significant improvements in asthma symptoms and decreased need for bronchodilator medication.[55] The effects, however, are small in most patients. In one striking study by Aubier et al, the use of nasal beclomethasone 400 μg decreased methacholine hyper-reactivity more than inhaled beclomethasone in the same daily dosage.[56] Such a finding seems to support strongly the contention that control of upper airway disease may be pivotal in the control of lower airway inflammation. However, before such counterintuitive results are accepted at face value, investigators must quantify the total corticosteroid burden and systemic absorption, not to assess the safety of the proposed regimen, but to ensure that the mechanism of the nasal corticosteroid is topical and not systemic.

Recommendation

Allergic rhinitis and chronic sinusitis commonly accompany asthma and may worsen asthma control or cause troublesome symptoms. Therapy of these nasal processes is worthwhile and appears to effect small improvements asthma outcomes (Level IB).

Disorders of Perception

Rubinfeld and Pain were the first to describe an abnormality of perception in patients with asthma.[57] In their seminal study, they used methacholine to induce airflow obstruction in patients with known asthma while questioning patients about their symptoms. Approximately 15% of patients were unable to detect a forced expiratory volume in 1 second (FEV$_1$) as low as 50% of the predicted normal value. This observation gave rise to the concept of the "poor perceiver" whose asthma was dangerous because of a failure to respond to the early warning signs of worsening asthma, a theme that has found its way into studies of fatal and near-fatal asthma. Patients who are resuscitated from an episode of near-fatal asthma are found to have blunted perception of hypoxic and hypercapnic stimuli and, perhaps, blunted perception of resistive loading.[58] Studies by Burdon and colleagues suggest that patients who are most at risk of being poor perceivers are those whose disease is long-standing and poorly controlled.[59] From this perspective, poor perception of symptoms is a matter of psychophysiologic accommodation. However, inspiratory reflexes and chemoreceptor responses are also thought to be largely inherited characteristics. Thus, some patients may be innately at risk of failing to perceive the actual severity of their asthma. A frequent recommendation for patients who are thought to be poor receivers and whose clinical course is characterized by frequent, unanticipated crises is that they use in-home self-monitoring with peak-flow meters. There is a superficial rationale to such a recommendation, but it ignores findings that patients often fail to adhere to recommendations for home peak-flow monitoring.[60,61] The recommendation must be regarded as a plausible but unproven solution.

If poor or blunted perception of respiratory sensations can account for the clinical phenomenon of "poor perception," it seems plausible that some patients may suffer from "heightened perception." Such a patient may have relatively mild or controlled asthma but would complain of frequent symptoms and would appear to have responded poorly to therapy. This phenomenon has not been well studied or frequently reported but may account for the number of instances in which patients complain of frequent mild symptoms. Recent observations describe a population of heightened perceivers and suggest a relationship to personality type.[62]

Recommendation

When asthma appears unresponsive, clinicians should determine the relationship between patient symptoms and objective measures of lung function or disease severity. This may be accomplished formally or informally, but when disproportion is detected (poor perception or heightened perception), therapeutic goals must be adjusted accordingly and monitored by objective measures (Level IIIB).

Steroid-Resistant and Steroid-Dependent Asthma

Some patients with refractory asthma are unresponsive to oral and inhaled corticosteroids. If steroid resistance is suspected, the diagnosis is confirmed by means of an oral steroid trial (prednisolone 1 mg/kg/d for 2 weeks) or, mindful of the possibility of noncompliance, a steroid trial with depot corticosteroid. In the absence of tobacco smoking and other injuries that might cause permanent airflow limitation, a lack of improvement in FEV_1 is reasonable evidence of steroid resistance. The prevalence of steroid resistance in asthma has been estimated as 1 in 1,000 to 1 in 10,000, but the true prevalence is unknown without the widespread molecular testing. Steroid resistance has been attributed to postreceptor transcription problems. Patients with steroid resistance typically have normal circulating levels of endogenous cortisol and normal endocrine function; the defect appears to be in the anti-inflammatory response to corticosteroids. Glucocorticoid receptor binding is usually normal. The molecular basis of the problem appears to be impaired communication between normal glucocorticoid receptors and deoxyribonucleic acid (DNA). Patients with steroid resistance have elevated basal levels of the transcription factor AP-1, a protein that may consume or bind to glucocorticoid receptors.

Steroid-dependent asthma is asthma controlled only with continuous use of oral or parenteral corticosteroids. Unlike steroid-resistant patients, there is a clinical response to corticosteroids. However, attempts to discontinue or lower the dosage of the oral steroid are met by asthma worsening. For some such patients, an underlying vasculitis or allergic bronchopulmonary aspergillosis will become manifest after a period of observation, and the reason for the steroid dependence will become known. In other patients, the phenomenon appears to be part of the spectrum of steroid resistance and may occur by similar mechanisms. One suggestion is that these patients develop relative steroid resistance secondary to asthmatic inflammation. Inflammatory cytokines such as interleukin-1 and tumor necrosis factor-α could activate transcription factors such as AP-1, which then bind to glucocorticoid receptors, thus reducing the number of receptors available for activation by glucocorticoids. It has also been suggested that β_2-agonists may cause relative glucocorticoid resistance by activating a transcription factor (cyclic adenosine monophosphate [AMP] response element binding protein [CREB]) that interacts directly with the glucocorticoid receptor in the same way as AP-1. This hypothesis is supported primarily by in vitro evidence. Anecdotal reports that troublesome asthma is improved by β_2-agonist withdrawal have never been substantiated by adequate controlled trials.[63]

When asthma appears to be unresponsive to conventional therapy, a trial of systemic corticosteroids may identify the patient's disease as being "steroid-resistant" or "steroid-dependent." As this categorization does not yet identify a specific disease mechanism and does not lead to a new therapeutic approach, the value of this assessment is unclear and cannot be recommended routinely (Level IIIC).

Brittle Asthma

The term "brittle asthma" has been coined to describe patients with characteristic patterns of uncontrolled disease.[64] These are syndromes rather than clearly defined entities with an established pathophysiology; it is not clear that these syndromes are different from the many other types of unresponsive asthma described elsewhere in this chapter.

Type I brittle asthma describes patients who have marked peak-flow variability in a constant and chaotic pattern.[65] Diurnal fluctuations in peak flow may average 40% and respond poorly to inhaled corticosteroid therapy, long-acting inhaled bronchodilators, and other conventional therapies. Patients with this pattern of uncontrolled asthma often have associated psychologic problems, and it is unclear whether these are the cause or consequence of the difficulties in controlling asthma. Continuous subcutaneous infusions of terbutaline have been used to treat the problem with some success but at the cost of great inconvenience and problematic muscle cramping with elevations of skeletal muscle enzymes.

Type II brittle asthma is characterized by sudden and unexpected attacks of life-threatening asthma against a background of relatively good disease control and relatively normal lung function.[65] Some such patients may suffer from disorders of perception as described above. A high prevalence of food allergy has been described in patients with type II brittle asthma. This observation and the finding that some patients have poor responses to inhaled bronchodilators has led to the suggestion that patients with type II brittle asthma may have some form of allergic airway edema or airway anaphylaxis, rather than asthma with smooth muscle constriction and eosinophilic airway inflammation. Self-administered epinephrine appears to be the recommended treatment of choice—an expert recommendation rather than a recommendation based upon controlled clinical trials.

Recommendation

The use of the term brittle asthma cannot be recommended. Although the term is a convenient shorthand that describes two patterns of poorly controlled asthma, there is no evidence at present that these patterns represent distinct pathophysiologic processes (Level IIIC).

Vasculitis and Allergic Bronchopulmonary Aspergillosis

An unknown proportion of patients with asthma who are apparently dependent upon oral corticosteroids will be found to have underlying vasculitis or allergic bronchopulmonary aspergillosis (ABPA). The exact prevalence of each disorder is unknown, and it seems likely that these diagnoses can be overlooked for prolonged periods of time. Modern asthma management guidelines recommend prompt treatment of exacerbations by systemic corticosteroids, a potentially life-saving approach that can mask an underlying vasculitis or ABPA. Indirect evidence of such underdiagnosis is suggested by the recent observation that some patients with troublesome asthma manifested unsuspected Churg-Strauss vasculitis after successful zafirlukast treatment allowed withdrawal of their chronic oral steroid treatment.[66]

Atypical clinical features should prompt consideration of these entities in patients with unresponsive asthma. Fleeting infiltrates on chest radiographs, chronic or recurrent sputum production, and proximal bronchiectasis are clinical features characteristic of ABPA and should prompt a further assessment with serum IgE assay, skin testing for aspergillus, and assessment for aspergillus precipitins. The presence of elevated IgE and IgG specific for aspergillus is said to be essential to the diagnosis of this entity.[62] If steroid-dependent asthma is accompanied by fleeting infiltrates on chest radiographs or signs of organ injury, as might occur with vasculitis, such a systemic illness should be considered and appropriate therapy administered promptly.

The exact prevalence of these entities in the population of patients with unresponsive asthma is unknown, but neither vasculitis or ABPA is considered common. It seems unlikely that routine serum IgE assay or vasculitis serology is warranted as part of the investigation of unresponsive asthma.

Recommendation

Atypical radiographic or clinical features in a steroid-dependent patient with asthma should prompt consideration of underlying vasculitis or ABPA (Level IIIC).

SUMMARY

"Difficult asthma" or "refractory asthma" is a common clinical problem that has been poorly addressed by clinical research. We lack a unifying definition for asthma that is unresponsive to usual therapy. As a result, our approach to this problem has been piecemeal. A review of the available literature suggests that causes of asthma that are unresponsive to usual therapy include misdiagnosis (eg factitious asthma, COPD), problems of health care delivery (eg noncompliance, poor inhaler technique), complicating factors (eg chronic sinusitis), and possibly subcategories of asthma with unique pathophysiology (eg steroid-resistant asthma). For clinicians who seek an approach to the patient with unresponsive asthma, it would appear wise to reconfirm the diagnosis by objective means and then to address common problems in management such as suboptimal compliance with prescribed therapy. When all such factors have been addressed, the clinician must turn his or her attention to issues that are suggested by the patient's history or pattern of disease and investigate each potentially causative factor until the asthma is controlled or the reason for the poor control is positively identified. Such an approach is empiric and the area of unresponsive asthma demands comprehensive and well-designed research programs.

REFERENCES

1. Rebuck AS, Chapman KR. Asthma: 2. Trends in pharmacologic therapy. Can Med Assoc J 1987;136:483–8.
2. Hargreave FE, Dolovich J, Newhouse MT. The assessment and treatment of asthma: a conference report. J Allergy Clin Immunol 1990;85:1098–111.
3. Boulet LP, Becker A, Berube D, et al. Summary of recommendations from the Canadian Asthma Consensus Report 1999. Can Med Assoc J 1999;161:S1–12.
4. Speight AN. Is childhood asthma being underdiagnosed and undertreated? Br Med J 1978;2:331–2.
5. British Thoracic Society. The British guidelines on asthma management 1995 review and position statement—introduction. Thorax 1997;52:S1–21.

6. Sheffer AL, Bousquet J, Busse WW, et al. International consensus report on diagnosis and management of asthma. Bethesda (MD): U.S. Department of Health and Human Services; 1992 Publication No.:92-3091.

7. Kesten S, Chapman KR. Physician perceptions and management of COPD. Chest 1993;104:254–8.

8. Chapman KR, Senathirajah N. The impact of pulmonary function testing on the diagnosis of asthma by primary care practitioners [abstract]. Am J Respir Crit Care Med 1999;155:A889.

9. Joyce DP, Chapman KR, Kesten S. Prior diagnosis and treatment of patients with normal results of methacholine challenge and unexplained respiratory symptoms. Chest 1996;109:697–701.

10. Dzyngel B, Kesten S, Chapman KR. Assessment of an ambulatory care asthma program. J Asthma 1994;31:291–300.

11. Newman KB, Mason UG III, Schmaling KB. Clinical features of vocal cord dysfunction. Am J Respir Crit Care Med 1995;152:1382–6.

12. Murray DM, Lawler PG. All that wheezes is not asthma—paradoxical vocal cord movement presenting as severe acute asthma requiring ventilatory support. Anaesthesia 1998;53:1006–11.

13. Boulet LP. Perception of the role and potential side effects of inhaled corticosteroids among asthmatic patients. Chest 1998;113:587–92.

14. Bender B, Milgrom H, Rand C. Nonadherence in asthmatic patients: is there a solution to the problem? Ann Allergy Asthma Immunol 1997;79:177–85.

15. Rand CS, Wise RA, Nides M, et al. Metered-dose inhaler adherence in a clinical trial. Am Rev Respir Dis 1992;146:1559–64.

16. Simmons MS, Nides MA, Kleerup EC, et al. Validation of the Doser, a new device for monitoring metered-dose inhaler use. J Allergy Clin Immunol 1998;102:409–13.

17. Joyce DP, Chapman KR. The Diskus device—a novel multi-dose powder inhaler. Today's Therapeutic Trends 1998;16:213–35.

18. Chapman KR. The choice of inhalers in adults and children over six. J Aerosol Med 1995;8 Suppl 2:S27–36.

19. Epstein SW, Manning CP, Ashley MJ, Corey PN. Survey of the clinical use of pressurized aerosol inhalers. Can Med Assoc J 1979;120:813–6.

20. Hanania NA, Wittman R, Kesten S, Chapman KR. Medical personnel's knowledge of and ability to use inhaling devices: metered-dose inhalers, spacing chambers, and breath-actuated dry powder inhalers. Chest 1994;105:111–6.

21. Kesten S, Zive K, Chapman KR. Pharmacist knowledge and ability to use inhaled medication delivery systems. Chest 1993;104:1737–42.

22. Amirav I, Goren A, Pawlowski NA. What do pediatricians in training know about the correct use of inhalers and spacer devices? J Allergy Clin Immunol 1994;94:669–75.

23. Kelling JS, Strohl KP, Smith RL, Altose MD. Physician knowledge in the use of canister nebulizers. Chest 1983;83:612–4.

24. Chapman KR, Love L, Brubaker H. A comparison of breath-actuated and conventional metered-dose inhaler inhalation techniques in elderly subjects. Chest 1993;104:1332–7.

25. Kesten S, Elias M, Cartier A, Chapman KR. Patient handling of a multidose dry powder inhalation device for albuterol. Chest 1994;105:1077–81.

26. Crain EF, Kercsmar C, Weiss KB, et al. Reported difficulties is access to quality care for children with asthma in the inner city. Arch Pediatr Adolesc Med 1998;152:333–9.

27. Leickly FE, Wade SL, Crain E, et al. Self-reported adherence, management behavior, and barriers to care after an emergency department visit by inner city children with asthma. Pediatrics 1998;101:E81–8.

28. Call RS, Smith TF, Morris E, et al. Risk factors for asthma in inner city children. J Pediatr 1992;121:862–6.

29. Hong CY, Ng TP, Wong ML, et al. Lifestyle and behavioural risk factors associated with asthma morbidity in adults. Q J Med 1994;87:639–45.

30. van Leeuwen WS. Bronchial asthma in relation to climate. Proc R Soc Med 1924;17:19–26.

31. Simon H, Grotzer M, Nikolaizik WH, et al. High altitude climate therapy reduces peripheral blood T lymphocyte activation, eosinophilia, and bronchial obstruction in children with house-dust mite allergic asthma. Pediatr Pulmonol 1994;17:304–11.

32. Tovey ER. Environmental control. In: Barnes PJ, Grunstein MM, Leff AR, Woolcock AJ, editors. Asthma. Philadelphia: Lippincott Williams & Wilkins; 1998. p. 1883–904.

33. Kogevinas M, Antó JM, Sunyer J, et al. Occupational asthma in Europe and other industrialised areas: a population-based study. Lancet 1999;353:1750–4.

34. Blanc PD, Toren K. How much adult asthma can be attributed to occupational factors? Am J Med 1999;107:580–7.

35. Celli BR, Snider GL, Heffner J, et al. Standards for the diagnosis and care of patients with chronic obstructive pulmonary disease. Am J Respir Crit Care Med 1995;152(5 Pt 2):S77–121.

36. Chapman KR, Bowie DM, Goldstein RS, et al. Guidelines for the assessment and management of chronic obstructive pulmonary disease. Canadian Thoracic Society Workshop Group. Can Med Assoc J 1992;147:420–8.

37. Callaghan CM, Dittus RS, Katz BP. Oral corticosteroid therapy for patients with stable chronic obstructive pulmonary disease. Ann Intern Med 1991;114:216–23.

38. Hatton MQF, Allen MB, Vathenen SV, et al. Compliance with oral corticosteroids during steroid trials in chronic airways obstruction. Thorax 1996;51:323–4.

39. Bousquet J, Vignola AM, Chanez P, et al. Airways remodelling in asthma: no doubt, no more. Int Arch Allergy Immunol 1995;107:211–4.

40. Kennedy JH. Silent gastroesophageal reflux: an important but little known cause of pulmonary complications. Dis Chest 1962;42:42–5.

41. Irwin RS, Curley FJ, French CL. Difficult-to-control asthma. Contributing factors and outcome of a systematic management protocol. Chest 1993;103:1662–9.

42. Sontag SJ, O'Connell S, Khandelwal S, et al. Most asthmatic patients have gastroesophageal reflux with or without bronchodilator therapy [comments]. Gastroenterology 1990;99:613–20.

43. Sontag SJ, Schnell TG, Miller TQ, et al. Prevalence of oesophagitis in asthmatic patients. Gut 1992;33:872–6.

44. Field SK, Sutherland LR. Does medical antireflux therapy improve asthma in asthmatic patients with gastroesophageal reflux? A critical review of the literature. Chest 1998;114(1):275–83.

45. Teichtahl H, Kronborg IJ, Yeomans ND, Robinson P. Adult asthma and gastro-oesophageal reflux: the effects of omeprazole therapy on asthma. Aust N Z J Med 1996;26:671–6.

46. Nagel RA, Brown P, Perks WH, et al. Ambulatory pH monitoring of gastro-oesophageal reflux in "morning dipper" asthmatic patients. BMJ 1988;297:1371–3.

47. Larrain A, Carrasco E, Galleguillos F, et al. Medical and surgical treatment of nonallergic asthma associated with gastroesophageal reflux. Chest 1991;99:1330–5.

48. Meier JH, McNally PR, Punja M, et al. Does omeprazole (Prilosec) improve respiratory function in asthmatic patients with gastroesophageal reflux? A double-blind, placebo-controlled crossover study. Dig Dis Sci 1994;39:2127–33.

49. Gustafsson PM, Kjellman NI, Tibbling L. A trial of ranitidine in asthmatic children and adolescents with or without pathological gastro-oesophageal reflux. Eur Respir J 1992;5:201–6.

50. Ford GA, Oliver PS, Prior JS, et al. Omeprazole in the treatment of asthmatic patients with nocturnal symptoms and gastro-oesophageal reflux: a placebo-controlled cross-over study. Postgrad Med J 1994;70:350–4.

51. Goodall RJ, Earis JE, Cooper DN, et al. Relationship between asthma and gastro-oesophageal reflux. Thorax 1981;36:116–21.

52. Ekstrom T, Lindgren BR, Tibbling L. Effects of ranitidine treatment on patients with asthma and a history of gastro-oesophageal reflux: a double blind crossover study. Thorax 1989;44:19–23.

53 Yan K, Salome C. The response of the airways to nasal stimulation in athmatics with rhinitis. Eur J Respir Dis 1983;64:105–9.

54. Chan CS, Woolcock AJ, Sullivan CE. Nocturnal asthma: role of snoring and obstructive sleep apnea. Am Rev Respir Dis 1988;137:1502–4.

55. Watson WTA, Becker AB, Simons FER. Treatment of allergic rhinitis with intranasal corticosteroids in patients with mild asthma: effect on lower airway responsiveness. J Allergy Clin Immunol 1993;91:97–101.

56. Aubier M, Levy J, Clerici C, et al. Different effects of nasal and bronchial glucocorticosteroid administration on

bronchial hyperresponsiveness in patients with allergic rhinitis. Am Rev Respir Dis 1992;146:122–6.

57. Rubinfeld AR, Pain MC. Perception of asthma. Lancet 1976;1:882–4.

58. Kikuchi Y, Okabe S, Tamura G, et al. Chemosensitivity and perception of dyspnea in patients with a history of near-fatal asthma. N Engl J Med 1994;330:1329–34.

59. Burdon JG, Juniper EF, Killian KJ, et al. The perception of breathlessness in asthma. Am Rev Respir Dis 1982;126:825–8.

60. Côté J, Cartier A, Malo JL, et al. Compliance with peak expiratory flow monitoring in home management of asthma. Chest 1998;113:968–72.

61. Malo JL, Trudeau C, Ghezzo H, et al. Do subjects investigated for occupational asthma through serial peak expiratory flow measurements falsify their results? J Allergy Clin Immunol 1995;96(5 Pt 1):601–7.

62. Chetta A, Gerra G, Foresi A, et al. Personality profiles and breathlessness perception in outpatients with different gradings of asthma. Am J Respir Crit Care Med 1998;157:116–22.

63. Sears MR. Dose reduction of beta-agonists in asthma. Lancet 1991;338:1331–2.

64. Ayres JG, Miles JF, Barnes PJ. Brittle asthma. Thorax 1998;53:315–21.

65. Ayres JG. Classification and management of brittle asthma. Br J Hosp Med 1997;57:387–9.

66. Wechsler ME, Garpestad E, Flier SR, et al. Pulmonary infiltrates, eosinophilia, and cardiomyopathy following corticosteroid withdrawal in patients with asthma receiving zafirlukast. JAMA 1998;279:455–7.

67. Chanarin N, Howarth PH. Specific problems: allergic bronchopulmonary aspergillosis. In: O'Byrne PM, Thomson NC, editors. Manual of asthma management. London: WB Saunders Company Ltd.; 1995. p. 607–20.

CHAPTER 25

Measures of Outcome

Pierre Ernst, MD, MSc, FRCPC
Samy Suissa, PhD

This chapter discusses measures of respiratory health commonly used to assess the efficacy of interventions in asthma. These are the measures employed to provide the evidence for evidence-based evaluation of asthma management. Each measure has advantages and disadvantages (Table 25–1), and the choice of measure to be used in any given study will depend upon the research question, the study design selected, the practicality of each measure in a given population, as well as the resources available. The measures that will be discussed are related to each other in various ways. The validity of these outcome measures, that is, the extent to which each measures what it claims to measure, is judged according to the degree to which they are inter-related (concurrent criterion validity). They are, however, not interchangeable, and each one measures different aspects of the asthma syndrome. Each measure has a different responsiveness, defined as the ability to detect clinically important changes, to proposed or studied interventions as well as differences in the specificity of the response observed, that is, the degree to which changes in the measure actually reflect changes in the asthmatic condition. The methods also vary as to their degree of reproducibility and have undergone varying degrees of standardization. This has important consequences for the power of a study to demonstrate benefit or to be certain that a clinically significant benefit has not been overlooked. Such standardization also facilitates the execution of multicenter studies.

Symptoms reported by patients will be considered first alone and then as part of composite measures to assess the asthmatic state. A presentation of the different measures of airflow limitation will follow and will include the measurement of airway responsiveness to various nonspecific stimuli. Markers of airway inflammation, whether measured directly or indirectly, will then be considered. Measures of quality of life will be briefly introduced. Last, we will discuss measures of health care use, quality of care, and morbidity, which have been used as measures of outcome in population-based studies.

Before we describe in detail the various outcome measures, it is important to briefly review the different designs used to study the benefit of asthma interventions. Indeed, there is a strong natural link that has developed between study design and outcome. The nature of the outcome, the complexity of its measurement, and the frequency of its occurrence have essentially restricted the outcomes that can be used by certain study designs and the designs that can be used with certain outcomes.

STUDY DESIGNS IN ASTHMA RESEARCH

The randomized controlled trial (RCT) is one of the preferred research tools in the evaluation of asthma interventions. Because it is randomized, it will usually eliminate extraneous differences between the intervention groups being compared. It is noteworthy to mention that, by chance, randomization may lead at times to unequal groups on one or more factors, so that statistical adjustments must be used in data analysis.[1] This happened in a recent trial in which subjects randomized to the leukotriene receptor antagonist zafirlukast had a baseline forced expiratory volume in 1 second (FEV_1) of 55% of predicted, compared with 74%

Table 25–1 *Advantages and Disadvantages of Various Outcome Measures*

Outcomes	Advantages	Disadvantages
Symptom measures	Easily obtained Sensitive to changes Standardized instruments for epidemiologic studies	Daily measures are cumbersome Intermittent measures rely on recall Well-accepted validated instruments for use in clinical trials only available for quality-of-life measures
Spirometry	Well standardized, reproducible FEV_1 is objective, reflects clinical state, has prognostic value	Needs to be measured on site for optimal results Insensitive to improvement in airway responsiveness
Peak-flow monitoring	Easy, portable Multiple daily measures sensitive to airway responsiveness and variability of airflow limitation	Less reproducible than FEV_1; single measures less sensitive Cumbersome when measured daily
Airway responsiveness	Bronchoprovocation with methacholine is well standardized Sensitive measure of airway status	Difficult to interpret in face of changes in baseline airway caliber Time consuming
Sputum cell count and differential	Sensitive reflection of airway inflammation Recently standardized	Not yet generally available Clinical significance not demonstrated
Expired NO	Easy to measure	Reproducibility needs to be improved Clinical significance not demonstrated
Morbidity and use of health services	Obvious clinical and economic significance	Usefulness limited to large cohorts and prolonged clinical trials

FEV_1 = forced expiratory volume in 1 second.

for the placebo group.[2] This is rare in large trials but can occur in smaller-sized trials. Due to the need to control the clinical trial situation, randomized trials result in a rigid and unnatural health care context that differs from the real-life situation in which the interventions, especially medications, are used. Nevertheless, such tight control is essential to create the experimental conditions necessary to assess the benefit of an intervention under optimal conditions and to determine the maximal potential effect of the intervention. The major limitations of this design are the high cost and very substantial resources required to conduct such studies properly. Patients must be seen and evaluated every 2 to 4 weeks, undergo extensive physiologic tests, respond to long questionnaires, and complete demanding daily diaries. Because of these demands, such trials are usually conducted on, at most, 600 patients and rarely exceed 26 weeks in duration. Exceptionally, START, a clinical trial of inhaled steroid treatment as regular therapy in early asthma, plans to recruit more than 5,000 subjects and follow them for 3 years. The RCT typically employs measures of respiratory symptoms, air-flow limitation, bronchial responsiveness, and inflammation as outcomes to assess the effectiveness of an asthma intervention. These outcomes are the only ones that can be studied with such sample sizes and follow-up. The more infrequent but major outcomes such as asthma mortality and morbidity require randomized trials with such large sample sizes as to be rarely feasible. Indeed, if one wished to assess whether, compared with placebo, a drug decreases the rate of asthma death by 50% (from 10 to 5 deaths per 10,000 asthma patients per year), one would need a randomized trial of approximately 50,000 subjects per group followed for 1 year.* If the study aimed to reduce the rate of asthma hospitalization by 50% (from 5.0 to 2.5 hospitalizations per 100 asthma patients per year), 1,000 subjects per treatment arm would be required.* Only one such randomized trial has ever been conducted to address these types of infrequent outcomes.[3] It involved 25,180 patients randomized either to salmeterol (n = 16,787) or to a short-acting β-agonist (n = 8,393) taken on a regular basis.

Another class of designs used to study the effectiveness and risk of interventions in asthma are the nonexperimental or observational epidemiologic designs. Cohort or case-control or even cross-sectional studies have been used successfully in asthma research. The particularity of these designs is that they address issues not considered in clinical trials, namely, infrequent and severe asthma outcomes, longer-term effects, and, most importantly, the real-life context of asthma management. A series of case-control studies from New Zealand assessed whether certain asthma drugs were associated with asthma mortality.[4-6] The Saskatchewan Asthma Epidemiology Project used a cohort approach as well as a nested case-control strategy to reassess these same risks for fatal and near-fatal asthma.[7,8] That study also demonstrated the benefits of regular inhaled steroid use in reducing the risk of fatal and near-fatal asthma (Level IIA).[9] Recently, case-control and cohort designs using data from the United States and Canada were employed to demonstrate the effectiveness of inhaled corticosteroids in reducing the rate of asthma hospitalization (Level IIA).[10-12] A population-based case-control study from Quebec assessed the risk of intraocular hypertension or glaucoma associated with the use of high doses of inhaled corticosteroids (Level II).[13] A cross-sectional design was used in Australia to assess the risk of cataract associated with inhaled corticosteroids,[14] a finding later corroborated by another population-based case-control study from Quebec (Level II).[15]

Characteristics common to all these studies are that they were conducted in very large populations using existing data collected in the context of health insurance administration, hospital management, or national health surveys.

The major drawback of these nonexperimental study designs is that the lack of randomization makes the assessment of the effectiveness of a drug subject to bias. This bias arises from confounding by indication, that is, the more severe asthmatic patients are receiving the more potent drug, the greater number of different drugs, as well as the higher doses, as compared to those asthmatic patients whose disease is less severe. Thus, comparisons between drug groups are confounded by different levels of asthma severity. This was the case in all the previously mentioned studies of β-agonists and fatal or near-fatal asthma as was later demonstrated by the pattern of increasing use of β-agonists (increasing severity) over time prior to the fatal or near-fatal attack.[16] On the other hand, very effective drugs such as inhaled corticosteroids have been shown to withstand the problem of confounding by indication in such nonexperimental studies: despite the fact that they are given to more severe asthmatic patients, they reduce the rate of severe attacks even when compared to asthmatic patients with milder disease not receiving such therapy (Level II).[10-12]

It would be useful for the reader to keep in mind the distinctions in study designs while reading the description of the various outcome measures and the natural link that has developed between design and outcome measure.

---

*Sample sizes are estimated for a two-sided test assuming a power (β) of 80% and a type I error (a) of 5%.

RESPIRATORY SYMPTOM MEASURES

Respiratory symptoms were first assessed in a standardized manner by the British Medical Research Council studies of chronic bronchitis and coal workers' pneumoconiosis.[17] This was the birth of respiratory epidemiology.[18] Emphasis was placed on validation of the symptoms of excess mucous production, such as daily cough and phlegm, and on the assessment of persistent, as opposed to intermittent, dyspnea. This quesionnaire was extended and modified by Benjamin Ferris Jr and the group at Harvard and became the American Thoracic Society (ATS) respiratory symptom questionnaire, available in both pediatric and adult versions and translated into many languages.[19]

In response to perceived deficiencies in these instruments for the study of asthma, Burney, in collaboration with the International Union against Tuberculosis and Lung Disease (IUATLD), developed and attempted to validate an asthma symptom and history questionnaire,[20] which has since been used for studies of the frequency and determinants of asthma in general population samples in Europe and elsewhere.[21] Interestingly, questions were included as to the use of asthma medications, providing a glimpse of variations in asthma therapy across Europe.[22] Similarly, for children, Innes Asher and colleagues throughout the world developed a short questionnaire on asthma symptoms and history, as well as allergic rhinitis and eczema (International Study of Asthma and Allergies in Childhood, or ISAAC).[23] The aim was to have a simple standardized instrument and method of application that would permit a comparison of the prevalence of allergic disease around the world and lead to hypotheses concerning the **principle** etiologies of asthma and the reasons for the apparent worldwide increase in its impact and recognition. None of these instruments lend themselves readily for use in the evaluation of interventions for the management of asthma.

The symptoms of asthma are typically wheeze, cough, shortness of breath, and chest tightness, with wheeze and dyspnea most often predominating. Symptoms are often intermittent or vary in severity. Symptom information has been routinely collected in most intervention trials, and most often the subject has been asked to grade his symptoms considered together. This appears reasonable since it is assumed that patients entered into clinical trials of asthma interventions have met entry criteria, including a firm diagnosis of asthma, and that other causes of respiratory symptoms have been excluded. Such a composite index assumes equal weights or importance for each symptom, and there is evidence that such an assumption is not unreasonable.[24] Symptoms have commonly been graded on a scale from 0 to 3; 0 when symptoms are absent, 1 for mild symptoms that do not interfere with activities, 2 for moderate symptoms that interfere with daily activities, and 3 for severe symptoms that interfere with most or many of the day's activities. Sleep disturbance and exercise limitation are often assessed concomitantly. The validity of such scoring has scarcely been examined. Using information collected during clinical trials of a leukotriene receptor antagonist, Santanello et al examined the measurement characteristics of two asthma symptom scales, one for daytime symptoms (Figure 25–1) and the other to assess disturbance of sleep due to asthma.[25] Scores were averaged daily, and these were used to calculate average weekly scores. The scores related closely to other daily measures, such as those of peak flow, and less well with weekly measures of forced expiratory volume in 1 second (FEV_1). Reproducibility was excellent.

Daily measures, while providing accurate information on duration, frequency, and intensity, are difficult to maintain even when the study period is only 2 weeks;[26] they are likely more difficult to maintain if the interval between visits is prolonged. A baseline period is usually included, and patients are randomized only if their compliance with daily diary recordings has been adequate. While this is likely necessary if symptoms are to be used as an effective measure of outcome, applicability of the results to asthmatic patients in general, that is, to those who are less compliant, is compromised. Furthermore, there is no information on the respective importance of the components of symptom scales such as intensity, frequency, or duration.

How often did you experience asthma symptoms today?

0	1	2	3	4	5	6
None of the time						All of the time

How much did your asthma symptoms bother you today?

0	1	2	3	4	5	6
Not at all bothered						Severely bothered

How much activity could you do today?

0	1	2	3	4	5	6
More than usual activity						Less than usual activity

How often did your asthma affect your activities today?

0	1	2	3	4	5	6
None of the time						All of the time

Figure 25–1 Example of a daily symptom scale. (Reproduced with permission from Santanello NC, Barber BL, Reiss TF, et al. Measurement characteristics of two asthma symptom diary scales for use in clinical trials. Eur Respir J 1997;10:646–51.)

Periodic measures on the other hand must rely on recall by the patient or a parent, and such recall may be influenced by the efficacy of the intervention examined. If symptom severity is to be recalled, the patient is asked to integrate his experience over a certain time. It is unlikely that such recall would be accurate for a period of longer than a month, at least for the daily occurrence of individual symptoms. Over prolonged periods of study, Gold et al, however, found that periodic interviews provided more information on symptoms than daily diaries, especially in the second year of a 2-year follow-up.[27] On the other hand, a period of recollection that is too short would not be appropriate for a symptom or event that is infrequent in the population under study. Such low endorsement of an item would reduce the ability of a scale to detect differences between individuals and groups.

Gibson et al, as part of a method proposed to detect mild exacerbations of asthma during withdrawal of inhaled corticosteroids, assessed symptoms both on a weekly basis, using an administered questionnaire, and in a daily diary.[28] Each symptom (cough, chest tightness, breathlessness, and wheeze) was graded on a nine-point scale from unbearable to absent. In addition, subjects were asked to judge whether each symptom had improved or worsened and by how much. Both the weekly symptom score and the daily symptom diary were highly responsive with significant deterioration detectable much earlier than by monitoring of peak flows. The questionnaire and daily diary are somewhat cumbersome, and this likely explains why this method has not been widely adopted. Wasserfallen et al developed an asthma symptom score for use in clinical trials that also includes queries about symptoms of rhinoconjunctivitis.[29] The questionnaire is meant to be given intermittently at follow-up visits, and it gathers information on symptoms in the prior week.

Various asthma scores have used symptoms and impact on daily activities to classify patients according to the severity of their asthma in the prior months or by observing changes over time; they have not been used to examine how such an instrument might perform as a measure of the impact of an intervention.[24,30–32] Symptom intensity, frequency, and duration have a profound impact on the quality of life of the asthmatic patient as will be discussed later. The use of symptoms as an outcome measure appears to be even more problematic in very young patients, since asthma in the first few years of life is often intermittent and objective confirmation of the diagnosis or the severity of the disease is often not possible.[33]

Use of supplemental or rescue β-agonist is also usually recorded in the daily diary at the same time as symptoms. This is likely to have the same limitations as daily symptom recordings unless actual use is verified, at least partially, with a delivery device containing a dose counter or by weighing of canisters. Such dose counters are not always reliable.[34] Use of medications and symptoms may also be combined to obtain a severity score which may be followed up over time.[35,36] Another way of summarizing daily diary information is to count the number of days without reported symptoms or need for rescue β-agonist within a given time period. We used the number of "symptom-free days" to compare the efficacy of zafirlukast, a leukotriene receptor antagonist, to placebo.[2] The disadvantage of this measure is that subjects may consciously or unconsciously reduce their activities to avoid experiencing symptoms of asthma.

Clinical scores, whether based on symptoms alone or combined with other information, are ordinal scales that must meet simple methodologic rules to be of value.[37] There must be a clear hierarchy from one level to the next, and each level needs to be exclusive and clearly defined. The different levels must be meaningful in a clinical sense, that is, they must represent easily recognizable clinical states, and the patient group to which the measure is applied must be able to move along the scale in both directions, that is, both improvement and deterioration should be equally possible. Scales can be divided into single-state and transition scales. Single-state measures assess the subject's condition at one point in time (though the measure can be carried out at different points in time and changes over time examined). In such situations, it is critical that the groups being compared be similar at the baseline evaluation or, more appropriately, that adjustment for the initial measure be carried out when assessing change over time. Transition scales directly assess the change within an individual from one observation to the next, and the average change within individuals in different groups is compared.

When adopting a clinical scale for use, one needs to verify that it has been validated among similar patients. Measures developed for adults are unlikely to be directly applicable to children. Scales that are responsive to the effects of treatment in severe disease may not be sensitive to change in milder patients. Differences in language, education, and socioeconomic status are all factors likely to limit the applicability of clinical scores based on patients' reports from one group to another.

Measures of Airflow Limitation

Limitation of airflow from the lungs is the most important and characteristic feature of asthma and is most reliably evaluated with the help of a spirometer. The FEV_1 or forced expiratory volume in the first second of a maximal forced expiratory maneuver is reproducible, provides an excellent estimate of the degree of bronchial obstruction, and is responsive to changes in the subject's clinical condition (Level IIA).[38] The validity and importance of the FEV_1 has been demonstrated by its correlation with inflammatory and structural changes in the airways and, more importantly, by its strong relationship to prognosis.[39–41] It is commonly used to assess asthma severity at the baseline assessment carried out in clinical trials. Once the maneuver has been grasped by the patient with the help of a technician experienced in obtaining a maximal effort, the major determinants of FEV_1 and FVC (forced vital capacity) are age, gender, and height.[42] The relationship of spirometric measures to these determinants is accurately described in prediction equations obtained in healthy individuals from the general population, and the predicted values obtained are used to account for the most of the expected differences between individuals. Standards are widely available describing the equipment to be used, the method of testing, selection of the best results, and the variation in the measures to be expected within a day as well as for longer time intervals.[43-46] The responsiveness and reproducibility of FEV_1 make it an ideal effect measure to be followed at weekly or monthly visits common to most trials of asthma therapy. Reproducibility can be further enhanced by performing the test at the same time of day at each visit, performing the test after administration of a bronchodilator, and not having the patient undergo testing soon after exercise or after coming in from the cold.[47]

The FVC as a single measure adds little to the measure of FEV_1 in subjects with asthma, apart from allowing one to verify that the test has been done properly. The ratio of the two measures ($FEV_1:FVC$) is a more sensitive measure of airflow limitation, especially when the FEV_1 remains within the normal range; however, the possibility of change in either measure means that this ratio is not suitable for evaluating change over time in response to an intervention. The tracing of the forced expiratory maneuver can be expressed graphically as volume versus time (spirogram) or flow plotted against volume (flow-volume loop). Other measures can be calculated from either the spirogram or the flow-volume loop, for example, the mid-expiratory flow rate or flows at a given level of vital capacity are of little or no additional value, at least in adults, due to their poor reproducibility.[48] The change in FEV_1 in response to an inhaled short-acting β-agonist bronchodilator is often used as a way to diagnose asthma, as discussed in Chapter 4. It has not been used as a measure of effect in clinical trials and is unlikely to be a useful measure because of its dependence on changes in the level of FEV_1 itself. Measures of FEV_1 have been little used for ambulatory monitoring, largely due to the complexity and cost of the equipment required. This is likely to change in the near future with the advent of increasingly inexpensive and portable spirometers.

Ambulatory monitoring of airflow is most often done with inexpensive portable peak-flow meters, which have been available for almost 20 years.[49] Reliability of these inexpensive tools has only been tested extensively in the past few years, however.[50] The measure of peak flow obtained is significantly less reproducible than the FEV_1, principally due to the greater effort dependence of the maneuver.[51] Peak flow is also less responsive to narrowing of the airways, and this may be particularly problematic in muscular individuals who are able to achieve high intrathoracic pressures at the onset of the maneuver and if the subject coughs at the onset of expiration.[52] For this reason, it is preferable to measure FEV_1 at clinic visits and reserve peak flow for ambulatory monitoring.[53] Further reduction in unwanted variability in the measure of peak flow can be obtained by comparing the value obtained to the value measured with a spirometer at the same sitting. Daily recording of peak flow has similar limitations to the daily recording of symptoms, mainly poor patient adherence. Subjects are usually instructed to blow in to the meter maximally three times at any one sitting and to record the best value. Measures are carried out, at a minimum, first thing in the morning prior to taking inhaled medications, after use of a bronchodilator if one is required, and again at bedtime.[54] Circadian changes in airway tone, which are exaggerated in asthma, dictate that the lowest value of the day will be observed in the early morning with higher levels later in the day. The difference in peak flow within the day, or peak-flow variability, is a measure of asthma control, increasing with the onset of exacerbations and decreasing with control of inflammation in the airways. Such variability has been considered as a measure of asthma severity[55] but has been little used as a measure of effect in clinical trials. Variability in peak flows can be expressed in several ways, but the amplitude mean (within-day maximum minus minimum divided by the mean of the values and multiplied by 100) is reported most commonly.[50,56] The possible benefit of an intervention has been judged by single measures of peak flow measured at the clinic visit or, more often, the value obtained on arising, or by the average value of this measure recorded over a defined period of time. Multiple daily measures of peak flow provide a measure of the effectiveness of asthma medication around the clock, and this is especially relevant for medications designed to provide sustained control of asthma symptoms.

Most children can perform acceptable spirometry by 6 years of age, whereas reproducible FVC maneuvers are not possible in most children under the age of 5 years. Alternative methods such as partial-flow volume curves obtained by performing thoracoabdominal compression in sedated infants[57] or measuring respiratory oscillation mechanics during tidal breathing[58] are much more complex than spirometry, and have so far been applied principally to studies with small numbers of children.

AIRWAY RESPONSIVENESS

Asthma is characterized by an increased response of the airways to nonspecific stimuli, and various methods have been used to assess this airway hyper-responsiveness (AHR). The stimuli used can be divided into two categories, direct and indirect. Direct stimuli most commonly employed are histamine and the cholinergic agonist methacholine. The latter has been adopted more widely, especially recently, because of the ability to administer higher equivalent doses without unpleasant side effects such as flushing and headache, which are commonly encountered with high doses of histamine. After measurement of baseline FEV_1, subjects first inhale the diluent followed by increasing doubling concentrations or doses of the bronchoconstricting agent. The FEV_1 is measured at a fixed time after each dose, usually at 30 and/or 90 seconds, and the test is stopped after the FEV_1 has fallen 20% or more from the value obtained after inhalation of the diluent or until the last dose has been administered. This method of bronchoprovocation has been found to be safe in the hands of experienced personnel and has been carried out in the field without direct medical supervision. The bronchoconstrictor agent is usually not administered if a significant drop in FEV_1 has occurred with inhalation of the diluent isotonic saline. The principal danger arises from the possibility of inadvertently administering a higher dose than planned, and for this reason it has been recommended that the bottles containing the various concentrations be color coded. Furthermore, a bronchodilator is usually given after the test is completed to ensure that the FEV_1 has returned to within 90% of the baseline value.

Although various efforts at standardizing the method have been undertaken and published,[59,60] no one method has achieved overall favor. There are different ways of delivering the inhaled bronchoconstrictor, of measuring the response, and of expressing the results.[61] This markedly impairs the comparability between studies but poses less of a problem when examining the effects of an intervention, since the same methodology can be used throughout. Attention to technical detail remains essential, but difficult, as demonstrated by the unwanted variability that has been shown in multicenter studies using the same equipment and methods.[62]

The degree of airway hyper-responsiveness has most often been expressed as the concentration that results in a fall of 20% in the FEV_1 (PC_{20}). The doses of methacholine may have a cumulative effect with certain protocols, and the results have therefore also been expressed as the dose resulting in a 20% fall in FEV_1 (PD_{20}). This also requires a measure of nebulizer output. Practically speaking, there is little difference between these two measures. The PC_{20} (or PD_{20}) is an overall measure of airway responsiveness measuring both sensitivity, a leftward shift in the log dose-response curve, and reactivity, an increase in the slope of the relation between fall in FEV_1 and the log dose of the agonist. From a practical point of view, especially when examining the effects of interventions between groups, there is little to gain by separating the various components of airway responsiveness, which also include threshold, the dose at which the FEV_1 has decreased significantly from baseline, and the plateau or maximal response, which is difficult to identify safely in asthmatic subjects and may not be present in those with more than mild disease. In normal populations, less than 50% of subjects will have an identifiable PC_{20}, which is most easily calculated by interpolation of the two last points on the log dose-response curve. While this poses problems in epidemiologic studies,[61] this is of less concern in studies of subjects with asthma, since almost all subjects, by definition, will have AHR. While the degree of AHR relates acceptably to asthma severity and the degree of inflammation in the airways, it is strongly influenced by starting airway caliber. The test is therefore most useful in those without airflow obstruction, and for changes in AHR to be interpretable, the starting FEV_1 should not have changed from one time to another. The test is fairly reproducible, within one to two doubling doses from one time to another.[53] Increases of 1.5 to 2 doubling doses are associated with worsening of symptoms and an increase in airway inflammation.[63]

To compensate for the inability to identify a value for PC_{20} in normal subjects and in those whose asthma improves significantly either spontaneously or by intervention, as well as to provide a continuous response measure that is amenable to the usual techniques of linear regression, calculation of a log dose-response slope has been proposed. This is derived by taking the percentage fall in FEV_1 from the postsaline value to the last dose of methacholine delivered and dividing it by this last dose of methacholine and expressing it on a log scale.[64] This requires adding a constant to avoid negative values for mild degrees of airway responsiveness, but it provides a value for any subject who inhaled at least one dose of methacholine. The problem remains as to how to consider subjects who drop their FEV_1 significantly in response to the saline diluent, since it is likely they have marked AHR.

Abramson et al proposed a modification of O'Connor et al's method (just described[64]) that requires that the subject be able to complete at least two doses or concentrations of methacholine.[65] They used linear regression to calculate a least squares slope. As pointed out by Chinn,[61] this is equivalent to analyzing the PC_{20} using censored regression techniques (PC_{20} is considered to be a censored measure since its value, the maximum dose delivered, is known only to a certain point on the log dose scale). Variations in the calculation of slope have been proposed to render it more amenable to statistical analysis.[61]

Exercise is an indirect bronchoconstrictor, and the mechanisms involved are discussed in Chapter 19 by Mark Inman. It is commonly used as a measure of airway responsiveness in children. It is carried out either under carefully controlled conditions in the laboratory using a treadmill or, for epidemiologic studies, as a free running test. It is important to control the level of exercise as well as ambient temperature and humidity. The bronchoconstrictive response to exercise is more difficult to analyze, since only one dose of the bronchoconstricting stimulus is available. Exercise-induced bronchospasm is therefore usually considered to be either present or absent. Correlation with bronchial response to direct stimuli is incomplete and it is not uncommon for subjects, especially children, to react to one but not the other at any one time.[66] Another indirect, but pharmacologic, stimulus to airway narrowing that has enjoyed a revival recently is adenosine.[67] Adenosine is a purine nucleoside that appears to cause airway narrowing more specific to asthma than methacholine, which commonly causes narrowing of the airways in other chronic airway diseases in both adults and children. Adenosine-induced bronchoconstriction appears more sensitive to inhibition with bronchodilators and may be more sensitive to improvements in airway inflammation than methacholine or histamine. Isocapnic hyperventilation and induction of airway narrowing by breathing controlled amounts of cold air act by mechanisms similar to exercise but have the advantage that a dose-response relationship can be obtained. The equipment required is cumbersome and expensive and there has been limited adoption of these methods.

Due to the lack of acceptability of subjecting children to methacholine in field studies in certain countries, hypertonic saline has been used as an indirect stimulus to airway narrowing. An ultrasonic nebulizer is used to deliver 4.5% saline; the equipment is easily available and affordable, and the method is becoming standardized. A dose-response is calculated by plotting the FEV_1 versus the volume nebulized or, to provide a correction for size in children, the time of aerosol inhalation that resulted in a 15% fall in FEV_1 can be reported.[68]

Measures of airway responsiveness are most often used to confirm the diagnosis of asthma in subjects whose lung function is normal and who do not demonstrate a significant improvement in FEV_1 following inhalation of a rapidly acting bronchodilator. They have also been used as an outcome measure in intervention studies. Examples include improvements in AHR with allergen avoidance[69] and with treatment with inhaled corticosteroids.[70] Worsening AHR with regular use of short-acting bronchodilators has been proposed as a potential mechanism to explain diminishing asthma control with regular use of this class of medication.[71] The lack of an increase in AHR following allergen challenge has been proposed as a method to prove the efficacy of preventive therapy.[72] Loss of protection against methacholine- or adenosine-induced bronchospasm with use of long-acting β-agonists has been used as a marker of potential adverse effects of these medications.[73] Recently, protection against methacholine-induced bronchoconstriction has been proposed as a way to compare the relative potencies of inhaled β-agonists.[74]

MEASURES OF AIRWAY INFLAMMATION

It is now well recognized that inflammation with infiltration by eosinophils[75] is an important, and possibly the principal, determinant of the asthmatic diathesis. Attempts have therefore been made to identify and quantify this inflammatory process. Markers of inflammation can be categorized as those measured in body fluids distant from the lungs and those assessed directly from the airways.

Among the former are the measure of inflammatory leukotrienes in the urine, which is technically difficult, and the measure of eosinophils or their products such as eosinophilic cationic protein (ECP) in the blood.[76] Eosinophils may decrease in response to treatment, but changes in the number or proportion of these cells in peripheral blood are also characteristic of diseases other than asthma. Levels of ECP in the blood are widely distributed, and this is in part due to variations in the temperature at which the blood is taken. Specificity is also poor, with increases being observed with atopic dermatitis for example. Finally, while various cytokines can be detected in peripheral blood and may be increased in patients with asthma, variability is very high and correlation with airway inflammation uncertain,[77] thus severely limiting their use as outcome measures.

The significance of the inflammatory process in asthma became readily apparent when biopsies of bronchial mucosa obtained with a flexible bronchoscope demonstrated histologic evidence of airway inflammation even in mild asthmatic patients.[78] The number and type of airway cells observed in bronchoalveolar lavage (BAL) obtained in a similar manner was also found to reflect the presence and severity of eosinophilic inflammation characteristic of asthma.[75] Bronchoscopy remains, however, an invasive procedure not suitable for serial measurements of effect required by most intervention studies.[79]

Sputum examination has more recently been proposed as a method to assess airway inflammation directly, but in a noninvasive manner.[80] Sputum is usually induced by the inhalation of nebulized hypertonic saline, either in increasing concentrations or for increasing lengths of time.[80] Marked bronchoconstriction may result, and airway caliber needs to be measured initially and followed at intervals, usually with spirometry. The average fall in FEV_1 observed, mostly in mild asthmatic patients, has been 5 to 7%. It is recommended that the nebulization stop if the FEV_1 falls by 20% or more. The test is not felt to be safe in patients whose FEV_1 is less than 60% predicted. A rapidly acting inhaled $β_2$-agonist such as salbutamol is usually administered beforehand. The sample must be processed quickly to assure viability of the cells. Several techniques have been proposed. After verification of the quality of the specimen to assure its origin is the airway as opposed to saliva, the nature and number of the cells is assessed. The supernatant can also be examined for cellular products such as ECP. A number of soluble mediators such as cytokines can also be measured. The validity of the method is suggested by the ease with which asthma can be distinguished from other diseases of the airway and from normal; it also has a correlation, though far from perfect, with the results of BAL and bronchial biopsy specimens. This technique has also been shown to be sensitive to intervention with inhaled or oral corticosteroids, the mainstay of asthma therapy.[81] It may prove to be an important indicator of the effectiveness of treatment as suggested by the persistence of airway inflammation, despite improvements in other measures such as symptoms and lung function described, for example, in patients receiving long-acting β_2-agonists.[82] Validation of the method ultimately depends on the prognostic significance of the abnormalities described.

Nitric oxide (NO) is found in increased amounts in exhaled air collected from patients with asthma. In untreated patients, the levels correlate with the severity of asthma and other measures of inflammation in the airways. Levels drop precipitously with corticosteroid therapy, whether inhaled or systemic, so that even patients with severe oral corticosteroid-dependent asthma will have lower levels measured in expired air than a mild asthmatic treated with inhaled β_2-agonists alone. Large amounts of NO can also originate from the paranasal sinuses and from the esophagus. The amount of NO is dependent on expiratory flow rate. All this makes the measure of lower airway NO difficult and quite variable.[83] Recommendations for standardization of the method have been published,[84] but the prognostic value as well as the capacity to measure significant changes in the asthmatic diathesis remains open to question.

HEALTH-RELATED QUALITY OF LIFE

Full coverage of this topic would require a chapter in itself. Only a brief introduction is provided here. Detailed information on the concepts and a description of the various instruments can be obtained from the American Thoracic Society website at www.atsqol.org. Measurement instruments consisting mainly of questionnaires have been developed to assess the impact of disease on various aspects of a patient's life which are often poorly reflected by physiologic measures and reporting of specific symptoms. Such aspects of patients' lives include physical and social functioning, role limitations due to physical and emotional problems, pain, vitality, and overall perception of one's health. There are so-called generic instruments that may be used to evaluate the impact for the patient of different chronic diseases. Examples are the short form 36 (SF-36) from the Medical Outcomes Study[85] and the Sickness Impact Profile (SIP).[86] While such instruments can be applied widely, they may lack sensitivity to the problems patients with a particular disease frequently encounter. Disease-specific instruments have therefore appeared, and instruments designed specifically for the evaluation of interventions in patients with asthma have gained popularity over the past 10 years. Perhaps the best known is the Asthma Quality of Life Questionnaire (AQLQ) developed by Juniper et al at McMaster University in Hamilton, Canada.[87] This instrument takes approximately 15 minutes to administer and addresses four categories or domains of patient complaints: symptoms, emotions, the effects of exposure to environmental stimuli, and limitation of activities. Other disease-specific instruments commonly used in the evaluation of asthma therapy include the asthma quality-of-life questionnaire developed by Marks et al[88] and the St. George's respiratory questionnaire developed by Jones, which is used commonly in patients with both asthma and COPD.[89]

MORBIDITY AND USE OF HEALTH CARE

While symptoms and physiologic measures may provide a sensitive and, at times, precise reflection of the asthmatic condition in an individual patient, they are expensive and time consuming to assess. Furthermore, the results observed are not directly interpretable as to their importance and impact on the individual and society. Consequences are more readily deducible from the identification of events such as an asthma exacerbation, hospitalization,

318 Evidence-Based Asthma Management

and even death. These events are also more easily converted into costs to the individual and to the health care system. Such information is assuming increasing importance in decisions concerning the allocation of health care resources.

Since asthma is characterized by episodic worsening, the identification of such exacerbations is certainly pertinent. Exacerbations have been defined as a combination of increases in symptoms and need for rescue β-agonist, worsening airflow limitation as detected either by ambulatory measures of peak flow or fall in FEV_1 measured at a clinic visit, or the need for a course of systemic corticosteroids as assessed by the physician in charge of the patient.[90,91] When using measures that require subjective judgment, such as the need for corticosteroids or for hospital admission during an acute exacerbation, it is critically important that the decision be made without knowledge of the therapies the study patient is receiving. This strategy is exemplified by the double-blind, double-dummy, randomized clinical trial in which the active and placebo medications cannot be differentiated and neither the patient nor the physician or other study personnel is aware of the treatment group to which the patient has been allocated.

Identification of morbid events in this manner remains burdensome. Information on emergency department visits and hospitalizations is often routinely collected or can be deduced by examining charts, thus allowing collection of data retrospectively and at a lower cost. Such recorded data avoids the inaccurate recall by patients of all but recent events and the bias induced by the better recollection of events by those having experienced more extreme outcomes, whether good or bad.

The use of information gathered previously (and most often not for the purposes of research) has limitations, mostly related to the quality of the information, however. The accuracy of the diagnosis of asthma is often in doubt, since confusion among various obstructive airway syndromes is common in clinical practice. This is especially the case with extremes of age: bronchiolitis and asthma are often confused in infants, whereas the labels of asthma and chronic obstructive pulmonary disease are often used interchangeably in older individuals. The diagnosis of asthma inferred from information recorded in hospital charts or in administrative databases appears quite accurate for patients between 5 and 45 years. Similar arguments hold when using deaths from asthma as an outcome.[92] As discussed earlier, observational studies are subject to bias, especially indication bias, and such bias needs to be carefully looked for and considered as possible explanations for any association observed.

REFERENCES

1. Pocock SJ, Hughes MD, Lee RJ. Statistical problems in the reporting of clinical trials: a survey of three medical journals. N Engl J Med 1987;317:426–32.

2. Suissa S, Dennis R, Ernst P, et al. Effectiveness of the leukotriene receptor antagonist zafirlukast for mild-to-moderate asthma. Ann Intern Med 1997;126:177–83.

3. Castle W, Fuller R, Hall J, Palmer J. Serevent nationwide surveillance study: comparison of salmeterol with salbutamol in asthmatic patients who require regular bronchodilator treatment. Br Med J 1993;306:1034–7.

4. Crane J, Pearnce N, Flatt A, et al. Prescribed fenoterol and death from asthma in New Zealand, 1981–83: case-control study. Lancet 1989;1:917–22.

5. Pearce N, Grainger J, Atkinson M, et al. Case-control study of prescribed fenoterol and death from asthma in New Zealand, 1977–81. Thorax 1990;45:170–5.

6. Grainger J, Woodman K, Pearce N, et al. Prescribed fenoterol and death from asthma in New Zealand, 1981–7: a further case-control study. Thorax 1991;46:105–11.

7. Spitzer WO, Suissa S, Ernst P, et al. The use of β-agonists and the risk of death and near death from asthma. N Engl J Med 1992;326:501–6.

8. Suissa S, Ernst P, Boivin J-F, et al. A cohort analysis of excess mortality in asthma and the use of inhaled beta-agonists. Am J Respir Crit Care Med 1994;149:604–10.

9. Ernst P, Spitzer WO, Suissa S, et al. Risk of fatal and near-fatal asthma in relation to inhaled corticosteroid use. JAMA 1992;268:3462–4.

10. Donahue JG, Weiss ST, Livingston JM, et al. Inhaled corticosteroids and the risk of hospitalization for asthma. JAMA 1997;277:887–91.

11. Blais L, Ernst P, Boivin JF, Suissa S. Inhaled corticosteroids and the prevention of readmission to hospital for asthma. Am J Respir Crit Care Med 1998;158:126–32.

12. Blais L, Suissa S, Boivin JF, Ernst P. First treatment with inhaled corticosteroids and the prevention of admissions to hospital for asthma. Thorax 1998;53:1025–9.

13. Garbe E, LeLorier J, Boivin JF, Suissa S. Inhaled and nasal glucocorticoids and the risks of ocular hypertension or open-angle glaucoma. JAMA 1997;277:722–7.

14. Cumming RG, Mitchell P, Leeder SR. Use of inhaled corticosteroids and the risk of cataracts. N Engl J Med 1997;337:8–14.

15. Garbe E, Suissa S, LeLorier J. Association of inhaled corticosteroid use with cataract extraction in elderly patients. JAMA 1998;280:539–43.

16. Suissa S, Blais L, Ernst P. Patterns of increasing beta-agonist use and the risk of fatal or near-fatal asthma. Eur Respir J 1994;7:1602–9.

17. Medical Research Council's committee on the aetiology of chonic bronchitis. Standardized questionnaire on respiratory symptoms. Br Med J 1960;2:1665.

18. Samet JM. A historical and epidemiologic perspective on respiratory symptoms questionnaires. Am J Epidemiol 1978;108:435–46.

19. Ferris BG. Epidemiology Standardization Project (American Thoracic Society). Am Rev Respir Dis 1978;118(6 Pt 2):1–120.

20. Burney PGJ, Laitinen LA, Perdrizet S, et al. Validity and repeatability of the IUATLD (1984) Bronchial Symptoms Questionnaire: an international comparison. Eur Respir J 1989;2:940–5.

21. Burney PG, Luczynska C, Chinn S, Jarvis D. The European Community Respiratory Health Survey. Eur Respir J 1994;7:954–60.

22. Janson C, Chinn S, Jarvis D, Burney P. Individual use of antiasthmatic drugs in the European Community Respiratory Health Survey. Eur Respir J 1998;12:557–63.

23. Asher MI, Keil U, Anderson HR, et al. International Study of Asthma and Allergies in Childhood (ISAAC): rationale and methods. Eur Respir J 1995;8:483–91.

24. Steen N, Hutchinson A, McColl E, et al. Development of a symptom based outcome measure for asthma. Br Med J 1994;309:1065–8.

25. Santanello NC, Barber BL, Reiss TF, et al. Measurement characteristics of two asthma symptom diary scales for use in clinical trials. Eur Respir J 1997;10:646–51.

26. Hyland ME, Kenyon CA, Allen R, Howarth P. Diary keeping in asthma: comparison of written and electronic methods. Br Med J 1993;306:487–9.

27. Gold DR, Weiss ST, Tager IB, et al. Comparison of questionnaire and diary methods in acute childhood respiratory illness surveillance. Am Rev Respir Dis 1989;139:847–9.

28. Gibson PG, Wong BJ, Hepperle MJ, et al. A research method to induce and examine a mild exacerbation of asthma by withdrawal of inhaled corticosteroid. Clin Exp Allergy 1992;22:525–32.

29. Wasserfallen JB, Gold K, Schulman KA, Baraniuk JN. Development and validation of a rhinoconjunctivitis and asthma symptom score for use as an outcome measure in clinical trials. J Allergy Clin Immunol 1997;100:16–22.

30. Usherwood TP, Scrimgeour A, Barber JH. Questionnaire to measure perceived symptoms and disability in asthma. Arch Dis Child 1990;65:779–81.

31. Brooks SM, Bernstein IL, Raghuprasad PK, et al. Assessment of airway hyperresponsiveness in chronic stable asthma. J Allergy Clin Immunol 1990;85(1 Pt 1):17–26.

32. Rosier MJ, Bishop J, Nolan T, et al. Measurement of functional severity of asthma in children. Am J Respir Crit Care Med 1994;149:1434–41.

33. Wilson N, van Bever H. Overall symptom measurement: which approach? Eur Respir J 1996;23 Suppl:8–11S.

34. Tashkin DP. Microelectronic adherence monitors for metered-dose inhalers: who monitors the monitors? J Allergy Clin Immunol 1999;104:22–4.

35. Juniper EF, Kline PA, Vanzieleghem MA, Hargreave FE. Reduction of budesonide after a year of increased use: a randomized controlled trial to evaluate whether improvement in airway responsiveness and clinical asthma are maintained. J Allergy Clin Immunol 1991;87:483–9.

36. Aas K. Heterogeneity of bronchial asthma. Sub-populations—or different stages of the disease. Allergy 1981;36(1):3–14.

37. Mackenzie CR, Charlson ME. Standards for the use of ordinal scales in clinical trials. Br Med J Clin Res Ed 1986;292:40–3.

38. Dahl R, Martinati LC, Boner AL. Monitoring of bronchial asthma. Respir Med 1997;91:581–6.

39. Beaty TH, Newill CA, Cohen BH, et al. Effects of pulmonary function on mortality. J Chron Dis 1985;38:703–10.

40. Kellie SE, Attfield MD, Hankinson JL, Castellan RM. Spirometry variability criteria—association with respiratory morbidity and mortality in a cohort of coal miners. Am J Epidemiol 1987;125:437–44.

41. Peto R, Speizer FE, Cochrane AL, et al. The relevance in adults of air-flow obstruction, but not of mucus hypersecretion, to mortality from chronic lung disease: results from 20 years of prospective observation. Am Rev Respir Dis 1983;128:491–500.

42. Becklake MR. Concepts of normality applied to the measurement of lung function. Am J Med 1986;80:1158–64.

43. American Thoracic Society. Standardization of spirometry—1987 update. Am Rev Respir Dis 1987;136:1285–98.

44. American Thoracic Society. Lung function testing: selection of reference values and interpretative strategies. Am Rev Respir Dis 1991;144:1202–18.

45. Pediatric Working Group P. Standardization of lung function testing in infants, children and adolescents. Bull Eur Physiopathol Respir 1983;19:15–24.

46. Pennock BE, Rogers RM, McCaffree DR. Changes in measured spirometric indices. What is significant? Chest 1981;80(1):97–9.

47. Becklake MR, White N. Sources of variation in spirometric measurements. Identifying the signal and dealing with noise. Occup Med 1993;8:241–64.

48. Buist AS. Current status of small airway disease. Chest 1984;86(1):100–5.

49. Hetzel MR, Clark TJH. Comparison of normal and asthmatic circadian rhythms in peak expiratory flow. Thorax 1980;35:732–8.

50. Quanjer PH, Lebowitz MD, Gregg I, et al. Peak expiratory flow: conclusions and recommendations of a Working Party of the European Respiratory Society. Eur Respir J 1997;24 Suppl:2–8S.

51. Paggiaro PL, Moscato G, Giannini D, et al. Relationship between peak expiratory flow (PEF) and FEV1. Eur Respir J 1997;24 Suppl:39–41S.

52. Krowka MJ, Enright PL, Rodarte JR, Hyatt RE. Effect of effort on measurement of forced expiratory volume in one second. Am Rev Respir Dis 1987;136:829–33.

53. Enright PL, Lebowitz MD, Cockroft DW. Physiologic measures: pulmonary function tests. Asthma outcome. Am J Respir Crit Care Med 1994;149(2 Pt 2):S9–18.

54. Sears MR. Use of peak expiratory flow meters in adults: practical aspects. Eur Respir J 1997;24 Suppl:72–4S.

55. Quackenboss JJ, Lebowitz MD, Krzyzanowksi M. The normal range of diurnal changes in peak expiratory flows. Relationship to symptoms and respiratory disease. Am Rev Respir Dis 1991;143:323–30.

56. Siersted HC, Hansen HS, Hansen NC, et al. Evaluation of peak expiratory flow variability in an adolescent population sample. The Odense Schoolchild Study. Am J Respir Crit Care Med 1994;149(3 Pt 1):598–603.

57. Hammer J. Forced expiratory flow analysis in infants and children. In: Zach M, Carlsen K-H, Warner JO, Sennhauser FH, editors. New diagnostic techniques in paediatric respiratory medicine. Sheffield (UK): European Respiratory Society Journals; 1997. p. 1–26.

58. Marchal F, Loos N. Respiratory oscillation mechanics in infants and preschool children. In: Zach M, Carlsen K-H, Warner JO, Sennhauser FH, editors. New diagnostic techniques in paediatric respiratory medicine. Sheffield (UK): European Respiratory Society Journals; 1997. p. 58–87.

59. Juniper EF, Frith PA, Dunnett C, et al. Reproducibility and comparison of responses to inhaled histamine and methacholine. Thorax 1978;33:705–10.

60. Sterk PJ, Fabbri LM, Quanjer PH, et al. Airway responsiveness. Standardized challenge and testing with pharmacological, physical and sensitizing stimuli in adults. Report Working Party Standardization of Lung Function Tests, European Community for Steel and Coal. Official Statement of the European Respiratory Society. Eur Respir J 1993;16 Suppl:53–83.

61. Chinn S. Methodology of bronchial responsiveness. Thorax 1998;53:984–8.

62. Chinn S, Arossa WA, Jarvis DL, et al. Variation in nebulizer aerosol output and weight output from the Mefar dosimeter: implications for multicentre studies. Eur Respir J 1997;10:452–6.

63. Lotvall J, Inman M, O'Byrne P. Measurement of airway hyperresponsiveness: new considerations. Thorax 1998;53:419–24.

64. O'Connor G, Sparrow D, Taylor D, et al. Analysis of dose-response curves to methacholine. An approach suitable for population studies. Am Rev Respir Dis 1987;136:1412–7.

65. Abramson MJ, Saunders NA, Hensley MJ. Analysis of bronchial reactivity in epidemiological studies. Thorax 1990;45:924–9.

66. Haby MM, Anderson SD, Peat JK, et al. An exercise challenge protocol for epidemiological studies of asthma in children: comparison with histamine challenge. Eur Respir J 1994;7:43–9.

67. Polosa R, Holgate ST. Adenosine bronchoprovocation: a promising marker of allergic inflammation in asthma? Thorax 1997;52:919–23.

68. Riedler J. Nonpharmacological challenges in the assessment of bronchial responsiveness. In: Zach M, Carlsen K-H, Warner JO, Sennhauser FH, editors. New diagnostic techniques in paediatric respiratory medicine. Sheffield (UK): European Respiratory Society Journals; 1997. p. 115–35.

69. Studnicka MJ, Frischer T, Weiss ST, et al. Seasonal and allergenic predictors of bronchial responsiveness to distilled water. Am Rev Respir Dis 1993;148:1460–6.

70. Juniper EF, Kline PA, Vanzieleghem MA, et al. Effect of long-term treatment with an inhaled corticosteroid (budesonide) on airway hyperresponsiveness and clinical asthma in nonsteroid-dependent asthmatic patients. Am Rev Respir Dis 1990;142:832–6.

71. Bhagat R, Swystun VA, Cockcroft DW. Salbutamol-induced increased airway responsiveness to allergen and reduced protection versus methacholine: dose response. J Allergy Clin Immunol 1996;97(1 Pt 1):47–52.

72. Inman MD, Hamilton AL, Kerstjens HA, et al. The utility of methacholine airway responsiveness measurements in evaluating anti-asthma drugs. J Allergy Clin Immunol 1998;101:342–8.

73. Taylor DA, Jensen MW, Aikman SL, et al. Comparison of salmeterol- and albuterol-induced bronchoprotection against adenosine monophosphate and histamine in mild asthma. Am J Respir Crit Care Med 1997;156:1731–7.

74. Parameswaran KN, Inman MD, Ekholm BP, et al. Protection against methacholine bronchoconstriction to assess relative potency of inhaled beta2-agonist. Am J Respir Crit Care Med 1999;160(1):354–7.

75. Bousquet J, Chanez P, Vignola AM, et al. Eosinophil inflammation in asthma. Am J Respir Crit Care Med 1994;150(5 Pt 2):S33–8.

76. Bousquet J, Corrigan CJ, Venge P. Peripheral blood markers: evaluation of inflammation in asthma. Eur Respir J 1998;26 Suppl:42–8S.

77. Pizzichini E, Pizzichini MM, Kidney JC, et al. Induced sputum, bronchoalveolar lavage and blood from mild asthmatic patients: inflammatory cells, lymphocyte subsets and soluble markers compared. Eur Respir J 1998;11:828–34.

78. Beasley R, Roche WR, Roberts JA, Holgate ST. Cellular events in the bronchi in mild asthma and after bronchial provocation. Am Rev Respir Dis 1989;139:806–17.

79. Jeffery PK. Bronchial biopsies and airway inflammation. Eur Respir J 1996;9:1583–7.

80. Kips JC, Fahy JV, Hargreave FE, et al. Methods for sputum induction and analysis of induced sputum: a method for assessing airway inflammation in asthma. Eur Respir J 1998;26 Suppl:9–12S.

81. Hargreave FE. Induced sputum for the investigation of airway inflammation: evidence for its clinical application. Can Respir J 1999;6:169–74.

82. McIvor RA, Pizzichini E, Turner MO, et al. Potential masking effects of salmeterol on airway inflammation in asthma. Am J Respir Crit Care Med 1998;158:924–30.

83. Gustafsson LE. Exhaled nitric oxide as a marker in asthma. Eur Respir J 1998;26 Suppl:49–52S.

84. Kharitonov S, Alving K, Barnes PJ. Exhaled and nasal nitric oxide measurements: recommendations. The European Respiratory Society Task Force. Eur Respir J 1997;10:1683–93.

85. Ware JE, Sherbourne CD. The MOS 36-item short form health survey (SF-36). I. Conceptual framework and item selection. Med Care 1992;30:473–83.

86. Bergner M, Bobbitt RA, Carter WB, et al. The Sickness Impact Profile: development and final revision of a health status measure. Med Care 1981;19:787–805.

87. Juniper EF, Guyatt GH, Ferrie PJ, Griffith LE. Measuring quality of life in asthma. Am Rev Respir Dis 1993;147:832–8.

88. Marks GB, Dunn SM, Woolcock AJ. An evaluation of an asthma quality of life questionnaire as a measure of change in adults with asthma. J Clin Epidemiol 1993;46:1103–11.

89. Jones PW. Quality of life, symptoms and pulmonary function in asthma: longterm treatment with nedocromil sodium examined in a controlled multicentre trial. Nedocromil Sodium Quality of Life Study Group. Eur Respir J 1994;7:55–62.

90. Taylor DR, Sears MR, Herbison GP, et al. Regular inhaled beta agonist in asthma: effects on exacerbations and lung function. Thorax 1993;48:134–8.

91. Pauwels RA, Lofdahl CG, Postma DS, et al. Effect of inhaled formoterol and budesonide on exacerbations of asthma. Formoterol and Corticosteroids Establishing Therapy (FACET) International Study Group. N Engl J Med 1997;337:1405–11.

92. Ernst P, Habbick B, Suissa S, et al. Is the association between inhaled beta-agonist use and life-threatening asthma because of confounding by severity? Am Rev Respir Dis 1993;148:75–9.

Index